A History of Immunology

I fancy you as coming to the acquisition of the myriad facts of medicine with little to tell you of the intellectual forces and historical sequences by which these facts have emerged.

Christian A. Herter

A
History of
Immunology

ARTHUR M. SILVERSTEIN

The Wilmer Institute and The Institute of the History of Medicine
The Johns Hopkins University School of Medicine
Baltimore, Maryland

ACADEMIC PRESS, INC.
Harcourt Brace Jovanovich, Publishers
San Diego New York Boston
London Sydney Tokyo Toronto

ACADEMIC PRESS, INC.
San Diego, California 92101

United Kingdom Edition published by
ACADEMIC PRESS LIMITED
24-28 Oval Road, London NW1 7DX

Library of Congress Cataloging-in-Publication Data

Silverstein, Arthur M.
    A history of immunology / Arthur M. Silverstein.
      p.   cm.
    About half of the chapters were published in abbreviated form in
the journal Cellular immunology.
    Includes indexes.
    ISBN 0-12-643770-X (alk. paper)
    1. Immunology—History.   I. Title.
    [DNLM: 1. Allergy and Immunology—history.   QW 11.1 S586h]
QR182.S55   1988
616.07'9'09—dc19
DNLM/DLC
for Library of Congress   88-14538
                                       CIP

PRINTED IN THE UNITED STATES OF AMERICA
91 92 93 94 95   9 8 7 6 5 4 3

IN MEMORY OF JUDY

Contents

List of Plates

Preface

I have always derived great enjoyment from reading the old literature. More specifically, I wanted to know not only what the earlier giants of immunology had said in their publications, but also how they thought and by whom they were influenced. These ventures into the past were only an innocent hobby at first but became something more once I came into contact with students. The Johns Hopkins University has an active interdepartmental immunology program, which includes a regular Tuesday evening informal seminar attended by faculty, graduate students, and interested postdoctoral fellows from various clinical and basic science departments. As, week after week, I listened to and participated in discussions that ranged over all aspects of current immunological thought and practice, I slowly became aware of a troubling fact—most of the young scientists (and not a few of their elders!) appeared to believe that the entire history of immunology could be found within the last five years' issues of the most widely read journals. Little that went before this was cited, and one might have concluded that each current line of work or current theoretical interpretation had arisen *de novo* and without antecedents. But perhaps the single event that triggered my serious entry into the study of the history of immunology was the receipt of a manuscript for review from one of our leading journals. This was an elegant study of an important problem, using up-to-date techniques, but one that Paul Ehrlich had reported on 80 years earlier! Not only was the author unaware of Ehrlich's work, but he was also unaware that his data and conclusions

xi

differed little from Ehrlich's, despite the marvels of our newer technologies.

I began then to spend part time in Hopkins's Institute of the History of Medicine, exploring in a more consistent fashion the treasures housed in its Welch Medical Library. These historical excursions led to a series of presentations at the annual Johns Hopkins Immunology Council Weekend Retreat and were in fact labeled "The Lady Mary Wortley Montagu Memorial Lectures" by a feminist colleague then in charge of the program committee. These same lectures also have served as the basis of many of the chapters in the present volume.

This book, then, is primarily directed to young immunologists, to provide both a better understanding of where immunology is today and how it got there as well as an introduction to the many social, political, and interpersonal factors that have influenced more than a century of progress in immunology. Of course, the book is not forbidden to more senior investigators, who may enjoy being reminded of some of the twists and turns that our science has taken and of some of the grand debates and personalities that have so spiced its history. If, in addition, the book should serve to interest professional historians of medicine in this important branch of twentieth-century biomedical science (to correct with further research some of my more egregious errors), then it will have more than served its purpose.

The reader will note by the title that this book is *a* history of immunology and not *the* history of immunology. Each author will view and interpret the past differently, will be guided by a different background and different values in assigning importance to past events, and will emphasize some aspects more and others less. For my part, I have chosen to deal with the history of immunology in terms of what I consider its most important conceptual threads (whether or not they proved "useful" to future progress), attempting to trace each of these longitudinally in time rather than to present a year-by-year list of the minutiae of its progress. It is hoped, in utilizing this approach, that most of the important events and discoveries and most of the important names will appear at one place or another. The price of this approach, however, is that some significant technical advances may receive short shrift if they did not contribute significantly to the advance of a concept (a deficit that I attempt to redress in a final chapter devoted primarily to technologies). This approach also involves a certain amount of repetition, since certain discoveries or theories may have played a major role in the development of more than one important immunological idea. In this sense, each of the chapters is meant to be internally self-sufficient and may be read independently of the others, but taken together they should present a fairly complete intellectual history of the discipline of immunology.

The reader of this book should be aware of a final caveat. No history of a discipline as active as immunology is today can hope to be completely up to date; otherwise the arrival of each new number of a journal would require immediate revision of the text. This is especially true in dealing with the history of ideas in such a field, since so many of our modern concepts and even phenomenologies are still the subject of debate and subject to verification and the test of time. I have therefore drawn an arbitrary line at the early 1960s, which is the time when "modern" immunology entered the present biomedical revolution. Classical immunochemistry gave way then to modern immunobiology, a phase shift announced by Burnet's clonal selection theory. If later events and discoveries are mentioned, it is only to provide a context for the evaluation of or comparison with earlier events, or to provide an endpoint to illustrate the further consequences of those earlier developments.

I would like to express my deep thanks to the many individuals who helped me along the way. I owe a debt to Philip Gell for having helped to get me started on the historical path; to Noel Rose and Byron Waksman for their many helpful suggestions on the history of autoimmunity and immunopathology; to Fred Karush for helping to clarify many aspects of molecular immunology; and to Robert Prendergast, Rupert Billingham, and Leslie Brent for many valuable suggestions. I am indebted also to Anne-Marie Moulin for many interesting discussions and for having permitted me to read and benefit from the manuscript of her thesis on the history of immunology. Chapter 1 was originally written in collaboration with Alexander Bialasiewicz and Chapter 2 in collaboration with Genevieve Miller, both of whom have given permission to include their important contributions in this book. The appendix containing the biographical dictionary would not have been as complete or as useful but for the generous assistance and encouragement of Dorothy Whitcomb, Librarian at the Middleton Library of the University of Wisconsin, and of her assistant, Terrence Fischer.

The faculty of the Johns Hopkins Institute of the History of Medicine have been especially helpful, not only in providing space, but also in giving me an informal training in certain aspects of historiography and in putting up with my many questions of fact or technique. Among these are Lloyd Stevenson, Owsei Temkin, Gert Brieger, Jerome Bylebyl, Caroline Hannaway, and Daniel Todes. John Parascandola, Chief of the Division of the History of Medicine at the National Library of Medicine in Bethesda, contributed significantly to my understanding of Paul

Ehrlich's work and also made available to me the facilities and collections of the National Library. I heartily thank Irene Skop and Liddian Lindenmuth for their superb secretarial and editorial assistance. Finally, I thank Academic Press and Sherwood H. Lawrence, editor of *Cellular Immunology*, for permission to adapt for this book some chapters previously published in that journal.

On History and Historians

*History is not the study of origins; rather
it is the analysis of all the mediations by
which the past was turned into our present.*
H. Butterfield

THE WORKING scientist who entertains the notion
of writing a history of a discipline must do so with
diffidence and no little trepidation. While such a scientist may know
more of the facts and scientific interrelationships within his or her
specialty than does the professional historian, nothing in a scientist's
training or experience has prepared him or her to deal in the special
currencies so familiar to the historian in general and to the historian of
science in particular. If the aim is to write more than a mere encyclopedia of names, places, and facts—an unappealing venture—then such
unfamiliar concepts as the sociology and epistemology of science and
cultural relativism must be dealt with. Such recondite ideas rarely enter
into the formal training of the biomedical scientist, and never into a
scientist's practice. Indeed, if the scientist considers such concepts at all,
it is probably with suspicion and perhaps disdain, relegating them to that
special limbo maintained for the "impure" social sciences, firm in the
conviction that his or her science is a dependably precise "pure" science.

But this is not the most serious challenge to the practicing scientist-
turned-historian. Assuming that he or she has overcome the typical

scientist's feeling that Santayana's maxim, "Those who cannot remember the past are condemned to repeat it," applies only to politicians, diplomats, and economists, the scientist–historian has a yet more difficult preparatory task to come. This involves nothing less than a reexamination *and perhaps rejection* of some most-cherished beliefs— beliefs rarely stated explicitly, but so implicit in all of the scientist's training and education and so permeating the scientist's environment as to have become almost the unwritten rules of the game.

The first of the beliefs to be reexamined is that of *the continuity of scientific development*. By this I mean that most mature scientists, and all students and members of the novitiate, tend to suppose that all that has gone before in a field was somehow aimed logically at providing the base for current work in that field. Thus, there is a general view that the history of a discipline involves an almost inexorable progression of facts and theories leading *in a straight and unbroken line* to our own present view of the workings of nature. (Historians refer to this as "Whig history"[1] and condemn its practice.) Put in other terms, the scientist is tempted to regard the development of science in much the same way that most of us seem to regard the origin of species—as a sort of melioristic evolution, following a preordained path toward the acme of perfection and logical unity: in the one case humankind, and in the other our present science.

But this is not really surprising when we consider how most science is practiced and reported and especially how scientists are trained. In the first instance, the scientist chooses a problem to work on that could scarcely be justified as other than the next logical step in the progress of the discipline, that is, the next obvious question to be asked and problem to be solved. Then, having successfully seen the research to its conclusion, the scientist submits the work to the scientific literature (the unsuccessful excursions generally go unreported). Now, for a variety of reasons including ego, space limitations, and the implicit cultural view of how science *ought* to function, our author prepares the manuscript so that, not only is the work presented as internally logical and the result of an ordered sequence from start to finish, but the background introduction and its supporting references from past literature are carefully chosen to demonstrate that this work was eminently justified in its choice and in fact was the next obvious step forward in a well-ordered history. Each communication in the scientific literature thus contributes mod-

1. Butterfeld, H., "The Whig Interpretation of History," W. W. Norton, New York, 1965.

estly and subtly, *but cumulatively,* to a revision of the reader's understanding of the history of the discipline.[2]

There is in science, however, a far greater force which operates to impose an order and continuity on its history, manifested not only by an influence on the types of problems deemed worthy of pursuit, but more importantly in the ways young scientists are educated. There is in any scientific discipline, and there ought to be, a priesthood of the elite. There are the guardians of the scientific temple in which resides the current set of received wisdoms. These are the trendsetters and the arbiters of contemporary scientific values. They are also, not coincidently, the principal writers of textbooks and the most sought-after lecturers, as well as the principal researchers in whose laboratories young people serve their scientific apprenticeships. They are, in brief, the strongest and most vocal adherents of what Thomas Kuhn, in his provocative book *The Structure of Scientific Revolution,* [3] has called "the current paradigm." In Kuhn's usage, a paradigm in any field is the current model system and the accepted body of theories, rules, and techniques that guide the thinking and determine the problems within that field. Kuhn points out that, when a change in paradigm occurs within a discipline (he insists that this is inevitably the result of an abrupt revolution), the textbooks must be rewritten to reflect the new wisdom. This invariably involves a revision in the interpretation of what went before, so that the new paradigm can be shown to be fully justified as a step forward in scientific progress and worthy in all respects to command the attention of the current community of scholars. Since the object of a text is pedagogy, the facts many and the concepts complex, what went before must necessarily be winnowed, abstracted, and digested in order to provide the student with what is required to follow in the illustrious footsteps of the current priests. Therefore, the modest history that is included in most texts, and the routine appeals to the idols and heroes of earlier times, are more often than not subconsciously slanted to help justify the current paradigm and its proponents; they serve to reinforce the impression of a uniform continuity of scientific development. Assuming that one is a reputable member of a current scientific community, and thus a subscriber to the current paradigm, the

2. Julius H. Comroe's essay "Tell it like it was" speaks well to this point: Comroe, J. H., "Retrospectoscope: Insights into Medical Discovery," Von Gehr, Menlo Park, California, 1977, pp. 89–98.

3. Kuhn, R., "The Structure of Scientific Revolution," 2nd ed., University of Chicago Press, Chicago, 1970.

scientist-turned-historian must be especially on guard not to contribute also to a revisionist history of the field. One might then be rightly accused of *presentism*,[4] the interpretation of yesterday's events in today's more modern terms and context.

The second of the beliefs that requires reexamination—one also nurtured by our traditional system of scientific pedagogy—is that of *the logic of scientific* development. We have already seen that the investigator justifies the choice of a research problem (not only to scientific peers but also to the sources of financial support) by demonstrating its logic within the context of the accepted paradigm. This is, of course, eminently reasonable, since a paradigm lacking inner logic (i.e., unable to define the nature of the problems to be asked within its context or to assimilate the results obtained) would scarcely merit support. But the existence of a logical order of development during the limited lifetime of a paradigm is often extended to imply an overall logical development of the entire scientific discipline. Moreover, the concept examined above, a smoothly continuous maturation of a science, implies also that its progression has been logical—the step-by-step movement of fact and theory from A to B to C, as the Secrets of Nature are unfolded and Ultimate Truth approached. Indeed, to accuse science of illogic in its development would, to many, imply the absence of a coherent unity underlying the object of science's quest—the description and understanding of the physical world.

And yet, there is so much that is discontinuous and illogical in the development of any science. On the level of the individual research activity, much attention is paid to the beauty and strength of that eminently logical process, the inductive Scientific Method. The working scientist, however, who thinks about the course of his or her own research must wonder sometimes whether the description is apt. One of the few *biologists* who has reflected aloud on this problem is Sir Peter Medawar, in his Jayne Lectures before the American Philosophical Society. Following the lead of philosopher Karl Popper,[5] Medawar challenges the popular notion:

> Deductivism in mathematical literature and inductivism in scientific papers are simply the postures we choose to be seen in when the curtain goes up and the public sees us. The theatrical illusion is shattered if we ask what goes on behind the scenes. In real life discovery and justification are almost always different processes. . . . Methodologists who have no personal

4. See, for example, G. W. Stocking's editorial "On the limits of presentism and historicism . . .," *J. Hist. Behavioral Sci.* 1:211, 1965.
5. Popper, K., "The Logic of Scientific Discovery," Hutchinson, London, 1959.

experience of scientific research have been gravely handicapped by their failure to realize that nearly all scientific research leads nowhere—or if it does lead somewhere, then not in the direction it started off with. In retrospect, we tend to forget the errors, so that "The Scientific Method" appears very much more powerful than it really is, particularly when it is presented to the public in the terminology of breakthroughs, and to fellow scientists with the studied hypocrisy expected of a contribution to a learned journal. I reckon that for all the use it has been to science about four-fifths of my time has been wasted, and I believe this to be the common lot of people who are not merely playing follow-my-leader in research. . . science in its forward motion is not logically propelled. . . . The process by which we come to formulate a hypothesis is not illogical, but non-logical, i.e., outside logic. But once we have formed an opinion, we can expose it to criticism, usually by experimentation; this episode lies within and makes use of logic.[6]

Even this last concession to the logic and continuity of the scientific method may overstate the case somewhat. But in any event, it certainly must be restricted in its application to the microenvironment of the normative science of a given time—that is, to a working hypothesis developed within the context of the accepted beliefs (paradigm) of the day. Within the macroenvironment of a scientific discipline in transition, these rules often fail. Not only may bold new formulations be insusceptible of formal "proof" by logical application of the scientific method, but the bases for their acceptance or rejection by individual members of the community are generally anything but logical: witness, in chemistry, the transition from the phlogiston theory to Lavoisier's oxygen theory (Priestley went to his grave denying that oxygen was a separate entity); in optics, the transition from corpuscular to wave theory to an ineffable something in between; or in bacteriology, the century-long dispute between believers in spontaneous generation and those who claimed *omnis organismus ex organismo* (Pasteur carried the day less by the compelling logic of his experiments—most had been done before him—than by his reputation and forceful disputation). In the field of dynamics also, it is difficult to subscribe to the idea that Newtonian theories represented a smoothly continuous development over Aristotelian dynamics, or that Einstein's theories emerged smoothly and logically from Newtonian requirements. Again, in immunology, the transitions represented by Pasteur in 1880, by the conflict between theories of cellular and humoral immunity in the 1890s, and by Burnet and the onset of the immunobiological revolution in the 1960s were hardly smooth evolutions and perhaps not even logical progressions.

6. Medawar, P. B., "Induction and Intuition in Scientific Thought," American Philosophical Society, Philadelphia, 1969.

Many of the great advances in the sciences, whether arising from a new theoretical concept or from a discovery which redirects a discipline, are in fact quantum leaps—daring formulations or unexpected findings hardly anticipated or predictable within the context of the rules and traditions of the day. Kuhn makes the interesting suggestion that it is only when the normal state of affairs in a science becomes unsettled, when the accepted paradigm no longer provides satisfying explanations for new anomalies which perplex its theories, when, in fact, the paradigm may no longer even suggest the proper questions to be asked, that a crisis stage is reached and the old paradigm is likely to be replaced—abruptly and discontinuously—by a new one. And often the critical discovery or novel formulation is made by someone not committed to the old paradigm and to the old approaches and mindset that it enforced—by the uncommitted young, or the unconfined outsider from another discipline. At such times, the "old guard" seem to view their science through lenses ground during the previous era. One is reminded of the hero in Voltaire's *L'Ingénu* who, brought up in feral innocence, "made rapid progress in the sciences. The cause of the rapid development of his mind was due to his savage education almost as much as to the quality of his intellect; having learned nothing in his infancy, he had not developed any prejudices. He saw things as they are."

Here again, the scientist-turned-historian must modify the customary approach to a discipline and consider the significance of the blind alleys of research, of the premature discoveries, of the mistaken interpretations, and of the "erroneous" or supplanted theories of the past. Without these our history, while more concise, would lack some of those condiments that are so very important for its full flavor.

The final one of the cherished (but essentially implicit) beliefs of the scientist which requires reexamination concerns *the impetus for scientific development*. By this I mean those forces which act to determine not only the direction but also the velocity of scientific activity and discovery. Most scientists seem to feel that this impetus is inherent within their discipline—an imperative driving force that dictates at least the sequence, and perhaps even the rate of its development. Thus, the scientist is fond of the notion of the "idea (or experiment) whose time has come" and supports this with case histories of simultaneous and independent discoveries. To a certain extent, of course, this concept is apt, especially within the context of the current paradigm, as we saw above. But even leaving aside those major discontinuous and nonlogical advances already mentioned, we are still left with anomalous developments. How do we explain, for instance, a "premature" discovery whose significance goes unrecognized at the time (Spallanzani's refutation of spontaneous generation in the eighteenth century, Mendel's genetics, the Koch phenomenon)?

More interesting yet are those extrascientific forces which impose themselves upon the course of scientific discovery and development. All too familiar is the effect of war upon science—the development of radar, of nuclear energy theory and practice, of transplantation immunology, to name but a few. One need only recall the Church's view of the Galilean heresy, the serious economic plight of the French silk industry whose appeal helped to direct the course of Pasteur's future work, or the benevolent views of science by Bismarck in Prussia and by Congressman James Fogarty and Senator Lister Hill in America, which did much to establish the scientific leadership in their respective countries. The ability of the Prussian Minister Friedrich Althoff to recognize talent and to reward the Kochs, Ehrlichs, and Behrings with university professorships and with their own institutes was one of the chief factors in German preeminence in bacteriology and immunology in the late nineteenth century. By contrast, Pasteur in France was forced to build his institute himself through public subscription, and later the operating funds of the Institut Pasteur came in no small part from its herd of horses and the commercial sale of antitoxins. The development of a yellow fever vaccine certainly owes much to the American occupation of Cuba after the Spanish–American war and to the building of the Panama Canal. Similarly, not the least contribution to the development of the polio vaccine was the affliction of Franklin D. Roosevelt, while the critical choice between a killed versus an attenuated virus vaccine was made for mainly political reasons by a nonscientist, Basil O'Connor, Director of the Polio Foundation. Finally, when an American president and Congress declare a "war on cancer" or on AIDS and appropriate massive funds in its support, all of science changes in both direction and velocity.

These are but a few of the well-explored and documented instances of profound sociopolitical influences upon the course of scientific development, but there are many others deserving of the attention of the historian (and scientist), and some will be found in the text that follows. No history of a science would be complete or even fully comprehensible without their inclusion, and they add spice to what might otherwise be a rather dull and tasteless fare.

1

Theories of Acquired Immunity

Blut ist ein ganz besonderer Saft.
—Goethe

T HE LATIN words *immunitas* and *immunis* have their origin in the legal concept of an exemption: initially, in Rome, they described the exemption of an individual from service or duty and, later, in the Middle Ages, the exemption of the Church and its properties and personnel from civil control. In her impressive review of the *History of Concepts of Infection and Defense,*[1] Antoinette Stettler traces the first use of this term in the context of disease to the fourteenth century, when Colle wrote *"Equibus Dei gratia ego immunis evasi"* in referring to his escape from a plague epidemic.[2] But long before that, poetic license permitted the Roman Marcus Annaeus Lucanus (A.D. 39–65) to use the word *immunes* in his epic poem "Pharsalia" to describe the famous resistance to snakebite of the Psylli tribe of North Africa. While the term was employed intermittently thereafter, it did not attain great currency until the nineteenth century, following the rapid spread of Edward Jenner's smallpox vaccination. Immunity was thus an available and apt term to apply during the 1880s and 1890s to the phenomena described by Pasteur, Koch, Metchnikoff, von Behring, Ehrlich, and other investigators. But long before any specific term such as immunity was applied and 1500 years before an explanation of it would be advanced, the phenomenon of acquired immunity was described.

Originally written in collaboration with A. A. Bialasiewicz.

1

Throughout recorded history, two of the most fearful causes of death were pestilence and poison. With great frequency, deadly epidemics and pandemics beset cities and nations, with great economic, social, and political consequences.[3] Despite a lack of knowledge of their origin, their nature, or even of their nosological relationship to one another, the keen observer could not help but notice that often those who by good fortune had survived the disease once might be "exempt" from further involvement upon its return. Thus, the historian Thucydides, in his contemporary description of the plague of Athens of 430 B.C., could say: "Yet it was with those who had recovered from the disease that the sick and the dying found most compassion. These knew what it was from experience, and had now no fear for themselves; for the same man was never attacked twice—never at least fatally."[4] The identity of this "plague" that killed Pericles and perhaps one-fourth of the population of Athens has been much disputed, and it is uncertain whether it was due to *Pasteurella pestis*. However, some thousand years later, a pandemic of what is more likely to have been bubonic plague occurred in A.D. 541 and is known as the plague of Justinian after the Byzantine emperor of that time. In his history, Procopius said of the plague: "it left neither island nor cave nor mountain ridge which had human inhabitants; and if it had passed by any land, either not affecting the men there or touching them in indifferent fashion, still at a later time it came back; then those who dwelt roundabout this land, whom formerly it had afflicted most sorely, it did not touch at all."[5] And after a further millennium, Fracastoro (1483–1553) felt free to offer the following tantalizing comment in his book *On Contagion*:[6] "Moreover, I have known certain persons who were regularly immune, though surrounded by the plague-stricken, and I shall have something to say about this in its place, and shall inquire whether it is impossible for us to immunize ourselves against pestilential fevers."[7] Unfortunately, Fracastoro, despite his promise to return to this intriguing suggestion, fails to do so later in the book.

Man's continuous experience with poisons has also had a far-reaching influence on the development of concepts of disease and immunity.[8] During Roman times, Mithridates VI, king of Pontus, described in his medical commentaries (which his conqueror Pompey thought worthy of translation) the taking of increasing daily doses of poisons to render himself safe from attempts on his life. This immunity (or adaptation) had far-reaching influence throughout the Middle Ages, when complicated mixtures for this purpose were universally known as the Mithridaticum or theriac. Indeed, as I shall show later, its influence was felt as late as the 1890s, when an adaptation theory of immunity was advanced, based upon Mithridatic principles.

Even more important was the centuries-long belief that many diseases were due to poison, known universally by its Latin name *virus*. (The Greek word *pharmakeia* still means poisoning, witchcraft, or medicine.) In the absence of knowledge of etiology or pathogenesis, the causative agent was long considered to be the *virus,* connoting not only poison but also the slime and miasma from which the poison was thought to originate. Even into the early twentieth century, the term virus was used almost interchangeably with bacterium to describe the etiological agent of an infectious disease. When in 1888 Roux and Yersin isolated diphtheria toxin,[9] and in 1890 von Behring and Kitasato described antitoxic immunity to diphtheria and tetanus,[10] it appeared for a brief period that almost 2000 years of interest in poison as the proximate cause of disease and in antidotes (German *Gegengifte*) had been vindicated. But the discovery soon thereafter of numerous diseases whose pathogenesis was based upon neither an exotoxin nor an endotoxin led to an early correction of this overgeneralization, although not before Paul Ehrlich had done his classic studies on immunity to the plant poisons abrin and ricin.[11]

Most textbooks of immunology begin with a short historical review, mention variolation and Jenner's vaccination against smallpox, but imply that theories of acquired immunity had to await Pasteur's germ theory of disease[12] and his first demonstration in 1880 of acquired immunity in the etiologically well-defined bacterial infection of chicken cholera.[13] This treatment may be due in part to the surprising absence of any hint of speculation in Jenner's writing on what he thought was the mechanism of vaccination in providing immunity to smallpox. Le Fanu suggests[14] that Jenner might have been influenced by the belief of his famous teacher John Hunter[15] that two diseases cannot coexist in an individual, or that perhaps he took seriously Hunter's advice in an earlier letter to Jenner on another subject: "I think your solution is just, but why think? Why not try the experiment?"[16]

A "modern" theory of acquired immunity would seem to require as minimal prerequisites: (1) the concept of an etiological agent; (2) a concept of transmission of this agent; (3) an understanding of the specificity and general reproducibility of a disease; and (4) some concept of host–parasite interaction. But, as Stettler points out, there were earlier theories of acquired immunity. These appear to have required an awareness of only two factors: a recognition of the phenomenon of inability to succumb twice during the course of a pestilence, and some concept, however primitive, of disease pathogenesis (plus, of course, a speculative mind). I shall, in this chapter, expand upon Stettler's list and examine these imaginative theories within the context of their times.

Magic and Theurgic Origin of Disease

As Sigerist points out in his *History of Medicine*,[17] there is only a nebulous border between magic and religion among primitive peoples. In the most primitive societies, both man and nature are thought to operate under the control of magical influences governed by spirits and demons.[18] These become formalized into sets of taboos and totems, followed often by the development of complex pantheons and occasionally by a monotheistic unification. It is only natural then, as Temkin[19] indicates, that in ancient civilizations such as Egypt, India, Israel, and Mesopotamia, disease came to be considered a punishment for trespass or sin, ranging from the involuntary infraction of some taboo to a willful crime against gods or men. The wearing of amulets, the chanting of incantations, and the offering of sacrifice were common measures to neutralize "black" magic, to ward off demonic disease, or to propitiate the gods, and such practices persist to the present time, even among "advanced" peoples.

Throughout recorded history, every civilization has recognized the theurgic origin of disease. The Babylonian epic of Gilgamesh, about 2000 B.C., records visitations of the god of pestilence; and in Egypt the fear of Pharaoh was compared with the fear of the god of disease during a year of severe epidemics. Throughout the Old Testament, God visits disease upon those who deserve punishment, including both His own people and those who oppose them. Thus, God through Moses smote the Egyptians (Exodus 9:9), the Philistines for their seizure of the Ark of the Covenant (I Samuel 5:6), and the Assyrians under King Sennacherib for invading Judea (Isaiah 37:36), but God equally brought down a pestilence that killed 70,000 people as punishment of David's sin of numbering the people (II Samuel 24). In ancient Greece, Sophocles records in "Oedipus the King" that the Sun god Phoebus Apollo caused the plague of Thebes because it had been polluted by the misdeeds of Oedipus, while the historians record that Apollo fired plague arrows upon the Greek host before Troy because their leader Agamemnon had abducted the daughter of his priest. Among the Hindus, sin, the breaking of a norm, the wanton cursing of a fellow man, and similar transgressions result in illness, for the gods and particularly Varuna, guardian of law and order, punish the offender.

With the concept of a vengeful deity, and especially with the rise of a belief in the hereafter, in which a life of earthly suffering might be followed by everlasting peace, the view of the nature of disease and of resistance to it underwent a significant change in early Christian times. While the opening of Pandora's box might only have released disease-as-punishment into the world, Eve's eating of the forbidden fruit did more: it permitted redemption. Now not only did God punish the sins of man with disease, but He could also employ it to purge and cleanse man of his sins. Thus, St. Cyprian, Bishop of Carthage (?200–258) could write of the plague then raging: "Many of us are dying in this mortality, that is many of us are being freed from the world . . . To the servants of God it is a salutary departure. How suitable, how necessary it is that this plague, which seems horrible and deadly, searches out the justice of each and every one."[20]

A theurgic view of disease has interesting implications for the immunologist. If throughout early history disease was considered as a punishment by the spirits or demons or gods for vice and sin, then being spared the initial effects of a raging pestilence or other disease (i.e., *natural immunity*) should automatically have been viewed as the inevitable result of having led a clean and pious life. Moreover, once disease came to be viewed as an expiation and purgative, the recovery from a deadly plague would imply not only that the sins of that individual had been minor but further that he had been cleansed of those sins and thus did not merit further punishing disease when the plague returned (*acquired immunity*). Such concepts may have been so implicit in the religiosity of the times as not to warrant explicit statement.

It is true, of course, as Edelstein[21] and others point out, that despite the common tendency among the ancients to consider a magical or religious origin of disease, physicians (and especially the Greeks) were in general rational and empirical, rejecting magic and any religious mysticism. Rationalism and empiricism were the greatest of the contributions of the Hippocratic school of Greece, a tradition that was maintained in the East by Islamic physicians and in the West throughout the Middle Ages and Renaissance until modern times. But it is difficult to know how such a rational approach might influence the thinking of physicians about so arcane a subject as infectious disease and resistance. While the officials of many cities were instituting the important public health measure of quarantine (French, 40 days) against infectious disease, influenza was ascribed to the *influence* of the stars and *mal-aria* to bad air. Again, the same Fracastoro who devised such "modern" theories of contagion could in the same book ascribe the appearance of syphilis in Europe to an earlier evil conjunction of Mars, Saturn, and Jupiter. Two hundred years earlier, these same planets had been universally held responsible for the Black Death that ravaged Europe and the East.

But the belief in astrological and theurgic bases for disease was not confined to "less advanced" times—it persists even today. In his description of the cholera epidemics of the nineteenth century, Rosenberg[22] points out that few medical men then believed that cholera was a contagious disease but thought (with Sydenham) that its cause lay in some change in the atmosphere. During the early days of the 1832 epidemic, the New York Special Medical Council announced "that the disease in the city is confined to the imprudent and intemperate," while the governor of New York proclaimed that "an infinitely wise and just God had seen fit to employ pestilence as one means of scourging the human race for their sins," and he found support for this stand in a newspaper report that of 1400 "lewd women" in Paris, 1300 had died of cholera!

Expulsion Theories of Acquired Immunity

From the time of the Hippocratic school in ancient Greece until its challenge by the rise of scientific medicine in the nineteenth century, most disease (whatever its provenance) was thought to reflect a disturbance of the four humors—blood, phlegm, yellow bile, and black bile—whence the terms sanguine, phlegmatic, choleric, and melancholic. During the earlier period, it was supposed that disease was due to a quantitative imbalance among the humors, and this belief led to widespread use of therapies that included bleeding, cupping, leeches, and purgatives and expectorants of many types. A further refinement (due in part to Galen, A.D. 130–?200) held that disease might also be caused by qualitative changes in the humors, involving changes in their temperature, their consistency, or even their fermentation or putrefaction. For example, smallpox was long considered to have a special affinity for the blood and to involve its fermentation. Given such a pathogenetic mechanism for this disease and an increasing understanding of its symptomatology and course between the fifth and tenth centuries A.D., it is not surprising that most early theories of acquired immunity would be formulated in the context of smallpox.

RHAZES

One of the most famous of the Islamic physicians was Abu Bekr Mohammed ibn Zakariya al-Razi (880–932), known in the West as Rhazes. In his *Treatise on the Smallpox and Measles*,[23] he not only gave the first modern clinical description of smallpox but also indicated very clearly that he knew that survival from smallpox infection conferred lasting immunity (although he did not employ this term). More than that, he provided a remarkable explanation for why smallpox does not occur twice in the same individual, the first such theory of acquired immunity that we have been able to find in the literature.

Like his contemporaries, Rhazes believed that smallpox affects the blood and is due more specifically to a fermentation of the blood that is permitted by its "excess moisture." He considered the pustules that form on the skin and break to release fluid as the mechanism by which the body expels the excess moisture contained in the blood. Drawing a parallel between the change in the blood during the development of man and the change in wine from its initial production by the fermentation of grape juice (must) to its spoiling, he wrote:

I say then that every man, from the time of his birth till he arrives at old age, is continually tending to dryness; and for this reason the blood of children and infants is much moister than the blood of young men, and still more so than that of old men . . . Now the smallpox arises when the blood putrefies and ferments, so that superfluous vapors are thrown out of it and it is changed from the blood of infants, which is like must, into the blood of young men, which is like wine perfectly ripened; as to the blood of old men, it may be compared to wine which has now lost its strength and is beginning to grow vapid and sour; and the smallpox itself may be compared to the fermentation and the hissing noise which takes place in must at that time. And this is the reason children, especially males, rarely escape being seized with this disease, because it is impossible to prevent the blood's changing from this state into its second state, just as it is impossible to prevent must . . . from changing.

This remarkable theory accounted satisfactorily for everything that Rhazes knew about smallpox. First, it affects virtually everyone, and that during youth, since youths have very moist blood. Next, he pointed out that smallpox was then seldom seen in young adults and almost never in the aged, presumably because all had undergone the natural drying of the blood that accompanied the aging process. Finally, lasting immunity would follow from earlier infection, and a second experience of this disease would be impossible, since the "excess moisture" of the blood required to support the disease would have been expelled from the body during the first attack.

But there is another almost more interesting aspect of smallpox implicit in Rhazes' theory of pathogenesis and acquired immunity. He presented smallpox as an almost benign childhood disease and as a salutary process that he apparently felt assisted the maturation from infancy to adulthood. Certainly no such theory could have been advanced by so astute an observer as Rhazes to explain the deadly disease that we know smallpox to be in modern times. Yet, this benign view of smallpox persisted into the seventeenth century in Europe, despite the ravages it was observed to inflict upon virgin Amerindian populations in the New World immediately following the Spanish conquests. One must wonder where virulent smallpox was in the tenth century, or whether the pathogen underwent some subsequent change in its virulence.[24]

GIROLAMO FRACASTORO, 1546

It was Fracastoro who first gave formal currency to the ideas not only that disease was caused by small seeds (*seminaria*) but that the contagion might spread directly from person to person, indirectly by means of infected clothing, etc., or even at a distance. Although Fracastoro thought that these seminaria might arise spontaneously within an individual or from air or earth or water, yet he believed that they would reproduce truly and transmit the same disease from one person to another. He thought that all seminaria had specific affinities for certain things—some for plants, some for certain specific animals—and in this way he explained "natural immunity" to certain diseases. Some seminaria had an affinity for certain organs or tissues, or for one or another of the humors. The seminaria of smallpox, he felt, had an affinity not only for blood, as Rhazes had suggested, but more specifically for that trace of menstrual blood with which each of us was supposed to be tainted *in utero* and which thenceforth contaminates our own blood. In this, Fracastoro picked up and expanded upon an idea advanced early in the eleventh century by Avicenna (Abu Ali al-Husein ibn Sina, 980–1037[25]). Fracastoro held that, following infection by smallpox seminaria, the menstrual blood would putrefy, rise to the surface beneath the skin, and force its way out via the smallpox pustules. In his own words:

> the pustules presently fill up with a thin sort of pituita and matter, and the malady is relieved by these very means . . . for this ebullition is a kind of purification of the blood; nor should we scorn those who assert that infection contracted by the child from the menstrual blood of the mother's womb is localized by means of this sort of ebullition and its putrefaction, and the blood is thus purified by a sort of crisis provided by nature. That is why almost all of us suffer from this malady, since we all carry in us that menstrual infection from our mother's womb. Hence this fever is of itself seldom fatal, but is rather a purgation . . . Hence when this process has taken place, the malady usually does not recur because the infection has already been secreted in the previous attack.

As with Rhazes' theory, that of Fracastoro appeared to explain all of the known phenomena associated with smallpox, with acquired immunity in this case resulting from the expulsion during the first illness of the menstrual blood contaminant without which clinical disease could not recur. Again, it is worth noting that six centuries after Rhazes, Fracastoro could still refer to smallpox in Italy as an essentially benign and almost beneficial process, apparently ignorant of its lethal effects upon the Mayan and Incan civilizations from 1518 on (see ref. 3). But Fracastoro's menstrual blood theory did not long survive critical evaluation, since Girolamo Mercuriali (1530–1606) certainly did know about the effects of smallpox on Amerindian populations. Mercuriali pointed out[26] that if the menstrual blood theory were correct and universally applicable, then smallpox should have preexisted in America rather than being carried over by ship-laden miasmas, and that indeed the disease should have afflicted Cain and Abel rather than its first appearance being recorded about the time of the Arabs. He also questioned why smallpox was restricted to mankind, since all other mammalian young should also possess a menstrual contaminant and thus be subject to the disease. But most interesting was his objection that if smallpox, measles, and leprosy were all due to menstrual blood, as many physicians maintained, then affliction with one of these diseases should protect against the others, since their common substrate would have been expelled. Such cross-immunity was, of course, contrary to observed fact.

We may add to the list of theories of acquired immunity in smallpox several minor variants on the menstrual blood expulsion theme. Thus, Antonius Portus[27] maintained that it was not menstrual blood but amniotic fluid that contaminated the fetus *in utero* and served after birth as the target for attacks by smallpox. In typical humoralist terms, amniotic fluid was supposed to undergo putrefaction, to rise to the surface, and to be expelled from the body of the smallpox victim by way of the pustules. Here, too, recurrence of the disease was held to be impossible because the host no longer possessed the amniotic fluid substrate that permitted infection to manifest itself in typical clinical symptoms. Similarly, the theory was held by some Chinese physicians that it was the contaminating remnants of umbilical blood in the newborn rather than menstrual blood or amniotic fluid that was responsible for the development of smallpox, and that it was the expulsion of putrefied umbilical blood upon which lasting immunity depended.[28] Indeed, they recommended the careful squeezing out of the blood from the umbilicus prior to ligation as a means of preventing smallpox.

A Distention Theory: Iatrophysics

The Renaissance that had so great an effect on the arts and literature during the fourteenth and fifteenth centuries did not significantly affect the sciences until 200 years later. Thus, during the sixteenth and seventeenth centuries, physics and astronomy came alive in the hands of

Copernicus, Galileo, Brahe, Kepler, and Newton; a new mathematics was developed by Napier, Descartes, Newton, and Leibnitz; the beginnings of modern chemistry could be seen rising from the occult practices of medieval alchemists, stimulated in great measure by Robert Boyle; and great contributions to medicine were made by Paracelsus, Vesalius, Paré, Fallopio, Harvey, and Sydenham.

The new physical sciences had important implications for contemporary medical thought and affected the manner in which diseases were viewed and their therapies formulated. Two new schools of medicine arose as a result of the scientific advances, each vying to apply its theories and its therapeutic regimens to the diseased patient.[29] On the one hand was the iatrochemical school, which interpreted all of physiology as the product of chemical reactions. This approach originated with Paracelsus and was developed and strongly espoused by van Helmont, who in the early seventeenth century could make the very modern-sounding comment about acquired immunity to reinfection: "He who recovers from this disease possesses thenceforth a balsamic blood, which makes him secure from this disease in the future."[30] What van Helmont meant by "balsam" is unclear, but he seems to imply a chemical–physiological rather than a vitalistic interpretation. As may be seen, most theories of acquired immunity conform, more or less, to iatrochemical ideas.

One theory of acquired immunity was advanced, however, that was based not upon iatrochemical ideas but upon the foundations of the second major school of medical thought, that of iatrophysics. These iatrophysical (or iatromechanical) concepts stemmed from Descartes's teaching that all bodily processes are mechanical in nature. The body was held to be a machine, and disease explicable in purely physical terms.

JAMES DRAKE, 1707

The English physician James Drake was of the iatrophysical persuasion. In his book *Anthropologia Nova: Or, a New System of Anatomy*, he suggested that smallpox was caused by a "feverish disposition of the blood," whereby "peccant matter was concocted" and could only escape by forcing its way through the skin with the formation of pustules.

> I conceive therefore that the Alteration made in the Skin by the *Small-Pox*, at whatever Age it comes, is the true Reason why the Distemper never comes again. For the distention, which the *Glands* and Pores of the Skin suffer at that time, is so great that they scarce ever recover their *Tone* again, so as to be able any more to arrest the Matter in its Course outward long enough, or in such quantity, as to create those *Ulcerous Pustules* which

are the very *Diagnosticks* of the *Small-Pox*. For tho' the same *Feverish Disposition* shou'd, and may again arise in the Blood, yet, the Passages thro' the Skin being more free and open, the Matter will never be stopt so there, as to make that appearance, from whence we denominate the *Small-Pox*. . . What has been said of the *Small-Pox*, will suffice to solve the *Phaenomena* of the *Measles, Scarlet Fever,* and *Erysipelatous Inflammation*.[31]

Thus, Drake stays well within the humoralist boundaries of his time but, by superimposing his mechanistic approach, is able to come up with a quite remarkable theory of acquired immunity. Unlike earlier expulsion theories or later depletion theories, Drake would permit smallpox infection to recur in the same individual and indeed to "concoct new peccant material" from the blood. But in an interesting and not uncommon identification of the symptoms with the disease itself, he maintained that the morbid matter would escape through the now-distended pores and glands of the skin as fast as it was formed, so that the symptoms (and thus the disease) could not appear a second time in the same individual. Again, Drake's theory implied a cross-immunity between smallpox and other exanthematous diseases, in apparent ignorance of Mercuriali's objections of 100 years earlier.

In fairness to Drake, I should point out that he advanced this interesting theory with great modesty and diffidence, writing: "Why the *Small-Pox* seldom visits any Person more than once in his Lifetime, has been a famous *Problem* much agitated with very little Success; & therefore if I succeed in my Attempt to resolve this no better than others have done before me, I shall not think it any Loss of Reputation, but shall freely wish others more Happy in theirs, when they undertake to reform my Notions."

Drake's iatrophysical theory of smallpox immunity was taken up by Clifton Wintringham some years later.[32] Wintringham proposed that the "contagious matter" causes a coagulation of the blood, which "increases the Bulk of its constituent Particles," thus obstructing "the ultimate and perspirable vessels," leading to pustule formation. These vessels are left dilated, so that new disease (symptoms) cannot reappear.

Depletion Theories

By the end of the seventeenth century, smallpox had become the serious disease in Western Europe that it was to remain until modern times (see ref. 24). However, in 1714 new attention was directed not only at smallpox but also at acquired immunity to this disease by a series of letters to the Royal Society of London by two Greek-Italian physicians, Emanuele Timoni and Jacob Pylarini, who for the first time brought to the official attention of Western medicine the Eastern practice of variolation, then currently popular in Constantinople. This procedure involved the establishment of a mild infection by the insertion of crusts derived from the pustules of "favorable" cases of active smallpox. The practice had apparently become a very widespread part of the folk medicine of many peoples, since reports soon emerged of its use not only in the Middle East, but in other parts of Asia, in Africa, in rural parts of Western Europe, and even in England. The practice was almost universally known as "buying the smallpox." Indeed, the Chinese, who may have originated the practice, refined it by blowing the infected matter into the nose through a silver tube, employing the left nostril for males and the right for females.[33]

As Genevieve Miller so well describes, smallpox inoculation very rapidly became popular in England, thanks in part to the efforts of Lady Mary Wortley Montagu, wife of the British Ambassador to Constantinople. However, Miller suggests elsewhere[34] that the role of Lady Mary, given great prominence by Voltaire in his *Lettres sur les Anglais*, was exaggerated and that more credit is due to the Royal Experiment, conducted in 1721–22 and followed avidly by the entire populace (see Chapter II). This experiment involved nothing less than the first clinical trial in immunity, in which the efficacy of inoculation was tested first upon condemned prisoners and then upon a group of orphans, in order that the prince and princess of Wales might be reassured and permit the inoculation of their children, which in fact took place in 1722 following the successful clinical trial. It is thus not surprising that the eighteenth century would be rich in both interest in and speculation about smallpox, inoculation, and the mechanism of the acquired immunity that inoculation furnished.

One of the most interesting examples of the general popularity of inoculation practices is furnished by Dühren in his diverting book, *The Marquis de Sade and His Time*.[35] In a section entitled "The Bawdy House of Madame Gourdan," he describes the medical (and other) practices of that most famous of eighteenth-century Paris bordellos. Madame Gourdan apparently retained the services of a Dr. Guilbert de Préval, one of France's most notorious charlatans, who possessed a most remarkable *spécifique* that was a true wonder drug. When injected into the skin, it was held not only to immunize the recipient against syphilis, but even to effect the cure of preexisting disease. Further, Madame Gourdan herself injected it into newly arrived girls as a diagnostic, to assure that they were free of syphilis. As Dühren exclaims, "Imagine, a sexual tuberculin in the 18th century. There is nothing new under the sun!"

Cotton Mather (1663–1728) was one of the remarkable figures of Colonial America. A man of great religiosity, he had played an active part in the Massachusetts witchcraft trials, but he also found time to pursue an impressive range of other interests. He regularly received the *Proceedings of the Royal Society of London* and thus quickly became aware of the communications of Timoni and Pylarini about inoculation. When, in 1721, a smallpox epidemic descended upon Boston, Mather was alone in urging the practice of variolation on the Boston physicians, and finally he convinced his friend Dr. Zabdiel Boylston to undertake this practice. Mather transmitted the Boston results to the Royal Society in several quite scholarly communications, and in 1724 published his *Angel of Bethesda,* the first medical book published in the American colonies.[36] In this remarkable book is a lengthy chapter entitled "Variolae Triumphatae, or the Small-Pox Encountred," in which Mather not only advanced a theory of acquired immunity in natural smallpox infection but also explained (in florid prose) why variolation is effective in inducing lasting immunity:

> Behold, the Enemy [smallpox] at once gott into the very *Center* of the Citadel: And the Invaded party must be very Strong indeed, if it can struggle with him, and after all Entirely Expel and Conquer him. Whereas, the *Miasms* of the *Small-Pox* being admitted in the Way of *Inoculation,* their Approaches are made only by the *Outerworks* of the Citadel, and at a Considerable *Distance* from the Center of it. The Enemy, tis true, getts in so far as to make Some Spoil, yea, so much as to satisfy him, and leaves no *Prey* in the Body of the Patient, for him ever afterwards to seize upon. But the *Vital Powers* are kept so clear from his Assaults, that they can manage the *Combats* bravely and, tho' not without a *Surrender* of those Humours in the Blood, which the Invader makes a Seizure on, they oblige him *to march out the same way he came in,* and are sure of never being troubled with him any more.

Thus, Mather does not view the inoculated material as being in any sense attenuated but considers that the milder disease results only from a peripheral infection, in contrast to the natural infection that gains deadly access to "the very Center of the Citadel." In both cases, however, he views the infection as acting upon some type of substrate (unidentified) that is depleted in the process, thus leaving "no Prey in the Body of the Patient" upon which subsequent infection can act. The similarity between this and other depletion theories, and those described earlier as expulsion theories, will be evident. In the one case the target or substrate

of the infection is used up in the process, while in the other it is expelled
from the body.

THOMAS FULLER, 1730, AND THE INNATE SEED

The seventeenth and eighteenth centuries saw the development of many
interesting notions about the etiology and pathogenesis of infectious
disease. Perhaps none was quite as fanciful as the concept of the "innate
seed," whose fertilization was thought to give birth to the disease process
itself. In the context of smallpox and of acquired immunity, it was
presented most elegantly by Thomas Fuller:[37]

> Nature, in the first compounding and forming of us, hath laid into the
> Substance and constitution of each something equivalent to Ovula, of
> various distinct Kinds, productive of all the contagious, venomous Fevers
> we can possibly have as long as we live. Because these Ovula are of distinct
> Kinds . . . as Eggs of different Fowls are from one another; therefore every
> sort of these Ovula can produce only its own proper Foetus . . . and
> therefore the Pestilence can never breed the Small Pox, nor the Small Pox
> the Measles . . . All Men have in them those specific Sorts of Ovula which
> bring forth Small Pox and Measles, and therefore we say that all Men are
> liable to them . . . The Ovula always lie quiet and unprolific, till impreg-
> nated, and therefore these Distempers seldom come without Infection,
> which is as it were the Male, and the active Cause. The Ovula of each
> particular Fever, are all, and every individual one of them, usually
> impregnated at once . . . And when these have been impregnated, and
> delivered of their morbid Foetus, there is an End of them . . . Upon this
> Account no Man can possibly . . . be infected with any of the respective
> Distempers any more than once.

Fuller's argument speaks elegantly for itself and would appear to
explain all of the known phenomenology of smallpox. Contagion and a
specific etiological agent are represented by the male element that comes
from without and specifically fertilizes the female elements (the ovula)
that reside innately within each of us. As with all seeds, once germinated
and sprouted, the specific seeds of that disease are depleted, and
thenceforth new etiological agents will fall upon sterile soil.

JAMES KIRKPATRICK, 1754

Kirkpatrick was a physician from Charleston, South Carolina, who, after
an early experience with variolation in America, went to London, where
he became one of the principal proponents of the practice. He, too,
espoused a theory that something was depleted from the blood during

the course of smallpox infection, whose absence thenceforth prevented a recurrence of the disease.[38] He postulated the existence of a "pabulum" in the blood, with which contagious variolous "primordia" from the outside united. By the time the disease had run its course, the pabulum had been used up, and thus both natural infection and that following variolation were followed by long-standing acquired immunity. As Kirkpatrick said of reinfection, "Its Seeds were sown in an exhausted Soil."

Elsewhere in the same book Kirkpatrick was guilty of a curious but prescient inconsistency. He suggested, without further amplification, that smallpox "left some positive and material quality in the constitution" that was responsible for prolonged immunity to reinfection. In this he may only have been parrotting an earlier suggestion by the famous Boerhaave (1668–1738), who made the casual suggestion that "people who have smallpox must have something remaining in their body which overcomes subsequent contagious infection."[39] In any event, such suggestions had been made often and were all but ignored during the eighteenth century, except for the occasional sarcastic reference such as was made by the antiinoculator Legard Sparham:[40] "Unless we could suppose some singular Virtue to remain in the Blood as a proper Antagonist, it would be absurd to think them secure from a second Infection, any more than that the Transfusion of the Blood or Matter of a venereal pocky Person into a sound Habit, should secure him from any future Amour with Impunity."

The view that acquired immunity is due to the depletion of a substrate necessary to the action of the pathogen was repeated often during the eighteenth century and became popular in France, following the English lead. Thus, the famous physician de la Condamine favored it in his communications to the Royal Academy of Sciences,[41] and his translator Maty injected the following personal footnote (p. 32) into de la Condamine's book: "I lately tried this experiment (inoculation) upon myself . . . and it had no effect upon my blood, as it had been sufficiently *defecated* 15 years before."

A similar view was repeated in 1764 by the remarkable Italian physician Angelo Gatti,[42] who for a time joined the *philosophes* in Paris to become one of the chief proponents of inoculation in France. In a book notably in advance of its times in its view of infection, resistance, and disease and in its attempt to cut through the often meaningless jargon of contemporary medicine, Gatti compared smallpox infection and acquired immunity to a body that a single spark can set afire, but that has thenceforth become "incombustible" although surrounded by flames. As he says, "In like manner, when you have seen the smallest variolous atom, by its bare application, infecting a human body, and afterwards behold the same body covered with the same kind of matter, and not in the least affected by it, will you not conclude that it is no longer susceptible of infection, and, if I may so say, that it is become invariolable?"

LOUIS PASTEUR, 1880

The rise of modern bacteriology in the 1870s, thanks principally to the studies of Pasteur and Robert Koch, provided for the first time a well-established etiological agent for infectious diseases, which could be studied both *in vivo* and *in vitro*. No sooner had he announced his epoch-making results on the induction of acquired immunity to fowl cholera using attenuated organisms than the exuberant Pasteur, never at a loss for ideas, theories, or biting repartee, advanced a theory to explain this phenomenon to the Academy of Sciences.[43] He pointed out that it was a frequent observation that bacteria grown in culture would initially multiply in great numbers; within days, however, the growth would slow down and finally cease. When these cultures were filtered, it was often found that while reseeding with unrelated bacteria might result in appreciable growth, reintroduction of the same bacteria would almost invariably lead to no new growth at all. Pasteur suggested that this phenomenon was due to the very highly specialized nutritional requirements of each species of organism; as long as the nutrients peculiar to a given organism remained in the solution, growth could proceed, but upon depletion of these special nutrients growth would cease and could not resume thereafter. Pasteur likened the body to an artificial culture medium in which only limited quantities of these special nutrients were present. Following natural infection, or artificial inoculation with attenuated organisms, the preexisting supply of these nutrients would be depleted so that the body could not support renewed growth following reinfection. Thus, prolonged immunity could be induced with great specificity, given the highly specialized nutritional requirements of each pathogen.

Pasteur's theory of depletion did not long survive the rapid advance of bacteriology that took place in the 1880s, and Pasteur, ever the realist, quickly dropped it. But the theory was taken up and pursued for a very long time by no less a figure than Paul Ehrlich. Ehrlich very early developed a keen interest in cancer, and as the result of experimental studies on the inability of certain tumors to grow in some animal species and on the regression of tumors, he formulated a theory of tumor immunity to which he applied the term *atrepsie*. He argued this theory

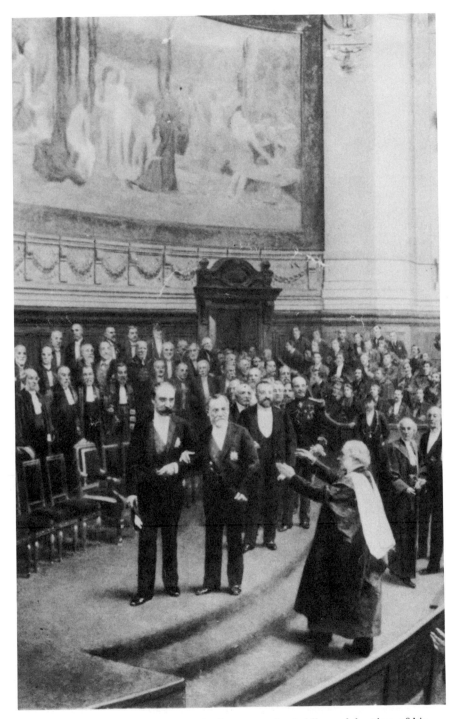

Louis Pasteur, honored at the Sorbonne at the Jubilee celebration of his seventieth birthday in 1892. (Courtesy National Library of Medicine)

elegantly and forcefully as late as 1907, in his Harben lecture before the Royal Institute of Public Health in London.[44] Paying due respect to Pasteur's depletion theory (which the Germans called *Erschöpfung*, "exhaustion"), Ehrlich suggested that just as bacteria might have special nutritional requirements, so also might different cancers. Thus, he thought that a tumor would fail to grow in a host lacking those special nutrients that it required or would regress when it had depleted the host of them. Being still much involved in elaborations of his side-chain receptor theory of antibody formation, he suggested that both bacteria and tumor cells might possess specific "chemoreceptors" that enable them to bind and then ingest those nutrients necessary to their growth. Ehrlich suggested that Pasteur need not have insisted upon complete depletion of a vital nutrient in the host—this he thought improbable. It may suffice either that the nutrient is reduced below a critical level or, more possibly, that the pathogen has lost the ability (receptors) to utilize that nutrient—a sort of atrophy of specific receptors!

The Retention Theory and Other Concepts

In the 10 years between Pasteur's first experimental demonstration of active acquired immunity and the discovery of antibody and of passive immunity by von Behring and Kitasato, rapid advances in the young field of bacteriology and the nascent field of immunology were matched only by the creativity of the investigators seeking explanations for their observations. All of these were, like Pasteur's depletion theory, couched in terms of the action of bacterial pathogens. However, they, like all earlier theories, were classified by Sauerbeck in his 1909 book on *The Crisis in Immunity Research*[45] as "passive" theories, in which the pathogen acts by itself to produce immunity in an otherwise inert host. With the exception of Metchnikoff's cellular (phagocytic) theory, originating in a zoological rather than a human disease context,[46] "active" theories of immunity involving host response awaited the discovery of antibody and complement.

THE RETENTION THEORY

Just as early experiments on the growth of pure cultures of the newly discovered bacteria led to Pasteur's depletion theory, so they also provided information upon which a diametrically opposite theory was formulated. Observations were made by numerous investigators that the growth of bacteria was accompanied by the formation of a variety of substances such as phenol, phenylacetate, skatol, and other aromatic compounds. It was von Nencki who apparently first noticed that the growth of bacteria in culture might be inhibited by these and other products of their own metabolism. This led him to formulate the so-called retention theory of acquired immunity,[47] in which it was postulated that during the course of an infection, the initial bacterial growth in the body would result in the buildup of high concentrations of these chemical inhibitors. This process would lead not only to cessation of growth during the initial infection but also to lasting immunity as a result of the retention of these inhibitors in the host. The specificity of this immunity was explained by assuming that each species of pathogen produced substances peculiar to its own metabolism and to whose inhibitory effect they alone were sensitive. This theory was taken up and championed before the French Academy of Sciences by Chauveau, Director of the Veterinary School at Lyon.[48] In studies of anthrax infection of Algerian sheep, Chauveau observed that the offspring of ewes infected during pregnancy, and especially shortly before parturition, showed an increased resistance to anthrax infection. Chauveau suggested that this increased immunity was due to the retention of inhibitory substances within the body of the infected mother and their transmission across the placenta to the fetus *in utero*. Little more was heard of the retention theory following the discovery of antitoxic and other antibacterial antibodies in the early 1890s.

OSMOTIC AND ALKALINITY THEORIES

The rapid progress made in physical chemistry toward the end of the nineteenth century had a strong influence on contemporary medical thought and practice. This influence was reflected in the famous dispute[49] between Paul Ehrlich on the one side and Jules Bordet and Karl Landsteiner[50] on the other, about whether antigen–antibody–complement reactions more closely resembled firm chemical unions or weaker "colloidal" interactions. Similarly, the new physicochemical concepts found their way into several early theories of acquired immunity.

Two years before his discovery of antitoxic antibodies, von Behring drew a parallel between blood alkalinity and bactericidal action.[51] He supposed that bacterial growth and the tissue changes that accompany it resulted in an increase in the alkalinity of the body to the point where bacterial growth was suppressed and presumably could not be later reinitiated. This is, in a sense, analogous to the retention theory described earlier and did not long survive further experimental work; indeed, von Behring himself helped to lay this theory to rest.

The osmotic theory was advanced by the prominent pathologist

Baumgarten[52] and was based on the suggestion that bacteria were destroyed in the body by osmotic rupture of their membranes. Again, it was supposed that bacterial growth resulted in the production of an increasingly less favorable osmotic environment that would presumably persist even after the initial infection had been cleared. Baumgarten maintained this view for many years and through many editions of his *Textbook of Pathogenic Microorganisms;* he held that the only function of antibodies was to render bacteria more susceptible to osmotic shock.

ADAPTATION THEORY

As I noted earlier, disease was long associated with the action of poisonous miasmata. Among adherents of the concept of contagion, many followed the lead of Boerhaave in ascribing disease to "venomous corpuscles" that not only were transmissible but also could reproduce their own kind and thus poison the humors of the infected individual to induce putrefaction, inflammation, and disease. Since Mithridatic adaptation to various poisons was common knowledge, it is not surprising to find hints of an adaptation theory of acquired immunity to infectious disease throughout these times. But it remained for von Behring to state this theory explicitly in his second paper on diphtheria immunity, if only to disprove it.[53] After recounting his elegant experiments demonstrating immunity to diphtheria toxin, he says, "One might at first think that the resistance to poison described here depends upon an adaptation to that poison (*Giftgewöhnung*) in the sense that it is employed among alcoholics or morphine- and arsenic-eaters . . . in short, that it is essentially a question of training or inurement." Von Behring then goes on to show that such an explanation is impossible in the present instance, because normal mice who have never encountered diphtheria toxin can be protected against lethal doses of it by passive immunization; indeed, the toxin can be neutralized *in vitro* with the serum of immune animals. Although the word *virus* continued to be applied nonspecifically to all pathogens for many years until its usage was restricted to the ultrafilterable and ultramicroscopic agents, and although it might even have retained its connotation as "poison" to some, the advances of the late nineteenth and early twentieth centuries largely demystified and even detoxified many diseases. Concepts such as those outlined in this chapter could not long survive the new knowledge derived from bacteriology, immunology, and experimental pathology.

I have concluded this review of theories of acquired immunity just short of those "modern" concepts that guide investigators today. In contrast to the theories described in this chapter in which the infected host was generally portrayed as a passive receptable in which disease ran its course and immunity might be established, current theories involving antibodies, complement, macrophages, and lymphocytes speak of host–parasite *inter*actions to which the infected or immunized individual makes an active contribution. I shall review in Chapter 3 the early history of modern humoral and cellular theories of immunity and the nature and implications of the early controversy that raged in the late nineteenth century between protagonists of these two concepts.

It will be apparent that throughout history there has been at least a rough consistency in the evolution of the concept of immunity, such as is found in the history of most ideas. At each stage, the contemporary understanding of the nature of immunity was very much a product both of its previous history as well as of contemporary developments in medicine in particular, and in the sciences and philosophy in general. Thus, no matter how improbable or inadequate these theories might appear today, whether derived from magic–theurgic principles, from post-Hippocratic humoralist doctrines, from later iatrochemical or iatrophysical teachings, or even from the early insights of modern bacteriology, they were all very much the product of their times. Each of them, if only transiently, appeared to explain satisfactorily the known phenomena of its day.

NOTES AND REFERENCES

1. A. Stettler, *Gesnerus* **29,** 255 (1972).

2. Colle, Dionysius Secundus; quoted in Stettler, note 1.

3. W. H. McNeill, *Plagues and Peoples.* Doubleday, New York, 1976.

4. Thucydides, *The Peloponnesian War* (Crawley, trans.), p. 112. Modern Library, New York, 1934.

5. Procopius, *The Persian War* (H. B. Dewing, trans.), Vol. I. Heinemann, London, 1914.

6. Girolamo Fracastoro, *De Contagione et Contagiosis Morbis et Eorum Curatione,* 1546 [W. C. Wright trans. (with Latin text), pp. 60–63. Putnam, New York 1930]. See also C. Singer and D. Singer, *Ann. Med. Hist.* **1,** 1 (1917).

7. The translator has here been perhaps too modern in his rendition. Fracastoro nowhere employs the word *immunis,* but rather "*et utrum consuescere pestilentiis possimus,*" which is perhaps better translated "whether it is possible to accustom ourselves to pestilences."

8. L. G. Stevenson, *The Meaning of Poison.* University of Kansas Press, Lawrence, 1959; L. Hopf, *Immunität und Immunisirung: eine medicinische-historische Studie.* Pietzker, Tübingen, 1902.

9. E. Roux and A. Yersin, *Ann. Inst. Pasteur, Paris* **2,** 629 (1888).

10. E. von Behring and S. Kitasato, *Dtsch. Med. Wochenschr.* **16,** 1113 (1890).

11. P. Ehrlich, *Dtsch. Med. Wochenschr.* **17,** 976, 1218 (1891).

12. L. Pasteur, J. Joubert, and C. Chamberland, *C. R. Hebd. Seances Acad. Sci.* **86,** 1037 (1878).

13. L. Pasteur, *C. R. Hebd. Seances Acad. Sci.* **90,** 239, 952 (1880).

14. W. R. Le Fanu, personal communication, 1977.

15. J. Hunter, *A Treatise on the Blood, Inflammation, and Gun-shot Wounds.* Webster, Philadelphia, Pennsylvania, 1823.

16. J. Baron, *Life of Edward Jenner.* Colburn, London, 1838. See also W. R. Le Fanu, *Edward Jenner.* Harvey & Blythe, London, 1951.

17. H. E. Sigerist, *A History of Medicine,* Vol. I, Chap. 2. Oxford University Press, New York, 1951. See also J. Procope, *Medicine, Magic, and Mythology.* Heinemann, London, 1954.

18. L. Thorndike, *A History of Magic and Experimental Science,* Vol. I, Chap. 1. Macmillan, New York, 1923. See also W. H. R. Rivers, *Medicine, Magic, and Religion.* Harcourt Brace, New York, 1927.

19. O. Temkin, Health and disease. In *Dictionary of the History of Ideas* (P. P. Wiener, ed.). Scribner's, New York, 1973.

20. Cyprian, *De Mortalitate* (M. L. Hannon, trans.), pp. 15–16. Catholic University, Washington D.C., 1933.

21. L. Edelstein, *Bull. Inst. Hist. Med.* **5,** 201 (1937).

22. C. Rosenberg, *The Cholera Years.* University of Chicago Press, Chicago, Illinois, 1962. See also E. H. Ackerknecht, *Bull. Hist. Med.* **22,** 562 (1948).

23. Rhazes, *A Treatise on the Small-Pox and Measles* (W. A. Greenhill, trans.). Sydenham Society, London, 1848.

24. A. E. Carmichael and A. M. Silverstein [*J. Hist. Med. Allied Sci.* **42,** 147 (1987)] have speculated that in fact only a mild form of smallpox, akin to *Variola minor,* existed in Europe prior to the seventeenth century.

25. *Avicennae Arabum Medicorum Principis,* Latin translation by Gerard of Cremona, Vol. II, pp. 72–73. Venice, 1608.

26. Hieronymus Mercurialis, *De Morbis Puerorum,* Book I, pp. 17–21. Basel, 1584.

27. Antonius Portus, quoted in G. Miller, *The Adoption of Inoculation for Smallpox in England and France,* p. 244. University of Pennsylvania Press, Philadelphia, 1959.

28. J. Kirkpatrick, *The Analysis of Inoculation,* p. 41. London, 1754.

29. F. H. Garrison, *An Introduction to the History of Medicine.* Saunders, Philadelphia, Pennsylvania, 1917. See also A. Castiglioni, *A History of Medicine.* Knopf, New York, 1947.

30. J. B. van Helmont, De Magnetica Vulnerum Curatione. In Sylvestre Rattray, *Theatrum Sympatheticum Auctum,* p. 477. Nuremberg, 1662.

31. J. Drake, *Anthropologia Nova: Or, a New System of Anatomy,* Vol. I, p. 25. London, 1707.

32. C. Wintringham, *An Essay on Contagious Diseases.* York, 1721.

33. Another method of immunization employed by primitive peoples is that against pleuropneumonia of cattle. De Rochebrun [*C. R. Hebd. Seances Acad. Sci.*

100, 659, (1885)] mentions that the Moors and the Pouls of Senegambia in Africa have a custom "whose origins are lost in the obscurity of history," in which a knife is plunged into the lung of an animal that died of the disease and then used to make an incision in the skin of healthy animals. "Experience has demonstrated the success of this protective operation."

34. Miller, G., Putting Lady Mary in her place: a discussion of historical causation. *Bull. Hist. Med.* **55,** 2 (1981).

35. E. Dühren (pseudonym of Iwan Bloch), *Der Marquis de Sade und seine Zeit,* pp. 123, 213. Barsdorf, Berlin, 1900.

36. C. Mather, *The Angel of Bethesda* (G. W. Jones, ed.). Am. Antiquarian Soc., Barre, Massachusetts, 1972. See also O. T. Beall and R. H. Shryock, *Cotton Mather: First Significant Figure in American Medicine.* Johns Hopkins University Press, Baltimore, Maryland, 1954.

37. T. Fuller, *Exanthematologia: or, an Attempt to give a rational account of Eruptive Fevers,* pp. 175 ff. London, 1730.

38. Kirkpatrick, ref. 28, p. 37.

39. H. Boerhaave, *Praxis Medica,* Vol. V, p. 308. Petavii, 1728.

40. L. Sparham, *Reasons Against the Practice of Inoculating the Small Pox,* p. 20. London, 1722.

41. C. M. de la Condamine, *A Discourse on Inoculation* (M. Maty, trans.). Vaillant, London, 1755.

42. A. Gatti, *Réflexions sur les préjugés qui s'opposent aux progrès et à la perfection de l'inoculation.* Musier, Bruxelles, 1764. See also A. Gatti, *New Observations on Inoculations* (M. Maty, trans.). Vaillant, London, 1768.

43. L. Pasteur, C. Chamberland, and E. Roux, *C. R. Hebd. Seances Acad. Sci.* **90,** 239 (1880).

44. P. Ehrlich, *Experimental Researches on Specific Therapeutics.* Lewis, London, 1908.

45. E. Sauerbeck, *Die Krise in der Immunitätsforschung.* Klinkhardt, Leipzig, 1909.

46. E. Metchnikoff, *Lectures on the Comparative Pathology of Inflammation.* Keegan, Paul, Trench, Trübner, London, 1893. [Reprinted by Dover, New York, 1968.]

47. M. von Nencki, *J. Prakt. Chem.* May (1879); cited in Sirotinin, *Z. Hyg.* **4,** 262 (1888).

48. A. Chauveau, *C. R. Hebd. Seances Acad. Sci.* **89,** 498 (1880); **90,** 1526 (1880); **91,** 148 (1880).

49. See Chapter 5 and H. Zinsser, *Infection and Resistance.* Macmillan, New York, 1914.

50. P. M. H. Mazumdar, *Bull. Hist. Med.* **48,** 1 (1974). See also P. M. H. Mazumdar, Karl Landsteiner and the Problem of Species, 1838–1968. Thesis, Johns Hopkins University, Baltimore, Maryland, 1976.

51. E. von Behring, *Centralbl. Klin. Med.* **9,** 681 (1888).

52. P. Baumgarten, *Berl. Klin. Wochenschr.* **37,** 615 (1900).

53. E. von Behring, *Dtsch. Med. Wochenschr.* **16,** 1145 (1890). For an earlier version, see P. Grawitz, *Virchow's Arch.* **84,** 87 (1881).

2

The Royal Experiment
on Immunity, 1721–1722

BY THE middle of the seventeenth century, smallpox (along with typhus) had replaced the plague as the leading infectious disease causing death in the adult population of Europe.[1] Epidemics of smallpox appeared with increasing frequency[2] and were all the more noticed because, unlike many other contemporary diseases, they afflicted the rich and powerful as well as the poor.[3] Many feared the disease as much for the disfigurement suffered by its survivors as for its impressive mortality, which averaged some 15 to 20% of those infected.[4]

It is customary to credit Edward Jenner with the development of the first effective immunization procedure to protect against an infectious disease. But when Jenner first published his findings on the use of cowpox vaccination in 1798,[5] there already existed an equally effective and (for the times) reasonably safe immunization procedure. This was smallpox inoculation, involving the (usually) dermal infection of the subject with the wild virus, which most often resulted in a mild, transient illness that thenceforth protected the individual against more severe forms of the disease. Prior to Jenner's publication, this procedure had been practiced with generally favorable results for some three-quarters of a century in "polite" society in Europe, and long before that was employed in many countries as a standard practice in the folk medicine

Originally written in collaboration with Genevieve Miller.

24

of "more primitive" peoples. It was, of course, common knowledge in the eighteenth century (and earlier) that a case of smallpox conferred life-long immunity.

The manner in which the practice of smallpox inoculation was introduced into England, where it first attained broad recognition and application,[6] is of great interest in several respects. First, the story illustrates the role of the medical "establishment" in conferring dignity upon, and gaining acceptance for, a new procedure. Second, it highlights the interesting contrast between the prestige of the physician and scientist in eighteenth-century society and that accorded them in later centuries. Whereas a Pasteur, a Behring, or a Koch could feel free in the 1880s to introduce novel procedures to the practice of medicine with no appeal to other than his own authority, the physician of a century and a half earlier hesitated and felt impelled to appeal elsewhere for more powerful patronage and support. Third, the introduction of inoculation to England involved what was probably the first recorded clinical trial in the history of immunity. And finally, it involved the use of human guinea pigs chosen from among the underprivileged and "inferior" peoples, a common practice that has persisted well into the present century and that has only recently begun to be questioned.

The Introduction of Inoculation to England

In Boswell's *Life of Johnson*, the learned doctor is recorded as suggesting that it was foolish to send Radcliffe traveling fellows to the Continent in order to add to medical knowledge; they should rather go "out of Christendom" and visit "barbarous nations."[7] This attitude was a common sentiment of his day, when the accounts of travelers to distant parts were eagerly read by an interested public, and when it was often stated that every single effective new remedy, such as cinchona or ipecacuanha, stemmed from its use among primitive peoples. It was, however, often easier to learn about such foreign arts and inventions than to introduce them and gain their acceptance by a basically conservative society. This resistance was especially true of medical innovation in the early eighteenth century, since not only was the general view of disease and of therapy tradition-bound to 2000-year-old concepts but also its practitioners had not yet become the independent social innovators that the following century would witness.

The Royal Society of London was established in 1660 for the promotion of learning, and by 1700 it had already achieved a prominent position as a clearinghouse for communications of scientific and medical interest from all parts of the world. It was common for Fellows of the

Royal Society to receive letters from individuals at some distant outpost, relaying new information or sending interesting specimens for study. One such communication, dated January 5, 1700, came to Dr. Martin Lister, a prominent London physician and Fellow of the Royal Society, from an East India Company trader stationed in China.[8] This letter reported "a Method of Communicating the Small Pox," involving "opening the pustules of one who has the Small Pox ripe upon them and drying up the Matter with a little Cotton . . . and afterwards put it up the nostrils of those they would infect." This procedure was preferable to natural infection, because the patient could be prepared for the illness and it could be done at an appropriate age and season for an optimal outcome. Apparently Dr. Lister did not relay this information further, but by a curious coincidence this Chinese practice was reported to the Royal Society at its February 14, 1700, meeting by Dr. Clopton Havers,[9] even before the letter to Lister could have reached its destination.

There is no evidence that this initial notice excited any attention within the medical establishment, and nothing more was heard of it in London for 13 years. Then, on May 27, 1714, Dr. John Woodward reported to the Royal Society[10] extracts of a letter dated Constantinople, December 1713, "An Account, or History, of the Procuring the SMALL POX by Incision, or Inoculation; as it has for some time been practiced at Constantinople." The writer of the letter was a Dr. Emanuele Timoni, born in Greece of Italian parents, who had taken his medical degree at Padua, but also had a degree from Oxford and had been elected Fellow of the Royal Society in 1703. At the time that he wrote on smallpox inoculation, Timoni had been practicing medicine in Constantinople for some years and was in fact family physician to the British Ambassador to the Porte, Sir Robert Sutton, and to his successor Edward Wortley Montagu.

In the letter, Timoni described inoculation as a familiar practice "for about the space of 40 years among the Turks and others." He gave a careful description of the choice of an appropriate donor, of the manner in which the patient was to be inoculated, and of the clinical course of the resulting mild disease. He observed

> that altho' at first the more prudent were very cautious in the use of this Practice; yet the happy Success it has been found to have in thousands of Subjects for these eight Years past, has now put it out of all suspicion and doubt; since the Operation having been perform'd on Persons of all Ages, Sexes, and different Temperaments, and even in the worst Constitution of the Air, yet none have been found to die of the *Small-Pox;* when at the same time it was very mortal when it seized the Patient in the common way, of which half the affected dy'd.

The Timoni report provoked several discussions of inoculation at the Royal Society meetings, resulting in a motion to instruct the Secretary to obtain further information on it from the British Consul at Smyrna. Two years later, the Royal Society reprinted in full a more extensive description of smallpox inoculation,[11] a report prepared by Dr. Jacobo Pylarini, then serving in Smyrna as Venetian Consul. Pylarini also testified to the efficacy and relative safety of the inoculation procedure. However, despite the widespread publicity given the practice of inoculation in the *Philosophical Transactions of the Royal Society* and in other leading scientific periodicals of the day, there seemed to be little inclination on the part of a cautious medical profession to adopt the practice. Physicians were apparently afraid to risk their reputations by testing this novel procedure.

But two individuals (neither, significantly, a physician) did independently undertake to popularize inoculation. One was Cotton Mather of Boston, who sent a letter in July of 1716 to Dr. John Woodward of the Royal Society, asking why the practice of inoculation had not been tried in England and stating that he intended to persuade the Boston physicians to employ it the next time that smallpox entered the city.[12] He was as good as his word, and during the smallpox epidemic of 1721 in Boston, he persuaded Dr. Zabdiel Boylston to undertake inoculation and later speculated on the nature of acquired immunity in smallpox infection.[13]

The second individual who espoused the doctrine of smallpox inoculation was Lady Mary Wortley Montagu, wife of the British Ambassador to Constantinople. It is not clear that Lady Mary was aware of the Timoni and Pylarini reports, but she soon learned of the local custom of smallpox inoculation, or ingrafting, and it made a great impression upon her. As she wrote in a letter to her friend Sarah Chiswell in April 1717:

> I am going to tell you a thing that I am sure will make you wish yourself here. The small-pox, so fatal, and so general amongst us, is here entirely harmless by the invention of *ingrafting* . . . I am patriot enough to take pains to bring this useful invention into fashion in England; and I should not fail to write to some of our doctors very particularly about it, if I knew any one of them that I thought had virtue enough to destroy such a considerable branch of their revenue for the good of mankind . . . Perhaps, if I live to return, I may, however, have courage to war with them.[14]

Lady Mary had obviously not much respect for the medical profession. She was, however, a firm convert to inoculation, and in March 1718 had her six-year-old son inoculated by Charles Maitland, surgeon to the Embassy.[15]

Lady Mary returned to London in 1719, but apparently did little to advance the cause of inoculation over the next two years, until the deadly smallpox epidemic of 1721 stimulated her to action. She thereupon sent for Maitland (who by this time had retired to a small town near London) and requested him to see to the inoculation of her three-year-old daughter Mary. Maitland was somewhat hesitant to perform this Eastern practice in London and insisted that outside physicians be called in as witnesses—he appeared to be reluctant to accept sole responsibility for the procedure. But finally, in late April of 1721, the young Montagu child was successfully inoculated. When the pocks appeared, three members of the College of Physicians examined her separately, and one of them was so convinced by what he saw that he had Maitland inoculate his own son, the only one of his children who had not yet already succumbed to the disease.

The impact of Lady Mary's demonstration of inoculation on the events that followed is not entirely clear. Undoubtedly it aroused considerable professional interest, although it was not reported in the newspapers of that time. History has usually credited Lady Mary with the dominant role in the introduction and acceptance of inoculation in England, an attribution based primarily on Voltaire's effulgent praise and his report that she enjoyed the close friendship of the Princess of Wales;[16] but this explanation has recently been opened to question.[17] Be that as it may, the groundwork had been laid for further experimentation with the inoculation procedure, and the currently raging smallpox epidemic, which was exacting a heavy toll among the upper classes, provided excuse enough to exploit any hopeful approach.

The Royal Experiment

One of the remarkable figures of eighteenth-century England then emerged as a champion of smallpox inoculation. This was Sir Hans Sloane, Bart., President of the Royal College of Physicians of London, one of the two Secretaries to the Royal Society (to whose presidency he would succeed Isaac Newton in 1727), and court physician first to Queen Anne and then to the current ruler, George I. Sloane had an inquiring mind and was interested in everything. (His personal library of over 50,000 books and his vast collection of botanical specimens, coins, and antiquities would later be sold to the nation to form the core of the British Museum.[18]). Sloane was thus in an excellent position to advance the cause of smallpox inoculation, both directly and indirectly.

During the height of the smallpox epidemic in early May 1721, the youngest child of the prince and princess of Wales fell ill with what was at first thought to be smallpox but later provided to be a milder ailment. Whether this was the spark that stimulated the interest of the intellectually and scientifically oriented Princess of Wales, Caroline of Ansbach, in the new procedure of inoculation is uncertain, but she must have feared for her children.

It is not clear exactly who was responsible for the royal interest in inoculation. Voltaire's candidate was Lady Mary Wortley Montagu. A contemporary account published by a German visitor maintained that it was Maitland who appealed to the princess for permission to experiment further with the procedure,[19] while Sloane's own "Account of Inoculation," written some 15 years after the event (and, unaccountably, not published until 1756) held that Princess Caroline, "to secure her other children, and for the common good, begged the lives of six condemned criminals . . . in order to try the experiment of inoculation upon them."[20] But Sloane's retrospective account contains other inaccuracies, and perhaps it does not do justice to his own role in the affair, as one of the most powerful promotors of the new scientific movement in England.

In any event, within a month of the illness of the royal child, the newspapers recorded that "some physicians" had made a representation to the king, to obtain permission to carry out experiments on condemned criminals in Newgate Prison, on condition that the prisoners receive subsequent pardon.[21] The king apparently acquiesced, for on June 14 the Secretary of State, Lord Townsend, addressed a letter to the attorney and solicitor generals, asking them to advise the crown "Whether His Majesty may by Law Grant his Gracious Pardon to two Malefactors under Sentence of Death upon Condition that they will suffer to be try'd upon them the Experiment of Inoculating the Small pox."[22] Three days later, an opinion was returned that "the Lives of the persons being in the power of His Majesty, he may Grant a Pardon to them upon such lawful Condition as he shall think fit; and as to this particular Condition We have no objection in point of Law, the rather because the carrying on this practice to perfection may tend to the General Benefit of Mankind."[23]

This interest in science on the part of George I was not surprising, and the new scientific movement in England, exemplified by the Royal Society, was fortunate in finding itself under Hanoverian rule. Before becoming George I of England, the elector of Hanover had patronized learning by supporting men like Leibnitz; and once in England, both he and the prince of Wales, later George II, had maintained their interest in science. They attended lectures on experimental philosophy, studied Newtonianism, and sponsored experiments in mechanics at Hampton Court. Indeed, Princess Caroline's intellectual curiosity led Voltaire to refer to her, after her husband ascended the throne, as the "*Philosophe aimable sur le Trône.*"

Whether Sir Hans Sloane was instrumental in prompting the initial appeal to the king is not known, but it was he who asked Maitland to perform the experiments upon the condemned criminals, and it was he who sought additional confirmation of the efficacy of the inoculation practice. Under the supervision of the two royal physicians, Sir Hans Sloane and Dr. John George Steigherthal, three male and three female prisoners were inoculated by Maitland at Newgate Prison on the morning of August 9, 1721. The importance of the proceedings and the significance of the royal patronage is attested to by the extensive coverage that the experiment received in the press and by the fact that it was witnessed by no less than 25 physicians, surgeons, and apothecaries, including eminent members of the College of Physicians and of the Royal Society.[24]

Incisions for the insertion of the smallpox pus were made on the arms and right legs of the convicts. Because, on August 12, the incisions were not as inflamed as expected, Maitland obtained sufficient fresh donor pock material to repeat the operation on five of the patients. Symptoms appeared on the next day in all but one man, and after a brief illness of varying severity, each of the patients recovered. (The one prisoner who never showed any reaction was found to have had smallpox the previous year.) Interest in these experiments was maintained, and the patients were visited almost daily by physicians and other interested persons. In addition, the newspapers continued their coverage of the experiments, and even reprinted the original Timoni description of five years earlier.

Shortly after the initial experiments, another prominent London physician, Dr. Richard Mead, obtained permission to try the Chinese method of inoculation on a young female prisoner. This procedure involved intranasal administration of matter from a favorable case of smallpox. In this case, the usual symptoms of smallpox appeared promptly, and although the woman was more seriously ill than any of the others, she recovered fully.[25] As agreed, all of the convicts who had been involved in these experiments were pardoned by the king and his council and were released from Newgate on September 6, 1721.

While the Newgate experiment convinced most people that smallpox inoculation was safe, there was still the question of its efficacy in preventing subsequent attacks of the natural disease. Some claimed that inoculation gave not true smallpox but chickenpox or swinepox, and that it would not confer immunity. To test this, Sloane and Steigherthal arranged, at their own expense, to send one of the pardoned women to a small town near London where Maitland lived in retirement and where a very severe smallpox epidemic was then raging. Under Maitland's supervision, the 19-year-old was ordered "to lie every Night in the Same Bed [with a 10-year-old smallpox victim], and to attend him constantly from the first Beginning of the Distemper to the very End." For a period of about six weeks, she was exposed to the most serious form of the disease, without contracting it herself, a fact to which numerous witnesses testified.[26]

To further confirm the original experiment on the safety of smallpox inoculation, Maitland successfully inoculated an additional six persons the following February, again under royal sponsorship. In this instance, the experiment was announced officially from Whitehall, and it was stated that "the Curious may be further satisfied by a Sight of those Persons at Mr. Forster's House in Marlborough Court at the Upper-End of Poland-street and Berwick-street in Soho, where Attendance is given every Day from Ten till Twelve before Noon, and from Two till Four in the Afternoon."[27]

Not satisfied with the inoculation experiments on adults, the newspapers announced in the middle of November that instructions had been given by Princess Caroline to draw up a list of all orphan children in St. James Parish, Westminster, who had not yet had smallpox, so that they might be inoculated at her expense. Although by this time Maitland had successfully inoculated several children in private, it was apparently felt that a public demonstration of the safety of the procedure in children was also necessary. Here again, the role of the royal advisors is well illustrated by a letter from the Royal Surgeon Claude Amyand to the Royal Physician Sir Hans Sloane in which, commenting on the availability of orphan children, Amyand wrote, "What I thought proper to urge was, that these fresh instances might reconcile those that were yet diffident about the success of the inoculation . . . The princiss will be glad to know wuther you think these wanting, and Therefore came to waite on you on this account."[28] Five orphan children were inoculated successfully in March, and once again the newspapers published the details and indicated where interested persons might view the patients.

Primarily as a consequence of these inoculation experiments, confidence in the new method had mounted by April of 1722 to the point where several prominent political figures called on Maitland to inoculate their children. Finally, on April 17, 1722, the prince and princess of Wales, after consultation with Sir Hans Sloane, had the operation performed on two of their daughters, 11-year-old Princess Amelia and

9-year-old Princess Caroline. While Sloane was hesitant to urge inoculation of the royal children, neither would he attempt to dissuade Princess Caroline "in a matter so likely to be of such advantage." Caroline resolved to have the inoculation performed and sent Sloane to the king to obtain his permission. Sloane advised the king that "it was impossible to be certain but that raising such a commotion in the blood, there might happen dangerous accidents not foreseen." The King replied that such accidents might happen from being bled or taking *any* medicine, no matter how much care was taken, and gave the royal consent to proceed (see ref. 20). The princesses were thereupon inoculated by Amyand, with the assistance of Charles Maitland and under the supervision of the royal physicians Sloane and Steigherthal. So important an event was naturally mentioned in all of the newspapers and helped to ensure at least the temporary popularity of the inoculation procedure in polite society.

Discussion

OPPOSITION TO INOCULATION

Despite the success of the royal experiment and the prominent example set by the inoculation of the royal children, smallpox inoculation did not escape severe criticism at the time, nor did it become widely practiced. Indeed, in the seven years following the royal experiment, only 897 inoculations were reported in the British Isles, America, and Hanover.[29] Of these, 17 patients (2%) died. This figure was substantially confirmed in a 1759 pamphlet by one B. Franklin of Philadelphia, who argued forcefully nevertheless for the advantages of inoculation.[30] But even though the mortality that accompanied smallpox inoculation was appreciably less than the estimated 1 person in each 6 to 10 who might expect to die of natural smallpox (not to mention those who would be disfigured), it did indicate that the inoculation procedure was not without its hazards. In addition to citing the dangers of inoculation, including further spread of the infection by the inoculated individual, those opposed to the practice claimed variously that it did not give true smallpox; that it did not protect against subsequent disease; and, above all, that it went against both God and Nature.

The antiinoculation banner was raised as early as 1722 by the surgeon Legard Sparham in his "Reasons against the Practice of Inoculating the Small-Pox."[31] Among other concerns, Sparham argued against the insertion of "poisons" into wounds and held that "till now, [we] never dreamt that Mankind would industriously plot to their own Ruin, and barter Health for Diseases." Only a little later, the Reverend Mr. Massey preached from the pulpit of the Parish Church of St. Andrew's Holborn on "the Dangerous and Sinful Practice of Inoculation." Mr. Massey held that the power to inflict disease rests upon God alone and it is He who gives the power to heal. The fact that one possesses the physical power or knowledge to perform an act does not imply that one has the moral right to do so. "I shall not scruple to call that a *Diabolic Operation*, which usurps an Authority founded neither in the *Laws of Nature* or *Religion*, which tends in this case to anticipate and banish *Providence* out of the World, and promotes the encrease of Vice and Immorality."[32]

But if inoculation had its difficulties in England, it met with even greater opposition in France, where word of the London inoculation experiments soon arrived. Here, the medical establishment itself rose in opposition to inoculation. The Faculté de Médicine of the University of Paris was not only a teaching body but also supervised medical police measures, drug inspection, medicolegal questions, and various other aspects of public health. When in 1723 the Faculté sponsored a disputation on inoculation—and then voted in favor of the thesis that inoculation was a useless, uncertain, and dangerous practice, and should be condemned—it was clear that inoculation would face great problems of acceptance in France. In fact, the adoption of inoculation in France lagged some 40 years behind its introduction into England.[33]

In general, interest in smallpox inoculation in England waxed and waned in parallel with the comings and goings of epidemics of the disease. Thus, the return of epidemic smallpox to London in 1746 led to the founding of a Smallpox and Inoculation Hospital, established for the provision of free care for smallpox patients and to make inoculation more readily available. But the epidemic ran its course, and interest in inoculation decreased; consequently, after 10 years it could be reported that only 1252 inoculations had been given in the hospital.[34] Interest in smallpox inoculation persisted for many years, even surviving the introduction of Jennerian vaccination until, in 1840, an Act of Parliament outlawed the practice, in final recognition of the additional safety offered by Jenner's innovation.

HUMAN EXPERIMENTATION

Few persons would have dreamed in 1721 of raising any question of the ethics of employing human prisoners for the type of experiment I have described here—indeed, few voices were raised against similar practices even in the present century.[35] Two or three centuries ago, as in most of recorded history, it was implicitly accepted (and often explicitly stated) that a life was valued increasingly more as one ascended the social ladder; and numerous examples of these valuations may be found. Thus, the Wangensteens in their book *The Rise of Surgery* cite the experiments done in an attempt to find a cure for Louis XIV's anal fistula.[36] In 1686 the king's physician Guy Fagon recommended that the surgeon Charles-François Félix relieve Louis XIV of his distressing ailment by operation. Provision was made for Félix to obtain knowledge and deftness in the procedure at a Paris hospital, and patients afflicted with *fistula in ano* were sent there for surgery. These experiments went on for some months, until Félix felt ready to work on the king; and, as the Wangensteens point out, "tradition has it that a number of these did not survive Félix's operation, and that the bodies were disposed of at night and the deaths were attributed to poisoning." In the end, the experiments succeeded, and the King's discomfort was alleviated.

Another example of this approach may be found in a suggestion made by J. Bellers in 1714 that hospitals be established in Britain to improve the treatment of disease.[37] Bellers was obviously a humanitarian, but the times permitted him to suggest that "one Hospital should be more particularly under the Care and Direction of the QUEEN'S [Anne's] Physicians; that they may take into it such Patients whose Infirmities at any time our SOVEREIGN may be subject to."

The royal experiment of 1721–22 was not the only clinical trial of smallpox inoculation, nor was it the only one to use social inferiors as human guinea pigs. During the spring of 1751, the Geneva Council gave its permission to l'Hôpital Générale et de la Bourse Française to experiment with inoculation, using "subjects entirely dependent upon the Directors, and principally upon bastards;" 18 persons were successfully inoculated in these tests.[38]

ON THE VALIDITY OF EXPERIMENTAL EVIDENCE

The design of the royal experiment might surprise the modern investigator and would certainly fail to qualify it for publication in a modern journal. No controls were employed, and the initial experiment tested the safety of the inoculation procedure in only six individuals and its efficacy (in preventing subsequent infection) in only one. But these were simpler times, when a procedure or a phenomenon either worked or did not work in a clear-cut fashion; the concept of utilizing large numbers to establish statistical significance had not yet been introduced.

It is interesting, in the same connection, to examine the data in Edward Jenner's original publication, which introduced smallpox vaccination to the world. In all, Jenner published 23 case reports, only 7 of which involved inoculation of cowpox virus into normal human recipients, and only 2 individuals were subsequently challenged with the wild smallpox virus to assess efficacy. But it was not the limited numbers in Jenner's report that led members of the Royal Society to reject an earlier draft of the "Inquiry," "lest he damage his reputation."[39] Apparently, they simply did not believe Jenner's claims and their implications, thus depriving him of the prestige of publication in the *Philosophical Transactions of the Royal Society*. Jenner was thereupon forced to have his *Inquiry* published privately, with consequences that are history.

Why was it that the practice of inoculation made such slow progress despite its royal patronage, whereas vaccination gained substantially worldwide acceptance and use within a very few years, though lacking any official backing at the outset? There was, as we have seen, no substantial difference in the quality of the initial data on safety or efficacy, and indeed vaccination had many early opponents also. The difference may well rest less on the force of scientific evidence than on a variety of unrelated social factors, as is often true of medical vogues even today. In 1722 such measures as smallpox inoculation were restricted to a relatively small class of the educated and landed gentry that composed "Society," and knowledge of or interest in scientific advance was rare in the rest of the population. But throughout the eighteenth century, the concept of public health spread fairly widely, as was witnessed by the founding of many hospitals for the poor and of societies devoted to the health and welfare of the underprivileged. Indeed, inoculation itself helped pave the way for vaccination, since much of the population saw the latter technique as an improved version of one already in use. Thus, I suggest that by the start of the nineteenth century, society as a whole was better prepared than it had been 75 years earlier to accept what appeared to be a significant medical advance against the dread smallpox.[40]

NOTES AND REFERENCES

1. C. Creighton, *A History of Epidemics in Britain,* Vol. II. Cambridge, 1894. See also P. Kübler, *Geschichte der Pocken und der Impfung.* Berlin, 1901.

2. It has been suggested [A. E. Carmichael and A. M. Silverstein, *J. Hist. Med. Allied Sci.* **42,** 147 (1987)] that only a mild form of smallpox existed in Europe prior to the seventeenth century and that virulent *Variola major* substantially replaced it by the 1660s.

3. C. M. de la Condamine, *Mem. Acad. R. Sci.* p. 615 (1754). "It is especially in the towns and in the most brilliant Courts that one sees it [smallpox] exert its ravages."

4. J. Jurin, *An Account of the Success of Inoculating the Small-pox in Great Britain, for the Year 1724.* London, 1725. (Analogous reports were published for the following two years.)

5. E. Jenner, *An Inquiry into the Causes and Effects of the Variolae Vaccinae . . .* Sampson Low, London, 1798.

6. See, e.g., A. C. Klebs, *Bull. Johns Hopkins Hosp.* **24,** 69 (1913); R. P. Stearns and G. Pasti, *Bull. Hist. Med.* **24,** 103 (1950); G. Miller, *The Adoption of Inoculation for Smallpox in England and France.* University of Pennsylvania Press, Philadelphia, 1957.

7. *Boswell's Life of Johnson,* Vol. II, p. 551. Oxford University Press, London, 1946.

8. Lister MS. 37, fol. 15, Bodleian Library, Oxford; quoted in Stearns and Pasti, ref. 6, p. 107.

9. Journal Book IX, Royal Society Library, p. 194.

10. *Philos. Trans. R. Soc. London* **29**(339), 72 (1714).

11. *Philos. Trans. R. Soc. London* **29**(347), 393 (1716).

12. J. B. Blake, The inoculation controversy in Boston: 1721–1722. *N. Engl. Q.* **25,** 490 (1952). See also G. L. Kittredge, Introduction to Increase Mather's, "Several Reasons Proving that Inoculating or Transplanting the Small Pox, Is a Lawful Practice, and That It Has Been Blessed by God for the Saving of Many a Life" (1721). Cleveland, 1921.

13. C. Mather, *The Angel of Bethesda* (1724) (G. W. Jones, ed.). Am. Antiquarian Soc., Barre, Massachusetts, 1972. Mather's theory of acquired immunity in smallpox has been discussed in Chapter 1.

14. Lady Mary Wortley Montagu, *Letters and Works,* Vol. I, pp. 308–309; quoted in R. Halsband, *J. Hist. Med.* **8,** 390 (1953).

15. C. Maitland, *Account of Inoculating the Small Pox.* London, 1722.

16. Voltaire, Sur l'insertion de la petite vérole (1727). In *Lettres Philosophiques,* 3rd Ed., pp. 130–151. Gustave Lanson, Paris, 1924. "*Cette dame* [Lady Mary] *de retour à Londres fit part de son expérience à la Princesse de Galles*"

17. G. Miller, Putting Lady Mary in her place: A discussion of historical causation. *Bull. Hist. Med.* **55,** 2 (1981). See also Miller, ref. 6.

18. "Dictionary of Scientific Biography," Vol. XII, pp. 456 ff.

19. M. E. Boretius, Special-Nachricht von der neuen Invention der Inoculationis variolarum, oder des Blatter-Peltzens, wie solche in London exerciret worden. *Samml. Nat. Med. Gesch. (Leipzig und Bautzen)* **17,** 206 (1723).

20. H. Sloane, An Account of Inoculation by Sir Hans Sloane, Bart., given to Mr. Randy to be published, Anno 1736. Communicated by Thomas Birch, D.D. Secret R.S. *Philos. Trans. R. Soc. London* **49,** 516 (1756).

21. *Weekly J. or Br. Gazetteer* June 17, p. 1952 (1721); *Applebee's Orig. Weekly J.* June 17, p. 2087 (1721).

22. Hardwicke papers, Vol. 786, Add. MS. **36,** 134, f. 58, British Museum, London.

23. Hardwicke papers, ref. 22.

24. *Applebee's Orig. Weekly J.* Aug. 12, p. 2134 (1721); *Weekly J. or Br. Gazetter* Aug. 12, p. 1999 (1721); *Weekly J. or Saturday's-Post* Aug. 12, p. 844 (1721).

25. R. Mead, *A Discourse on the Small Pox and Measles*, pp. 88–89. John Brindley, London, 1748.

26. Reference 15, p. 20.

27. *London Gaz.* Mar. 6–10, No. 6040 (1722).

28. Sloane MSS, MS. 4076, f. 331, Mar. 14, British Museum, London, 1722.

29. J. G. Scheuchzer, *J.–Book R. Soc.* **XIII,** Mar. 27, 319 (1729).

30. B. Franklin, "Some Account of the Success of Inoculation for the Small-Pox in England and America." London, 1759. [Reprinted in L. H. Reddis, *"Edward Jenner and the Discovery of Smallpox Vaccination.* George Banta, Menasha, Wisconsin, 1930; also in *Mil. Surg.* **65,** 645 (1929).]

31. L. Sparham, "Reasons against the Practice of Inoculating the Small-Pox As Also a Brief Account of the Operation of This Poison, Infused after This Manner into a Wound," p. 26. London, 1722.

32. Edmund Massey, "A Sermon against the Dangerous and Sinful Practice of Inoculation. Preach'd at St. Andrew's Holborn, on Sunday, July the 8th, 1722." London, 1722.

33. Miller, ref. 6.

34. *Gentleman's Mag.* **28,** 41 (1758).

35. See articles by G. H. Brieger, A. M. Capron, C. Fried, and M. S. Frankel, in the section on human experimentation. In *Encyclopedia of Bioethics,* Vol. II, pp. 683–710. Free Press, New York, 1978.

36. O. H. Wangensteen and S. D. Wangensteen, *The Rise of Surgery,* p. 13. University of Minnesota Press, Minneapolis, 1978.

37. J. Bellers, "An Essay Towards the Improvement of Physick in Twelve Proposals," 1714; cited in J. Woodward, *To Do the Sick no Harm: A Study of the British Voluntary Hospital System to 1875.* Routledge & Kegan Paul, London, 1974.

38. Léon Gautier, "La Médecine à Genève jusqu'à la fin du dix-huitième siècle," Geneva, 1906; cited in Miller, ref. 6.

39. E. M. Crookshank, *History and Pathology of Vaccination,* Vol. I, pp. 250 ff. H. K. Lewis, London, 1889. Crookshank was, 90 years later, an anti-vaccinationist, so his account may be suspect—see anonymous contribution to the "Jenner Centenary Number," *Br. Med. J.* **1,** 1257 (1896).

40. The rapid spread of acceptance of vaccination throughout the world, and the resulting adulation of Jenner, can best be compared with the similar response to Pasteur's antirabies treatment of the 1880s. In both instances, the initial evidence on safety and efficacy was incomplete, but the world responded with alacrity and enthusiasm, and even their governments rewarded them. When Jenner interceded with the French on behalf of an English prisoner, Napoleon, then at war with England, remarked that he could not refuse anything to this great benefactor of mankind.

3

Cellular versus Humoral Immunity: Determinants and Consequences of an Epic Nineteenth-Century Battle

IN A major address to the congress of the British Medical Association in 1896, Lord Lister suggested that if ever there had been a romantic chapter in the history of pathology, it was certainly that concerned with theories of immunity. Lister's reference was to two epic but interrelated battles that had occupied pathologists, bacteriologists, and immunologists over the course of several decades—battles that saw opposing schools engage in passionate debate and a degree of vilification almost unknown in present-day science. When Lister spoke in 1896, the first of these great disputes was nearing its resolution. This one involved the question of the basic nature of the inflammatory reaction—whether inflammation is an abnormal response harmful to the host or a normal and beneficial component of its defensive armamentarium. However, the second of these battles had not yet been resolved and was still being fought in every journal and at every congress relating to the subject. Its focus was on the question of whether innate and acquired immunity to infection could be best explained by cellular or by humoral mechanisms. In that exciting decade when remarkable discoveries crowded close on one another's heels, when new mechanisms, new organisms, new diseases appeared with almost every issue of the journals, the protagonists from one or the other camp grasped each new item eagerly to bolster their own theory or to cast doubt upon that of the opposition.

The lines that divided the two camps were fairly sharply drawn. Conceptually, the cellularists argued that the chief defense of the body

38

against infection resided in the phagocytic and digestive powers of the macrophage and the microphage (the polymorphonuclear leukocyte). The humoralists claimed that only the soluble substances of the blood and other body fluids could immobilize and destroy invading pathogens. Geographically, the cellularists were predominantly French and rallied round Elie Metchnikoff at the Pasteur Institute in Paris. The humoralists were predominantly German and followed the leadership of Robert Koch and his disciples at Koch's Institute in Berlin.

An examination of the history of the cellular–humoral dispute illustrates several interesting points. First, it provides the historian of ideas with yet another example of how earlier and even outmoded concepts help to determine the structure and content of future thought and how the intransigent commitment to a scientific dogma often prevents timely and rational compromise. Second, it provides to the sociologist of science yet another striking example of the way in which nonscientific events may contribute importantly to both the direction and the velocity of scientific development. Finally, it provides to the modern immunologist the sobering caution that the triumph of one concept in such a dispute may for many decades stifle developments dependent upon the other concept, to the detriment of the scientific discipline.

Background to the Conflict

As is true of most conceptual advances in science, the theory of a cellular basis for immunity and the violent opposition it engendered arose, not in a scientific and cultural vacuum, but in an environment that largely defined the nature and direction of the subsequent debate. Among the determinants of the battle over the central nature of immunity, some may be traced back over 2000 years to the ideas of Hippocrates, some appeared only with the development of a true medical science and of Virchow's new pathology in the mid-nineteenth century, whereas some, surprisingly, were founded on the international politics and nationalistic rivalries of the contemporary era. It is only in the context of these background elements that the directions taken by this epic struggle, its intensity, and the full flavor of this "romantic chapter" may be fully appreciated.

THE NATURE OF DISEASE

For over 2000 years, following the teachings of Hippocrates, Celsus, and Galen,[1] disease was considered to be a maladjustment of the normal ratios of the four vital humors: the blood (*sanguis*), the phlegm (*pituita*), the yellow bile (*chole*), and the black bile (*melaine chole*). This humoral tetrad, almost a mystical part of a larger system that included Aristotle's four basic essences (earth, water, fire, and air) and the four primary qualities (hot, cold, wet, and dry), influenced medical theory and medical practice even into the nineteenth century,[2] despite the long-standing appreciation that some diseases were contagious, and despite the early recognition that prior exposure to a "plague" might protect the individual from the current contagion. Even into the early nineteenth century, cupping, purgatives, phlebotomy, and the application of leeches were still common practices applied to all types of disease, to restore the ill-humored to healthier proportions. Given a humoral theory of disease going back over 20 centuries, coupled with a humoral approach to prophylaxis and therapy of similar ancestry, it is not surprising that the mere name "humoral" as applied to a theory of immunity would carry with it much traditional respect and prestige. This situation was true even despite the serious criticism leveled at more modern humoralist offshoots, such as the hematohumoral theory of Rokitansky.[3]

It was only in 1858, about 25 years before Metchnikoff's first publication on the phagocytic theory, that Rudolph Virchow issued a comprehensive challenge to the remnants of the humoral theory of disease, in the form of a claim that all pathology is based upon the malfunction of cells rather than upon the maladjustment of humors.[4] Although Virchow's cellular pathology was widely acclaimed and respected, even a quarter-century later in the 1880s humoralism had not yet fully given way to Virchow's cellular concepts, upon which Metchnikoff based his theory of immunity.

Another factor important for an understanding of the nature of disease, and another example that ancient concepts die hard, was that involving etiology. Any precise concept of immunity had necessarily to be based upon the acceptance that infectious diseases are specific and reproducible. But only slowly did the medieval notion of ill-humors and miasmas give way to the recognition that each infectious disease is produced by its own specific pathogenic microorganism. The first barrier to be overcome in this acceptance was the old belief that the variety of microorganisms seen since the time of Leeuwenhoek were spontaneously generated and almost infinitely mutable. The concept of spontaneous generation should have been destroyed in the eighteenth century by the work of Spallanzani (1768) and others, but it persisted and was defended by prominent scientists even up to the 1860s and 1870s. It finally gave way, at least in France, before the brilliant experimentalism and, more decisively, the forceful argumentation of

Louis Pasteur.[5] Again, it was not until the late 1870s, barely five years before Metchnikoff advanced his new theory of immunity, that the germ theory of disease finally gained wide acceptance, due in part to its proclamation by Pasteur[6] and to Robert Koch's elegant description of the etiology of wound infections.[7]

One may thus conclude that the cellular theory of immunity advanced by Elie Metchnikoff in 1884[8] did not constitute just one further acceptable step in a well-established tradition; rather it represented a significant component of a conceptual revolution with which contemporary science had not yet fully learned to cope.

THE NATURE OF INFLAMMATION

It is important that the modern reader appreciate that at the time it was advanced Metchnikoff's theory of phagocytosis was less a contribution to immunological thought than to the field of general pathology, which for 30 to 40 years had been debating the nature of the inflammatory response. It will be recalled that at this point cellular pathology was only 25 years old, that a formal germ theory of disease was scarcely 5 years old, and that the demonstration by Louis Pasteur of a vaccine prophylaxis for chicken cholera (the first carefully designed scientific study that was to serve as the foundation for the new science of immunology) had appeared only 4 years earlier.[9]

Thus, there was little or no context of immunological thought in which to fit the Metchnikovian theory: neither Edward Jenner with smallpox nor Louis Pasteur with chicken cholera had understood the mechanism responsible for the immunity they were able to induce.[10] But there was a broad context in the general pathology of inflammation against which Metchnikoff's new theory could be measured, and here the phagocytic theory constituted a strong challenge to accepted dogma. The inflammatory reaction that accompanied infectious diseases and especially traumatic wounds had usually been considered deleterious to the host. This belief was perhaps understandable in the days before the concept of antisepsis, when the inflammatory response presented most often as a purulent and violent accompaniment of a wound, most often rendering an unfavorable prognosis. Even the repeated reference to a "laudable pus," most notably by that remarkable poet and scientist Erasmus Darwin (1731–1802) in his *Zoonomia* of 1801, did not seriously challenge the belief in the noxious contribution of the inflammatory response. With the rise of microscopy and anatomical pathology, purulent discharges were early associated with those inflammatory cells later named macrophages and microphages, and thus these cells were

indentified as the most obvious component of the deleterious inflammatory reaction. Moreover, it was generally thought by most pathologists of
the era that phagocytic cells actually provided an admirable means of
transport for infectious organisms in their dissemination throughout the
body.

It was in this context that Metchnikoff dared to suggest that the
phagocytic cells, far from being harmful, in fact constitute a first line of
defense in their ability to ingest and digest invading organisms. It is not
surprising, therefore, that when Rudolph Virchow visited Metchnikoff
in his laboratory in Messina in 1883, he advised Metchnikoff to proceed
with great caution in advancing his theories, since "most pathologists do
not believe in the protective role of inflammation."[11]

Metchnikoff's challenge to contemporary pathological thought,
however, was not limited to his iconoclastic view of the significance of the
inflammatory response. Indeed, he dared to challenge the current
concepts and authorities on the very nature of inflammation. Virchow
himself had formulated a concept of parenchymatous inflammation, a
concept invoking a disturbed nutrition and intensified local proliferation
of parenchymal cells due to injury by the pathologic agent, thus leading
to the *tumor,* which he considered the most significant component of the
process. Julius Cohnheim, on the other hand, concluded from his
famous experiments that inflammation was due primarily to lesions of
the walls of the blood vessels, a pathology permitting passive leakage of
all of the components (primarily humoral) then recognized in the
inflammatory response.[12] Thus, Cohnheim considered that the *rubor*
was the most significant sign of the inflammatory reaction. Even though
the field of general pathology was divided on which of these two
mechanisms was most important for the inflammatory reaction, almost
all agreed with these great pathologists that inflammation was a deleterious reaction of no benefit to the host—a purely passive response on
the part of the insulted organism. It is understandable that Metchnikoff's radical views would have a poor reception, because they not only
challenged the very foundation of then-current dogma, they also were
advanced by an individual who was (1) not a member of the confrater-
nity of pathologists (Metchnikoff was a zoologist); (2) not even a
physician (the chemist Pasteur had encountered similar problems); and
(3) a Russian (a people then traditionally considered somewhat backward by many Western Europeans).

INTERNATIONAL POLITICS

In 1888, the itinerant expatriate Metchnikoff took up permanent
residence in Paris as *Chef de Service* at the Pasteur Institute. His natural

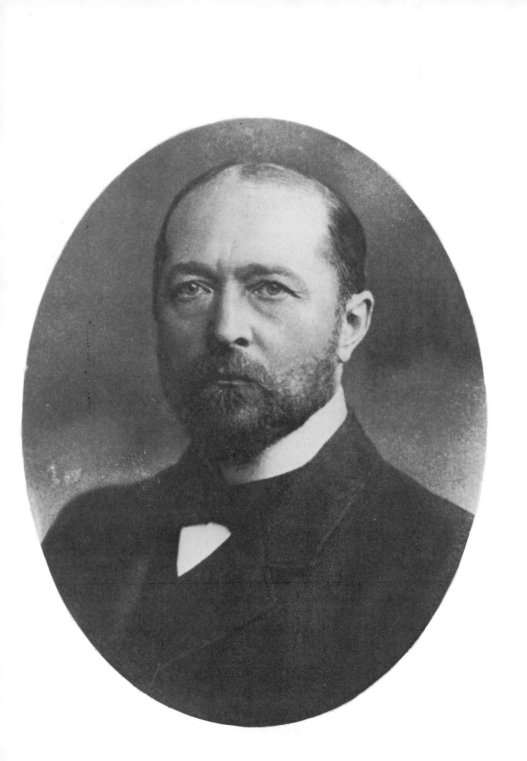

Emil von Behring (Courtesy National Library of Medicine)

inclinations, reinforced by the fervent patriotism of Pasteur, engendered in Metchnikoff a strong passion for his adopted homeland. Proponents of the cellular theory thus naturally looked to Paris and the Pasteur Institute for their leadership, and the cellularists were drawn, for the most part, from among French scientists. In Germany, however, Metchnikoff's theory came under severe attack at an early date, first by Baumgarten in Berlin and then by other German pathologists. This curious geographical partisanship was even more sharply defined by a division of sentiment within recently unified Germany itself. The most vocal opponents of the Metchnikovian theory, all from within Prussia, were Baumgarten, Bitter, Christmas-Dirckinck, Ziegler, Gaffky, and Emmerich, all of Berlin; Flügge of Göttingen; Weigert of Breslau; and Frank of Friedrichsheim. Of those Germans who spoke out on behalf of Metchnikoff, Hess was in Heidelberg, Ribbert in Bonn, and Buchner in Munich, all from regions of Germany that had historically resented Prussian power and hegemony. Elsewhere, Gamelaia and Banti in Italy and Calus in Vienna voiced their support of Metchnikoff.[13] British workers were in general neutral on the issue, with the notable exception of the francophile Lord Lister, who repeatedly acknowledged the debt that his antiseptic theories owed to Pasteur and Metchnikoff.

The principal division in the cellularist–humoralist battle was between France and Germany, a division that reflected the overall nationalistic tendencies of the time. England had for over 600 years been the traditional enemy of France, dating from the time that the descendants of the Norman conquerors of England laid claim to their old lands and even to the throne of France. Even after the English were expelled from the continent, the principal element of their foreign policy was to subsidize coalitions of the smaller states in Europe, including the German states, to neutralize a powerful France. The continuing French policy, on the other hand, was to prevent the development of a powerful continental opponent among the German-speaking peoples. The Germans, in their turn, had long resented the power of France and felt that French Alsace should be a part of a greater Germany. A tradition of enmity between France and the German states (and especially Prussia) thus matured over a long period of time and culminated in the ignominious defeat of the French and the loss of Alsace in 1870–71 at the hands of a Germany now unified under Prussian rule.

The phagocytic theory of immunity was not the only dispute in which objective science appeared to have been compromised by the aftereffects of the Franco-Prussian War. In the aftermath of the siege of Paris, Louis Pasteur, who in 1868 had received an honorary M.D. degree from the University of Bonn, returned his honors in anger. He wrote to the head of the Faculty of Medicine at Bonn that

Now the sight of that parchment is odious to me, and I feel offended at seeing my name, with the qualification of *virum clarissimum* that you have given it, placed under a name which is henceforth an object of execration to my country, that of Rex Gulielmus . . . I am called upon by my conscience to ask you to efface my name from the archives of your faculty, and to take back that diploma, as a sign of the indignation inspired in a French scientist by the barbarity and hypocrisy of him who, in order to satisfy his criminal pride, persists in the massacre of two great nations.

In response, Pasteur received a reply from the Principal of the Faculty of Medicine of Bonn, who "is requested to answer the insult which you have dared to offer to the German nation in the sacred person of its august Emperor, King Wilhelm of Prussia, by sending you the expression of its entire contempt" (see ref. 5). Ten years later, Pasteur and Robert Koch were engaged in violent debate about the etiology, pathogenesis, and prophylaxis of anthrax and other diseases, with unseemly and vituperative statements being issued from both sides. Indeed, the first volume of the Reports of the German Imperial Health Office in 1881 could almost have been subtitled "anti-Pasteur," containing as it did scathing criticisms of Pasteur's work by Koch and his students Löffler and Gaffky.[14] These authors declared that Pasteur was incapable of cultivating microbes in a state of purity, that he did not know how to recognize the septic vibrio (although he himself had discovered it!), and that many of his experiments were "meaningless." Pasteur, on his side, pursued the debate with his customary vigor, even going so far as to challenge Koch to face-to-face debate at the International Congress of Hygiene at Geneva in 1882. When, in the end, Pasteur's demonstration of the efficacy of anthrax vaccination was fully vindicated by the famous experiments at Pouilly-Le-Fort,[15] Pasteur rejoiced aloud that this great discovery had been a French one, and it is not difficult to define the alternative that he might have feared. It is interesting that yet another great immunological debate, concerning the nature of the antigen–antibody interaction, was carried on between Jules Bordet at the Pasteur Institute in France and Paul Ehrlich in Germany.[16]

It was in this environment, then, that the cellular-versus-humoral debate proceeded. As was appropriate for the halls and journals of science, few overt hints appeared that anything other than pure objective science determined this debate. One such instance, however, appeared in a paper by Abel,[17] which was highly critical of Metchnikoff; Abel made a statement about "interpretations which we on the German side cannot share." Metchnikoff was highly incensed by this statement, and in a later book called Abel to task for such unscientific nationalism.[18]

One may only wonder whether this debate would have been as vitriolic or protracted had the international political setting been different during the latter half of the nineteenth century. Paul de Kruif goes too far perhaps in suggesting in his book *Microbe Hunters*[19] that this epic struggle in immunology contributed to the start of World War I, but it does seem probable that, in a minor way at least, it did represent one of the continuing reverberations of the Franco-Prussian War of 1870.

Cellular versus Humoral Immunity

THE EARLY DEBATE

Ilya (later Elie) Metchnikoff was born in the Steppe region of Little Russia in 1845. He studied invertebrate zoology in both Russia and Germany and developed a keen interest in invertebrate embryology while working at Naples with the great Russian embryologist Kovalevsky. His work in this field was extremely productive; consequently, by the late 1870s he had established for himself a significant reputation in zoological circles. It was during this period that he developed an interest in the digestive processes of invertebrates and especially in the intracellular digestion exhibited by the wandering mesodermal cells of metazoans. This interest in digestion was to remain with Metchnikoff throughout his life and accounts for his zeal in the popularization of yogurt in Western Europe and for the prominent place that digestive disorders play in so many of his writings.[20]

It was while working in the Marine Biology Laboratory on the straits of Messina that Metchnikoff first conceived of the phagocytic theory. In one of those conceptual leaps that occur in a science, an investigator may look at an old phenomenon and suddenly gain a new insight. In his own words:

> One day when the whole family had gone to the circus to see some extraordinary performing apes, I remained alone with my microscope, observing the life in the mobile cells of a transparent starfish larva, when a new thought suddenly flashed across my brain. It struck me that similar cells might serve in the defense of the organism against intruders. Feeling that there was in this something of surpassing interest, I felt so excited that I began striding up and down the room and even went to the seashore in order to collect my thoughts. I said to myself that, if my supposition was true, a splinter introduced into the body of a starfish larva, devoid of blood vessels or of a nervous system, should soon be surrounded by mobile cells as is to be observed in the man who runs a splinter into his finger. This was no sooner said than done . . . I was too excited to sleep that night in the expectation of the results of my experiment, and very early the next morning I ascertained that it had fully succeeded. That experiment formed

the basis of the phagocytic theory, to the development of which I devoted the next twenty-five years of my life.[21]

While continuing his studies of phagocytic cells in invertebrates, Metchnikoff immediately realized the significance of his theory for human disease; and as early as 1884 he published a paper on the relationship of phagocytes to anthrax. He quickly followed this with studies on erysipelas, typhus, tuberculosis, and numerous other bacterial infections. In his 1891 book, *Comparative Pathology of Inflammation*, Metchnikoff formalized the statement of the phagocytic theory and demonstrated in detail its Darwinian evolutionary development.[22]

No sooner had the phagocytic theory appeared in the literature than it came under severe and protracted attack.[23] At the outset, these objections were of a quite general nature, as befitted a theory that flew in the face of so many conventional wisdoms. As the debate proceeded and as new experiments flooded the literature, both the claims for the phagocytic theory and the counterclaims against it assumed a more precise form. In retrospect, the objections to Metchnikoff's theory may be cataloged under the following headings: (1) the phagocytes fail to ingest one or another pathogenic organism; (2) even where organisms are ingested by phagocytes, those organisms either are not destroyed or had already come under humoral attack; and (3) even when phagocytes can be shown to be effective components of the immune response, their role is secondary to the earlier action of some humoral factor. (We will omit here a discussion of the criticisms of some of Metchnikoff's more exuberant claims, such as those that the phagocytes are the chief agents of the aging process, wherein active phagocytosis of neurons was claimed to contribute to senility and the phagocytosis of hair pigment to graying.)

It was not until 1888 that the opponents of Metchnikoff's cellular theory found a proper banner around which they could rally, and a phenomenology upon which to base a humoral alternative to the phagocyte. In that year Nuttall, during the course of experiments designed to put Metchnikoff's theory to the test, observed that the serum of normal animals possesses a natural toxicity for certain microorganisms.[24] This observation was quickly seized upon by many investigators, most notably by Buchner,[25] who not only was the first of the theoreticians of the humoral concept of immunity (without becoming anticellularist), but who also named the active bactericidal factor alexin (protective substance; Ehrlich later renamed it complement). It is interesting that this observation had almost been foretold a century earlier by John Hunter, the famous surgeon, naturalist, and teacher of

Edward Jenner in his *Treatise on the Blood, Inflammation, and Gunshot Wounds,* in which he noted that blood did not decompose as readily as other putrescible materials.[26] For a number of years after 1888, the scientific journals were filled with reports that the cell-free fluids of normal and especially of immunized animals could kill bacteria, so no recourse to Metchnikoff's phagocytic cells was needed to explain both natural and acquired immunity. This view received perhaps its most powerful support from the observation of Pfeiffer, who found that the injection of cholera vibrios into the peritoneal cavity of immune guinea pigs was followed by the rapid destruction of the vibrios.[27] This Pfeiffer phenomenon involved an early granular change and swelling of the organisms, followed soon after by complete dissolution and disappearance, i.e., the process of bacteriolysis. Moreover, it was soon shown that the Pfeiffer phenomenon could be passively transferred by injecting serum from an immunized guinea pig into the peritoneal cavity of a normal guinea pig—it was even shown that bacteriolysis would proceed *in vitro.* The humoralists claimed that on those occasions when microorganisms could actually be found within phagocytic cells, it was probably part of the cleanup operation of damaged bacteria.

In response to these strong attacks by the humoralist school, Metchnikoff and his students at the Pasteur Institute were by no means silent. In paper after paper, these investigators demonstrated that there is often no relationship between the natural bactericidal powers of the serum of different species and their susceptibility to infection by a given organism. Rather, as in the case of anthrax, the resistance of a species could often be directly correlated with the ability of its phagocytes to ingest this organism. (It is interesting that so many of Metchnikoff's telling experiments were performed using the anthrax bacillus. As Zinsser later pointed out (see ref. 16), this was a highly fortuitous choice, since the resistance of this bacillus to immune lysis is especially well marked and phagocytosis seems indeed to be the chief mode of bacterial destruction.)

A further method of investigation employed by Metchnikoff while endeavoring to prove his point was the attempt to demonstrate that virulent bacteria could be protected from destruction in the body of a resistant animal if the function of the leukocytes was inhibited. This prediction led to a number of ingenious experiments, such as the one performed by Trapeznikoff on anthrax infection of frogs.[28] Whereas anthrax spores injected subcutaneously were rapidly phagocytosed and destroyed, those introduced in little sacks of filter paper were protected from phagocytes and remained virulent, although bathed in the tissue fluids. (This experiment is very reminiscent of the Algire chamber that was employed over 60 years later to demonstrate that allograft rejection is based upon cellular rather than humoral mechanisms.[29]) Another of the interesting experiments of the era was that of Cantacuzène,[30] who showed that animals treated with opium are much more susceptible to infection than are normal controls, as the presumed consequence of the inhibition of motility of the drugged phagocytic cells. Finally, Metchnikoff showed repeatedly that the nonspecific creation of a macrophage-rich peritoneal exudate, with the attendant activation of those macrophages, would protect that host against intraperitoneal injection of lethal doses of bacteria. This technique was an early forerunner of another modern practice, that of nonspecific immunotherapy.[31]

The debate thus ebbed and flowed during the first decade following 1884, with the cellularists appearing at times to carry the day, and the humoralists claiming victory at other times. But slowly the tide appeared to turn against the phagocytic theory, forcing Metchnikoff, in his zealous defense of the phagocytic theory, to formulate rather extreme *ad hoc* hypotheses. When faced with increasingly convincing evidence of the bactericidal properties of immune serum, Metchnikoff postulated that immunization led to the formation of substances called "stimulins" that acted directly upon phagocytes to enhance their activity. Again, when evidence mounted on the important role of serum complement (thanks in no small measure to the work of Jules Bordet in Metchnikoff's own laboratory), the cellularists were forced back to the position that complement probably originates in any event from the destruction of blood macrophages during the clotting process. Still later, Metchnikoff felt forced to go to great lengths to show that his theory was not inconsistent with Ehrlich's side-chain concept.

THE GROWING HUMORAL TIDE

The most telling blow to the cellular theory of immunity came in 1890 with the discovery by von Behring and Kitasato that immunity to diphtheria and tetanus is due to antibodies against the exotoxins of these bacteria.[32] When, shortly thereafter, it was demonstrated that passive transfer of immune serum would protect the naive recipient from diphtheria, with no obvious intercession by any cellular elements,[33] the humoralists felt that they had been vindicated, and Koch felt free to proclaim the demise of the phagocytic theory at a congress in 1891. The discovery of antibodies against these exotoxins, and even against toxins of nonbacterial origin such as ricin and abrin,[34] supported the earlier

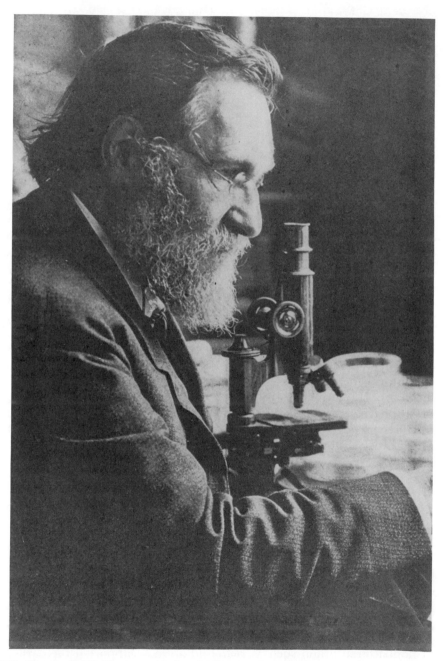

Elie Metchnikoff (Courtesy National Library of Medicine)

view that most infectious diseases were toxic in nature; thus, it could be claimed that protection was due in large part to humoral antitoxic antibodies. Although the discovery of the Pfeiffer phenomenon quickly corrected this generalization by showing that circulating antibody could induce direct bacteriolysis of cholera organisms, even this observation provided yet another strong support for the humoral concept. Bordet's demonstration[35] that even the erythrocyte could be lysed with antibody in the absence of phagocytes demonstrated the generality of this phenomenon and further reinforced the humoralists' claims.

As the decade of the 1890s progressed, new observations lent further weight to claims for the supremacy of the role of humoral antibody in the mediation of immunity. New antibodies against different microorganisms were reported regularly, and their specificities demonstrated. The discovery of the precipitin reaction[36] and Ehrlich's classic work on the titration of antidiphtheria antibodies and diphtheria toxin[37] (which did much to found the field of immunochemistry) demonstrated that antibody was more than a concept: it was a substance that one could see and feel and study in the test tube. And most immunologists were much more comfortable with antibody than they were with the difficult phagocyte. Discovery of bacterial agglutination[38] provided still another convincing demonstration of the importance of humoral antibody in defense against infection. It only remained for Ehrlich to provide a theoretical formulation in his side-chain concept of the functions of antibody, antigen, and complement[39] to make the antibody the principal object of interest to almost all immunologists. This victory was helped in no small measure by the pictures that Ehrlich published to illustrate his side-chain theory—pictures that made it easier to believe that antibodies and complement were "real substances" with comprehensible receptors and simple modes of action.

By the turn of the century, then, most active investigators favored one or another modification of a humoral theory to explain natural immunity and, certainly, acquired immunity. Metchnikoff was correct in receiving the impression at a congress in 1900 that his theory was not well understood, but he was perhaps too late in his attempt to rectify this situation by publishing a year later his famous book, *Immunity in the Infective Diseases*. Of course, the phagocytic theory continued to be referred to and was covered extensively in the textbooks of the day; but it was treated more as a general phenomenon of great biological interest and as a tribute to a tireless and personally highly respected worker than as a serious competitor among general theories of immunity. Even the discoveries of anaphylaxis,[40] of the Arthus phenomenon,[41] and of serum sickness[42] provided indirect support for the humoralists' view-

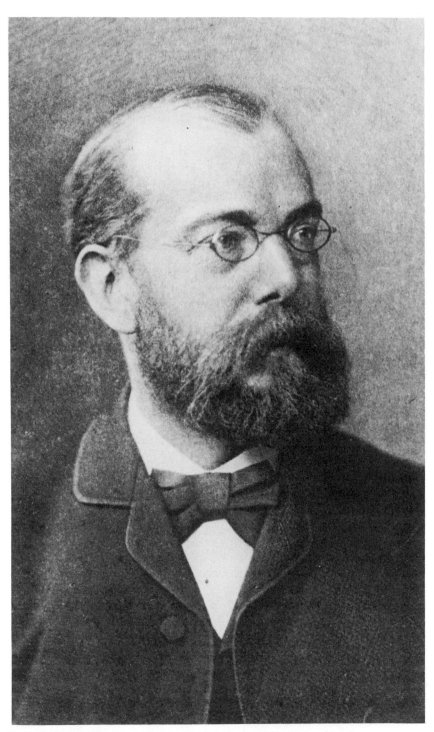

Robert Koch (Courtesy National Library of Medicine)

point. While no one at the time quite knew what the relationship was between immunity and these manifestations of allergy, it was clear that these were somehow immunological phenomena dependent upon humoral antibody for their attainment.

As is most often the case in scientific disputes such as that between the cellularists and humoralists, the triumph of one theory over another is not proclaimed by some impartial arbiter, to be followed by general public acquiescence. The best measure of outcome is an assessment of the influence of these theories on the active members of that scientific community, especially an assessment of the subjects of research among the younger scientists. A review of the literature of the early twentieth century shows that although the cellularist–humoralist debate appeared to be continuing—based upon what the older generation was *saying* in the literature—most scientists old and young were *doing* work on antibodies and complement rather than on cells. (Even later, as Brieger[43] points out, Metchnikoff's work was more revisited than extended.)

Two events occurred over the next few years to make it appear that the result of this silent vote in favor of the humoral theory of immunity was not widely appreciated. In 1908, the Swedish Academy conferred the Nobel prize in physiology or medicine jointly on Metchnikoff, the current champion of cellularism, and on Ehrlich, the then-leading exponent of humoralist doctrines, "in recognition of their work in immunity." While it is dangerous to speculate upon motives, one cannot help but feel that this joint recognition was an attempt to arbitrate the dispute between cellularists and humoralists. But to judge again from the literature, the decision came too late, since active research on the participation of cells in immunity continued to decline.

Another apparently belated attempt to mediate the cellularist–humoralist dispute and to rationalize their differences followed the naming and description of the mode of action of opsonin by Wright and Douglas in England.[44] These investigators claimed that both humoral and cellular functions were equally important and interdependent, in that humoral antibody interacts with its target microorganism to render it more susceptible to phagocytosis by macrophages. Upon this simple structure, Wright constructed an elaborate and extremely complicated therapeutic scheme involving the determination of "opsonic indexes" and the administration of autovaccines at certain critical periods during the course of the infectious process. This approach became so popular in early twentieth century England that Bernard Shaw, a close friend of Almroth Wright, used it as the subject of his play "The Doctors' Dilemma." In his otherwise scathing castigation of the medical profession, Shaw, the skeptic and therapeutic nihilist, summarizes Wright's approach in his "Preface on Doctors":

> Sir Almroth Wright, following up one of Metchnikoff's most suggestive biological romances, discovered that the white corpuscles or phagocytes, which attack and devour disease germs for us, do their work only when we butter the disease germs appetizingly for them with a natural sauce which Sir Almroth named opsonin . . . The dramatic possibilities of this discovery and invention will be found in my play. But it is one thing to invent a technique: it is quite another to persuade the medical profession to acquire it. Our general practitioners, I gather, simply declined to acquire it.

However, Shaw was wrong and Wright was too optimistic: many tried, but the techniques proved so difficult and unreproducible in practice as to become unfashionable within a decade (see ref. 16). In partial consequence of this, he came to be referred to (out of his hearing) as Sir Almost Right, but while Wright acquired a new nickname, the cellular theory of immunity lost its last opportunity for revival for many years to come.

Consequences of the Humoralist Victory

It is the central thesis of this chapter that the fall from favor of Metchnikoff's cellular (phagocytic) theory of immunity carried with it profound implications for future developments in the young discipline of immunology. The most imaginative and productive investigators working on the cutting edge of a science tend to choose their problems based upon what they (or their teachers) feel is most significant, rather than what is technically the easiest. Behind them come the less imaginative, content to follow the fashions of the day. During the early decades of the twentieth century, it was clear to most workers that antibody held the key to an understanding of immunity, and thus it constituted the natural choice for investigative work. Moreover, the direction of antibody research itself underwent a significant change that was detrimental to cellular studies, a change due to the decline of what has been called the Golden Age of bacteriology. As the discovery of new pathogens and new phenomena slowed around the turn of the century and as those infectious diseases amenable to immunological prophylaxis or therapy were satisfied, nascent immunology more and more turned away from medicine and biology and toward chemistry. This shift was initiated early on by the studies and theories of the ever chemically oriented Ehrlich and given a strong push by the famous chemist Svante Arrhenius.[45] This new direction was more than adequately reinforced during the 1920s and 1930s by the elegant work of Landsteiner on serological specificity[46] and of Heidelberger and his students on quantitative immunochemistry.[47] Leaving aside Pasteur himself (who, though trained as a chemist, was the quintessential biologist), it is interesting to note the number of workers trained in chemistry who became interested in immunology, including Arrhenius, Haurowitz, Heidelberger, and Linus Pauling.

But the failure of the cellularist doctrine to gain adherents in the scientific community meant also that many approachable problems in cellular immunology were neglected as being "uninteresting" in the humoralist context of the times. This statement is not meant to suggest that all of the important problems could have been solved, or even that many of the important questions could immediately have been posed: rather, one might reasonably have expected slow but substantial progress in cellular immunology over the next 40 to 50 years. Thus, instead of endless searches for circulating antibody associated with tuberculosis, the tuberculin reaction, and contact dermatitis, histopathological studies and their resultant conclusions might have been obtained many decades earlier rather than awaiting the important descriptions of Gell and Hinde,[48] Turk,[49] and Waksman[50] in the 1950s. Such studies might have pointed up much earlier the importance of the lymphocyte in immunological phenomena. Again, the phenomenological demonstrations of Mackaness,[51] Rowley,[52] and others on the critical role of cellular immunity in certain bacterial infections required few advances over the techniques available to Metchnikoff and could certainly have been pursued 50 years earlier had the cellularists still held sway. Finally (but by no means exhausting the potential list), the pioneering cell transfer experiments of Landsteiner and Chase,[53] establishing the critical role of mononuclear cells in cellular immunity, were well within the technical competence of investigators early in this century. But the notion of cellular immunity was out of favor, and few investigators in that environment were stimulated to pose the questions that might have led to such studies.

For a period of almost 50 years, few questions about cells in immunity were asked within a discipline comfortable with the dogma that circulating antibody would provide all essential answers to the problems of immunity and immunopathology. Only rarely during the first half of the twentieth century did an investigator think it worthwhile to study the role of cells in immunological phenomena or to explore the basis of "bacterial allergy" or "delayed hypersensitivity," as it was variously termed. In the 1920s and early 1930s, Zinsser[54] studied bacterial allergy, and Dienes and co-workers[55] studied delayed hypersensitivity to simple protein antigens injected into tubercles (the forerunner of the adjuvant), a possibility extended by Jones and Mote[56] and by Simon and Racke-mann.[57] In tissue culture experiments, Rich and Lewis[58] showed the importance of inflammatory cells in tuberculin allergy, and Harris, Ehrich, and co-workers carried on extensive studies of the role of the lymphocyte in antibody formation.[59] But these were isolated excursions out of the mainstream that made little impression upon immunological thought at the time. As late as 1951, in his classic book, *The Pathogenesis of Tuberculosis,*[60] Arnold Rich could conclude that little was known about the nature of bacterial allergy, its relationship to immunity, or even the extent to which the familiar macrophage and the ubiquitous but mysterious lymphocyte were involved in its development.

The study of delayed hypersensitivity only attained respectability and became an appropriate topic for immunological symposia[61] and books in the early 1960s, in conjunction with a shift in immunology from a chemical to a more biological approach. This radical change in emphasis can be traced directly to the development of the type of crisis in immunology that Thomas Kuhn has suggested is often responsible for major conceptual changes within a scientific discipline.[62] The new questions posed about the mechanism of allograft rejection, of immuno-logical tolerance, of immunity in certain viral infections, of the patho-genesis of autoallergic diseases, and of the phenomena associated with immunological deficiency diseases could no longer be answered within the framework of a classic theory based solely upon the functions of humoral antibody. Despite the hiatus of over 50 years, the explosion of activity in cellular immunology during the 1960s was such that many of the gaps in our knowledge about cell functions in immunity were rapidly filled; at least partial vindication could be claimed for Metchnikoff's cellular theory of immunity; and a new journal bearing the title *Cellular Immunology* could appropriately be started in 1970. It is still permissible, however, for one to wonder whether cellular immunology would be even further developed today, and even somewhat different, had the humoral theory of immunity not triumphed over the cellular theory in the late nineteenth century.

NOTES AND REFERENCES

1. H. E. Sigerist, *A History of Medicine*, Vol. II. Oxford University Press, New York, 1961.

2. E. H. Ackerknecht, *A Short History of Medicine.* Ronald Press, New York, 1955. See also A. Castiglioni, *A History of Medicine*, 2nd Ed. Knopf, New York, 1947.

3. R. J. Miciotto, *Bull. Hist. Med.* **52,** 183 (1978).

4. R. Virchow, *Die Cellularpathologie in ihrer Begründung auf physiologische und pathologische Gewebelehre.* Hirschwald, Berlin, 1858. [English edition: *Cellular Pathology.* Dover, New York, 1971.]

5. R. Vallery-Radot, *La Vie de Pasteur.* Hachette, Paris, 1901. [English edition: Dover, New York, 1960.] (For a comprehensive history of the spontaneous generation controversy, see J. Farley, *The Spontaneous Generation Controversy from Descartes to Oparin.* Johns Hopkins University Press, Baltimore, Maryland, 1974.)

6. L. Pasteur, J. Joubert and C. Chamberland, *C. R. Hebd. Seances Acad. Sci.* **86,** 1037 (1878).

7. R. Koch, *Untersuchungen über die Aetiologie der Wundinfectionskrankheiten.* Vogel, Leipzig, 1878.

8. E. Metchnikov, *Virchows Arch.* **96,** 177 (1884).

9. L. Pasteur, *C. R. Hebd. Seances Acad. Sci.* **90,** 239, 952 (1880).

10. W. Bulloch, *The History of Bacteriology.* Oxford University Press, London, 1938 (see also Chapter 10).

11. O. Metchnikoff, *Life of Elie Metchnikoff.* Houghton, Mifflin, Boston, 1921. See also the biography by his devoted student and co-worker A. Besredka, *Histoire d'une idée, L'oeuvre de E. Metchnikoff.* Masson, Paris, 1921.

12. J. Cohnheim, *Neue Untersuchungen über die Entzundung.* Hirschwald, Berlin, 1873.

13. The order of battle in this dispute is discussed by E. Ziegler, [*Beitr. Pathol. Anat. Jena* **5,** 419 (1889)].

14. *Mitt. Kaiserl. Gesundheitsamte* **1,** 4, 80, 134 (1881).

15. L. Pasteur, *C. R. Hebd. Seances Acad. Sci.* **84,** 900 (1877).

16. H. Zinsser, *Infection and Resistance.* Macmillan, New York, 1914. See also P. H. Mazumdar, *Bull. Hist. Med.* **48,** 1 (1974).

17. R. Abel, *Zentralbl. Bakteriol. Parasitenkd. Jena* **20,** 760 (1896).

18. E. Metchnikoff, *L'Immunité dans les Maladies Infectieuses.* Masson, Paris, 1901. [English translation: Macmillan, New York, 1905; reprinted by Johnson Reprint, New York, 1968.]

19. P. De Kruif, *Microbe Hunters.* Harcourt, Brace, New York, 1926.

20. E. Metchnikoff, *The Nature of Man.* Putnam, New York, 1903.

21. Metchnikoff, ref. 11, pp. 116–117.

22. E. Metchnikoff, *Lectures on the Comparative Pathology of Inflammation.* Keegan, Paul, Trench, Trübner, London, 1893. [Reprinted by Dover, New York, 1968.]

23. The most comprehensive criticism was by P. Baumgarten, *Z. Klin. Med.* **15,** 1 (1889).

24. G. Nuttall, *Z. Hyg.* **4,** 353 (1888).

25. H. Buchner, *Zentralbl. Bakteriol.* **6,** 561 (1889).

26. J. Hunter, *Treatise on the Blood, Inflammation, and Gunshot Wounds.* Webster, Philadelphia, Pennsylvania, 1823.

27. R. Pfeiffer, *Z. Hyg.* **18,** 1 (1895).

28. A. V. Trapeznikoff, *Ann. Inst. Pasteur, Paris* **5,** 362 (1891).

29. G. H. Algire, *J. Natl. Cancer Inst.* **15,** 483 (1954).

30. J. Cantacuzène, *Ann. Inst. Pasteur, Paris* **12,** 273 (1898).

31. Symposium on Immunotherapy of Tumours, in *Progress in Immunology*, Vol. III, pp. 559–605. Elsevier, New York, 1977.

32. E. von Behring and S. Kitasato, *Dtsch. Med. Wochenschr.* **16,** 1113 (1890).

33. E. von Behring and E. Wernicke, *Z. Hyg.* **12,** 10, 45 (1892).

34. P. Ehrlich, *Dtsch. Med. Wochenschr.* **17,** 976, 1218 (1891).

35. J. Bordet, *Ann. Inst. Pasteur, Paris* **12,** 688 (1899).

36. R. Kraus, *Wien. Klin. Wochenschr.* **10,** 736 (1897).

37. P. Ehrlich, *Klin. Jahrb.* **6,** 299 (1897).

38. M. Gruber and H. E. Durham, *Muench. Med. Wochenschr.* **43,** 285 (1896).

39. P. Ehrlich, *Proc. R. Soc. London, Ser. B* **66,** 424 (1900).

40. P. Portier and C. Richet, *C. R. Seances Soc. Biol. Ses Fil.* **54,** 170 (1902).

41. M. Arthus, *C. R. Seances Soc. Biol. Ses Fil.* **55,** 817 (1903).

42. C. von Pirquet and B. Schick, *Die Serum Krankheit.* Deuticke, Vienna, 1906. [English edition: *Serum Sickness.* Williams & Wilkins, Baltimore, Maryland, 1951.]

43. G. H. Brieger, Introduction. In *Immunity in Infective Diseases,* by E. Metchnikoff. Johnson Reprint, New York, 1968.

44. A. E. Wright and S. R. Douglas, *Proc. R. Soc. London, Ser. B* **72,** 364 (1903).

45. S. Arrhenius, *Immunochemistry.* Macmillan, New York, 1907.

46. K. Landsteiner, *The Specificity of Serological Reactions.* Harvard University Press, Boston, Massachusetts, 1945. [Reprinted by Dover, New York, 1962.]

47. E. A. Kabat and M. M. Mayer, *Experimental Immunochemistry,* 2nd Ed. Thomas, Springfield, Illinois, 1961.

48. P. G. H. Gell and I. T. Hinde, *Br. J. Exp. Pathol.* **32,** 516 (1951); *Int. Arch. Allergy* **5,** 23 (1954).

49. J. L. Turk, *Delayed Hypersensitivity.* Wiley, New York, 1967.

50. B. H. Waksman, *Int. Arch. Allergy Appl. Immunol.* **14,** Suppl. (1959). See also B. H. Waksman, in *Cellular Aspects of Immunity* (G. E. W. Wolstenholme and M. O'Connor, eds.), p. 280. Churchill, London, 1960.

51. G. B. Mackaness and R. V. Blanden, *Prog. Allergy* **11,** 89 (1967).

52. D. Rowley, *Adv. Immunol.* **2,** 241 (1962).

53. K. Landsteiner and M. W. Chase, *Proc. Soc. Exp. Biol. Med.* **49,** 688 (1942).

54. H. Zinsser, *J. Exp. Med.* **34,** 495 (1921); **41,** 159 (1925).

55. L. Dienes and E. W. Schoenheit, *Am. Rev. Tuberc.* **20,** 92 (1929).

56. T. D. Jones and J. R. Mote, *N. Engl. J. Med.* **210,** 120 (1934).

57. F. A. Simon and F. M. Rackemann, *J. Allergy* **5,** 439, 451 (1934).

58. A. R. Rich and M. R. Lewis, *Bull. Johns Hopkins Hosp.* **50,** 115 (1932).

59. T. N. Harris, E. Grimm, E. Mertens, and W. E. Ehrich, *J. Exp. Med.* **81,** 73 (1945).

60. A. R. Rich, *The Pathogenesis of Tuberculosis,* 2nd Ed. Thomas, Springfield, Illinois, 1951.

61. G. E. W. Wolstenholme and M. O'Connor, eds., *Cellular Aspects of Immunity,* Ciba Foundation Symposium. Churchill, London, 1960.

62. T. S. Kuhn, *The Structure of Scientific Revolutions,* 2nd Ed. University of Chicago Press, Chicago, Illinois, 1970.

4

Theories of Antibody Formation

a cis-immunologist will sometimes speak to a
trans-immunologist; but the latter rarely
answers.
—Niels Jerne

THE DISCOVERY of humoral antitoxic antibodies in the early 1890s[1] exerted a profound influence upon the future development of both immunological practice and immunological thought. On the practical level, the demonstration of the presence of specific agents in the serum of immunized animals opened the way for the prevention or cure of infectious diseases by passive-transfer serum therapy. Yet another direct consequence of this discovery was the development of serological tests such as agglutination, the precipitin reaction, and complement fixation, all of which contributed to a veritable revolution in infectious disease diagnosis during the following two decades. On the theoretical level, the discovery of circulating antibody provided a new and almost impregnable rallying point for those who argued that humoral factors rather than cellular mechanisms were all-important in explaining natural and acquired immunity. This was a battle whose outcome would direct the course of immunology for several generations.[2] But the discovery of antibody opened another theoretical door that would entrance immunologists for the next 80 years or so. Where and how were these antibodies formed within the immunized host, and how did they acquire the exquisite specificity so characteristic of the immune response?

Throughout the long and meandering history of this particular set of immunological ideas, several curious phenomena appear that deserve the attention of both the historian and the philosopher of science. These

59

phenomena may not be unique to immunology but may provide more general hints about how science and scientists operate.

1. Cis- and trans-immunology: problems in scientific communication. Niels Jerne has pointed out[3] that two competing schools of thought, each reflecting a different type of training and indeed a different worldview, long dominated immunological speculation. On one side were the cis-immunologists (the biologists), who attempted to define immunology by working forward from the first interaction of antigen with cell and who worried much about the implications of such biological phenomena as the booster antibody response, changes in the "quality" of antibody with repeated immunization, and the problem of immunological tolerance. On the other side were the trans-immunologists (the chemists), who worked backward from the antibody molecule itself and concerned themselves principally with quantitative relationships, the size of the antibody repertoire, and the structural basis of immunological specificity. As this chapter will demonstrate, these two groups might sometimes ask the same question but would invariably weigh the answer using different criteria, based upon the different aspects of the immune response that each felt to be critical. Thus, they would often argue not *with* one another, but *past* one another. Communication gaps such as this appear to have existed throughout science almost from its beginning. Among the more famous examples of this was the attempt to explain the basis of species evolution.[4] The field paleontologists and systematists studied populations and the phenotype and argued ultimate causes backward from the existing diversity of species, while the laboratory geneticists studied individuals and the genotype and argued proximate causes forward from the still hypothetical gene. For decades, the two schools did not appreciate the importance of one another's work. Again, a similar situation developed around the famous controversy about the age of the earth.[5] Neglecting the calculations of biblical fundamentalists, one saw the geologists and paleontologists of the late nineteenth century demanding immense spans of time for the gradual attainment of present conditions, while the physicists, led by Lord Kelvin, showed with forceful thermodynamic argument that the earth must have cooled from its initial high temperature in a far shorter time. It required the discovery of a new phenomenon, radioactivity, to resolve the issue.

2. The perseveration of ideas. In immunology, as in other scientific disciplines, one may note with interest how frequently an old concept, thought to have been rendered obsolete by the weight of countervailing data and/or a more satisfactory hypothesis, was revived. The revival is often advanced without adequate acknowledgment of its predecessors and almost invariably with a total disregard for the facts that contributed to the demise of that predecessor. Someone has said that good ideas must be rediscovered at least once in each generation. Is the timing similar, then, for bad ideas?

3. *The idea advanced "before its time."* The history of science is replete with instances of the publication of a new important concept that passes unnoticed at the time. This phenomenon happens occasionally because the idea may be "hidden away" in an obscure journal (like the genetic work of Gregor Mendel[6]), only to be discovered much later. More often, the failure occurs because the idea cannot be readily integrated into the governing rules and paradigms of the scientific discipline, and thus passes unnoticed. Only when the time is right will the "new" theory be acclaimed, often with little credit to its predecessors. Thus, in immunology, the antigen instruction theory of antibody formation is universally credited to Breinl and Haurowitz, Mudd, and Alexander and was rapidly and widely accepted in the early 1930s, although numerous instruction theories had been advanced previously, as I shall show. Again, Jerne's natural selection theory of antibody formation struck a sympathetic chord in 1955, although similar theories had been advanced at least twice in the preceding 60 years.

It will be the aim of this chapter on the history of theories of antibody formation to call attention to many long-forgotten contributions to its progress. I shall, however, also examine the general scientific contexts in which all these speculations were advanced and the mind-set of the speculators themselves, hoping to learn something from them about how science itself functions.

Antigen Incorporation Theories

BUCHNER, 1893

The noted German bacteriologist Hans Buchner was the first to confront the new conceptual problem posed by the discovery of antibodies. As early as mid-1893, in an address to the Medical Society of Munich on bacterial toxins and antitoxins, Buchner offered a simple solution to the problem. He proposed that the antitoxin was formed directly from the toxin itself, hinting at some fairly simple transformation. As he put it:

> Everything speaks also for the fact that the antitoxin contains a cell plasma substance of the specific bacteria, that accumulates in the immunized animal's body. We saw already earlier that toxalbumin must be considered as a specific product of the bacterial plasma. Toxalbumin and antitoxin should be, by their nature, very closely related, and even substances of the same specific kind, or perhaps they may even be different modifications of

one and the same substance. That one of these acts as a poison and the other not, I see therein no contradiction against this assumption, since we know that from almost non-poisonous choline, the very poisonous neurin arises by mere decomposition in water, or that poisonous peptone develops by simple digestion from fibrin derived from the circulatory system. On the other hand, however, a common origin of both substances from the bacterial plasma, the poisonous and the protective, opens directly a sure understanding of the specific nature of this protection.[7]

In an era when nothing was known about the chemical nature of toxins or antitoxins and little was known about the chemistry of biological macromolecules in general, it is not surprising that Buchner's hypothesis found such ready favor. It appeared to explain the mechanism whereby the antibody was endowed with specificity for the immunizing antigen, and it consigned to the antigen rather than to the host the primary role in antibody formation. Any requirement that the host contribute the new product would, as I shall show, raise more questions than it answered.

Even so, objections to Buchner's hypothesis were not long in coming. In the same year, Emile Roux, who had already made notable contributions to the study of toxins and antitoxins, showed with Vaillard that the continuous bleeding of a horse immunized with tetanus toxin did not diminish the antibody titer, even after the equivalent of its entire original blood volume had been removed.[8] How could antibody formation continue, without fresh supplies of antigen, if Buchner's view was valid? An even more telling blow against the antigen transformation (or incorporation) theory came with the work of Knorr, who showed that the injection of one unit of tetanus toxin into a horse might result in the production of as much as 100,000 units of circulating antitoxin.[9] The numbers appeared to argue too strongly against the theory; and despite a somewhat belated support for the theory provided by Metchnikoff in 1900,[10] Buchner's concept appeared already to have succumbed in the face of such strongly contradictory evidence.

HERTZFELD AND KLINGER, 1918

In a lengthy review entitled "The Reactions of Immunity,"[11] E. Hertzfeld and R. Klinger employed most of its 44 pages to muster support for "their own" theory of antibody formation. With scarcely a nod to Buchner, and with no mention of the data that had doomed his proposal several decades earlier, they refer repeatedly to "our theory," but explain it in words similar to those that Buchner had employed. "We shall explain, in what follows, that the essential in all immunization events depends upon the antigen being split up to a certain degree in the organism, from whose origin composite, yet still specific breakdown products are absorbed on the surface of appropriate colloidal proteins, and in this form represent 'antibody.'" And somewhat later they go on to say: "In order to make this type of specificity possible, the split products of the antigen still possess a characteristic chemical composition of their own, for were this not the case, then it would be impossible to understand why the antibody in question should react precisely only with this antigen, and not with a large number of others." It is interesting that this elaborately propounded theory, published as it was in so widely read a journal, should receive so little attention either then or later. It was scarcely mentioned at all, except somewhat obscurely, and when the antigen incorporation concept was revived a decade later, any credit that was given was to Buchner and not to Hertzfeld and Klinger.

MANWARING, RAMON, LOCKE, MAIN, AND HIRSCH, 1926–1930

In his presidential address to the American Association of Immunologists in 1926, W. H. Manwaring complained that Paul Ehrlich's immunology "constitutes today our most serious handicap to immunological progress, both in theoretical and in practical lines."[12] He insisted that the field was in desperate need of a new and consistent theory "to unravel the mystery of the origin and nature of antibodies." He did not have long to wait, for at the very same meeting a paper was presented by Locke, Main, and Hirsch,[13] proposing that specific antibody was nothing more than a derivative of antigen. "It is postulated that antibodies are composed of clusters—of relatively large dimension—in which an elementary, naturally occurring, protein substance is absorbed in preponderating amount on nuclei of a binding substance derived from the injected antigen, and that they owe their individual properties to the proportion and character of this binding substance." Three years later a similar theory was advanced, without reference to the others, by Gustave Ramon,[14] who was to contribute so much to the immunology of diphtheria. According to Ramon, "antitoxin and antibodies in general will find their origin in the formation of humoral complexes constituted of materials originating in the organism and of elements derived from the specific antigen, this by a physicochemical process in the case of antitoxins and, more simply, a physical process for the other antibodies." In each case, the earlier rise and the reason for the fall of Buchner's original suggestion were either entirely neglected or else given only slight attention.

While the others supported the antigen incorporation theory of antibody formation with data, Manwaring propounded it only with fervor. After a brief flirtation with an instruction theory involving enzymes,[15] antigen incorporation became a crusade in his hands. In flowery language not often matched in scientific journals, he celebrated the "Renaissance of Pre-Ehrlich Immunology,"[16] implying that Buchnerian immunology had been revived. He attributed the current parlous state of immunology to outdated physiological concepts and said: "Theoretical immunologists were soon convinced that there must be something radically wrong in their logic, but few of them dreamed that the error was not theirs, but in the basic mid-Victorian religio-physiology in which they placed such implicit faith." He saw salvation in a new immunology, based on the notion "that specific antibodies might not be hereditary specific antidotes, but might be retained, modified alien entities or partially dehumanized human proteins—hybridization products between toxic or infectious agents and host tissues."

If Buchner's original hypothesis had stimulated much experimental work to disprove it, then this reappearance of the same idea stimulated even more. The new wave of investigators seemed to be unaware of the earlier, similar studies. Now Heidelberger and Kendall[17] and Topley[18] showed, as had Knorr 32 years earlier, that the amount of antibody formed in the immunized animal was far greater than the amount of antigen utilized. Indeed, Hooker and Boyd pointed out, using Topley's data, that a single molecule of antigen might induce enough antibody to agglutinate 600 bacteria.[19] The same authors showed that anti-arsanilic acid antibody contained no arsenic,[20] and Berger and Erlenmeyer showed similarly the absence of arsenic in antibody against the atoxyl hapten.[21] Once again, the weight of all of this evidence that antigen could not possibly be incorporated, in whole or in part, into the antibody molecule was overwhelming, and the theory was laid to rest once again, this time apparently for good.

Ehrlich's Side-Chain Theory

In addition to his medical studies, Paul Ehrlich spent time in the laboratories of the famous organic chemist and enzymologist Emil Fischer. He brought from this experience a lifelong interest in the relationship between chemical structure and biological function.[22] This interest was reflected in all of his subsequent work as one of the founders of modern immunology and of chemical pharmacology as well. Ehrlich's debt to structural chemistry is perhaps nowhere better illustrated among his immunological publications than in his famous paper of 1897, describing how diphtheria toxin and antitoxin interact and the method of their measurement.[23] Not only did he postulate that immunological specificity was due to a unique stereochemical relationship between the active sites on antigen and antibody, he introduced also the concepts of affinity and of functional domains on the antibody molecule. This work provided the taproot from which the field of immunochemistry later grew; he would be famous for this contribution alone. But Ehrlich also appended to this study a theory of the basis for antibody formation, an inclusion that assured the report a unique position in the history of immunology.

Like Elie Metchnikoff's earlier phagocytic theory of immunity,[24] Paul Ehrlich's theory of antibody formation was based upon the process of intracellular digestion. He pointed out that many different types of nutrients were utilized, apparently specifically, in the metabolism of the cell; and he suggested that these nutrients could interact and be absorbed by the cell only if structurally specific receptors exist on the cell surface with which the nutrient molecules can react chemically. As Ehrlich put it, "The reactions of immunity, after all, represent only a repetition of the processes of normal metabolism, and their apparently wonderful adjustment to new conditions is only another phase of *uralte protoplasma Weisheit* [the ancient wisdom of the protoplasm]." Since certain toxins have a greater affinity for one organ than another, Ehrlich suggested that specific receptors for these toxin molecules also exist on the surface of certain cells. Like a nutrient, the toxin would bind to its specific receptor and thus be assimilated, following which the receptor would either be freed for renewed function or else be regenerated by the cell. When, however, large amounts or repeated doses of toxin were administered, then the cell would overcompensate for the loss of these side-chain receptors, producing so many that some would be released into the blood. Since they possessed complementary sites specific for the given antigen, these side chains would now function as circulating antibody. In this formulation, Ehrlich followed the lead of his cousin, the pathologist Carl Weigert, who had formulated a "law of overcompensation" to explain a variety of phenomena observed in general pathology.[25]

Ehrlich's side-chain theory contained all of the necessary elements to qualify as a true natural selection concept. Antibodies were *natural* constituents of the cell surface, formed within the cell. They possessed from the start the structural configuration that determined their specificity for a given antigen. The purpose of antigen was to *select* from among all of the side chains available only those able to interact specifically, and the cell was then caused to produce more of these specific molecules for export into the blood, requiring only the triggering effect of antigen. As I mentioned earlier, in 1897 Ehrlich's ideas were not yet bothered by the problem later posed by an overly large repertoire of antibodies. Furthermore, his suggestion that the specific side chain represented the shedding of a portion of some giant protoplasmic molecule was probably all that was permitted by the current state of knowledge of cells and macromolecules. But his prediction that the basis of immunological specificity resided in a unique three-dimensional configuration of the antibody molecule would later be verified; and his inspired suggestion that antibody formation was the cellular response to the interaction of antigen with cell-surface receptors would not be improved upon for over 60 years.

Instruction Theories

Despite the immediate and widespread success of Ehrlich's side-chain theory, some workers, following the lead of Jules Bordet, paid little attention to its explanation of *how antibodies are formed*. They attacked it, rather, because they considered it a too-complicated and erroneous explanation of *how antibodies function*. As Bordet said,

> Ehrlich's theory has exerted a quite grievous influence, in engendering a series of artificial conceptions . . . relating notably to the constitution and classification of antibodies, to the mechanism of fixation of complement, etc. By the abuse which it has made of graphic representations which translate the outer aspect of the phenomena without penetrating to their inner meaning, it has spread the acceptance of facile and premature interpretations.[26]

Other workers, however, voiced objection to the very basis of the theory. In 1897, when the theory was formulated, only a limited number of antibodies were recognized, specific for the toxins of pathogenic organisms. Thus, the known antibody repertoire was quite limited, and defensive antibody receptors on cells seemed a likely, if teleological, Darwinian explanation for their presence. The picture changed completely within only a few years, with the demonstration of antibody formation against isologous and heterologous erythrocytes, against spermatozoa and other cellular constituents, and against a wide variety of bland proteins.[27] These findings brought into question implicitly the *need* for such receptors and explicitly raised the doubt that the Ehrlich theory was tenable, in view of the growing size of the antibody repertoire. If, however, the information for so large a repertoire could not possibly arise from within the host, then it surely must be carried in from the outside. What else was there but antigen? As early as 1905, Karl Landsteiner (an avowed opponent of Ehrlich's) could say with M. Reich "that the activity of cells producing normal serum components . . . is altered following the stimulus of immunization, and so form differently constituted products."[28] This was the first time that anyone had suggested that antibody was a completely new substance.

DIRECT TEMPLATE THEORIES

Bail and Co-workers, 1909–1914. Oskar Bail spent most of his career at the German University in Prague, where he became chairman of the Department of Hygiene and Bacteriology. In a series of papers published before the First World War, he advanced an instruction theory of antibody formation that would be little improved upon over the next 40 years. This historically important contribution passed almost completely unnoticed by later theorists.

Bail and Tsuda[29] were troubled, as were others, by the great number of different side chains demanded by Ehrlich's theory. They suggested that antigen is not destroyed after its interaction with specific antibody but may release the latter and continue its function, which is to bind "natural antibodies" from normal blood, leaving the impress of its specificity upon the latter molecules. Working primarily with cholera vibrios, they pointed out that

> The reaction product between cholera substance and serum is able itself to function further as antigen, so that the quantitative relationship between the amount of immunizing antigen employed and the amount of antibody finally contained, will also be better understood . . . which of necessity must lead to a new view of antibody formation.

Bail and Tsuda were the first of many believers in the antigen-template theory of antibody formation to draw the obvious conclusion—that the process should work also *in vitro,* under appropriate conditions, and thus that antibody might be synthesized outside of the body.[30] Indeed, they claimed to have synthesized anticholera antibodies *in vitro.* As they summarized: "the principal result, the obtaining of a solution specifically active for cholera from a nonspecific normal serum with the help of cholera vibrios, is secure."

The theory was further supported and extended by Bail and Rotky in 1913[31] and by Bail alone in 1914.[32] They held that immunizing antigen persists in the body, it interacts with and impresses its specificity on normal human substances, and then gives these up into the circulation to continue its action, further enhancing the titer of specific antibody.

The Complement Theory of Thiele and Embleton, 1914. Thiele and Embleton were primarily interested in immune hemolysis and hemolytic antibody and in how antibody participates with complement in the destruction of erythrocytes. In a paper on "The Evolution of Antibody,"[33] they offered an instruction theory, suggesting that hemolytic antibody derives from complement by a series of "differentiation steps," under the influence of antigen. This contribution, quite out of the mainstream of immunological thought, received little attention and is included here only to illustrate the widely ranging formulations of early speculators.

Ostromuislensky, 1915. In the midst of the First World War, there appeared two remarkable papers in the obscure (to Western immunologists) *Journal of the Russian Physicochemical Society*.[34] These publications not only reported the *in vitro* production of specific antitoxins but also based this approach upon a theory of antibody formation that claimed that immunological specificity was due not to a particular chemical constitution of the molecule but to a special physical state of the colloidal antitoxin molecules that distinguishes antibodies from ordinary globulins. This special state is impressed upon an "ordinary" globulin by contact with the antigen molecule, which could then split off and repeat its function. Although he showed a wide familiarity with the Western literature, Ostromuislensky seems to have been unaware of the earlier work by Bail and co-workers, and thus we may credit him with an independent contribution to immunologic theory.

Haurowitz and Breinl, Topley, Mudd, and Alexander, 1930–1932. By 1930, it was understood that antibodies were globular proteins and that proteins were somehow built up of random arrangements of 20-odd different amino acids, the so-called building blocks of life. It was unclear, however, whether there was any regularity or reproducibility in the amino acid sequence of the polypeptide chain, or where and how the information for any particular sequence might be stored and retrieved. There were thus few restrictions during this period on the direction in which speculation might be carried in seeking an explanation of the basis for immunological specificity. Even so, the increasing knowledge of the chemistry of proteins demanded that henceforth any theory of antibody formation involve the basic mechanism of protein formation.

Based upon the then-reasonable assumption that the information for the universe of different antigenic determinants could not possibly be incorporated in the vertebrate genome, a wave of new instruction theories was proposed, since logic appeared to demand that each antigen must carry with it the information for its own immunological specificity. Instruction must now be on the level of antibody synthesis, however; and for the first time the notion of antigen-as-template became explicit.

The new theory was advanced almost simultaneously by Topley[35] and by Breinl and Haurowitz,[36] and independently also by Mudd[37] and by Alexander.[38] It took its most definitive form in the hands of Breinl and Haurowitz, who proposed that an antigen would be carried in the body to the site of protein formation, where it would serve as a template upon which the nascent antibody molecule might be constructed. Since the antibody molecule was to be synthesized upon the surface of the antigen, it seemed reasonable to propose a mechanism whereby the stereochemical structure of the antigenic site would determine a unique amino acid sequence on the antibody, thus accounting for the complementary and specific fit of antibody for antigen. Implicit in this theory, of course, was the requirement that antigen persist throughout the course of antibody formation.

This instruction template concept of antibody formation found broad acceptance in the chemically oriented immunology of the day, since it appeared to dispose of several conceptual dilemmas that had worried earlier immunologists. First, the new theory answered the objection of those who claimed that the body could not possibly have accumulated in evolution the information required to produce antibodies against the thousands of synthetic haptenic determinants that Landsteiner and others had shown to be immunogenic (i.e., it solved the antibody repertoire size problem). Second, the template theory accounted well for the repeated observation that many thousands of molecules of antibody might appear in the blood for each molecule of antigen injected. Finally, of course, it accounted in structural terms for immunological specificity. But one of the major shortcomings of the new theory, not even mentioned by its proponents, was its inability to explain why a second exposure to antigen should result in a much enhanced and more rapid booster antibody response.

It is worthy of note that none of these authors made any mention of the earlier instruction theories of antibody formation. This omission is especially interesting in the case of Breinl and Haurowitz, since they were then working in the department in Prague of the very same Oskar Bail who 20 years earlier had advanced an instruction theory of antibody formation substantially equivalent to their own.[39]

Pauling, 1940. The theory of interatomic and intermolecular forces that gained Linus Pauling his first Nobel Prize had important implications for an understanding of the specificity of many biological interactions. It was Pauling himself who applied these concepts to the antigen–antibody interaction, an interest that was stimulated by earlier conversations with Karl Landsteiner.[40] Pauling and his students, most notably David Pressman, showed formally that the specificity of the antibody–hapten interaction was due to the interaction of complementary three-dimensional configurations of atoms, as Paul Ehrlich had so long ago suggested. Their binding energy could also be well explained by a combination of ionic, hydrogen-bonding, and van der Waals interactions.

Always on the lookout for the important scientific challenges of the day, the imaginative Pauling speculated on how the antibody protein molecule could possibly acquire and maintain the unique three-dimensional configuration that would endow it with specificity for a given antigen.[41] The answer was typical of the Pauling approach; antibody specificity must be due to the unique tertiary structure of a given antibody molecule, achieved through a unique folding of its peptide chain. (In 1940, the individuality of the primary amino acid sequence of proteins was unknown, as was the influence of this sequence on tertiary structure.) Since he did not favor a mysterious process whereby antigen instructed the amino acid sequence of the antibody molecule, as postulated by Breinl and Haurowitz, Pauling presented a simpler and more chemically justifiable theory. Antigen would serve as the template for the final step of protein formation, in which the coiling of the nascent polypeptide chain of the antibody molecule would conform more or less precisely to the template offered by the surface determinant of the antigen molecule.[42] Once the appropriate configuration had been attained, it would be stabilized by familiar interatomic bonds and thus satisfy all of the requirements of specific antibody. Pauling's picture of this process is illustrated in Fig. 4.1.

A further elaboration of Pauling's concept was provided by Karush,[43] who pointed out a critical defect in the Breinl-Haurowitz formulation. Any template that determines primary amino acid sequence must be *linear,* and thus cannot also "provide directly information for the development of nonconvalent [tertiary] structure." The antigenic template must therefore act on the preformed chain, to permit it to fold uniquely into the antigen-specific complementary region required. Karush also proposed that this unique folding is stabilized thenceforth by multiple disulfide bridge cross-linkages and that antibody heterogeneity is determined by the extent of such cross-linking.

Like other chemically oriented instructionists before him, Pauling's

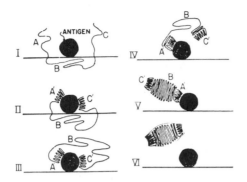

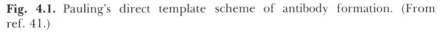

Fig. 4.1. Pauling's direct template scheme of antibody formation. (From ref. 41.)

chief concern was to explain specificity and repertoire size. The former area was his forte, and he could say of the latter: "The number of configurations accessible to the polypeptide chain is so great as to provide an explanation of the ability of an animal to form antibodies with considerable specificity for an apparently unlimited number of different antigens." He, like the others, did not demand of his theory an explanation of the more biological phenomenology of the antibody response.

Although Pauling's template theory of antibody production appeared to accord more than its predecessor with contemporary scientific theories, in fact all of these instruction theories shared much the same advantages and disadvantages. Indeed, Pauling's theory gained an additional defect, which was pointed up by newer data. While it had not yet been firmly demonstrated that the antibody molecule was multivalent, the very fact of the antigen–antibody precipitin reaction and the form of the percipitin curve led Marrack to suggest in 1934 that antibodies were at least divalent and possibly multivalent, thus enabling an antigen–antibody precipitin lattice to be established.[44] Furthermore, the repeated demonstration by Landsteiner that multiply substituted proteins could engage in precipitation with anti-hapten antibody suggested strongly that the antibody not only must be multivalent but also must have each of its active sites specific for the same grouping. In contrast, Pauling's theory implied that the specific sites on the antibody molecule were formed and stabilized at different areas on the surface of the antigen, thus implying that they ought in general to be heteroligating (i.e., to exhibit a different specificity at each of their reactive sites).

INDIRECT TEMPLATE THEORIES

The Adaptive Enzyme Theory of Burnet, 1941. F. Macfarlane Burnet brought to his interest in immunology a broad background in virology and experimental pathology. But of overriding importance for his future immunological theories was the fact that he was, like Bordet, an unabashed biologist who had little use for the purely molecular concepts of his chemically oriented predecessors. Thus, he faulted the template theory of Breinl and Haurowitz in his 1941 book, *The Production of Antibodies.*[45] In words that Jules Bordet might have used 40 years earlier, Burnet could say that "in the circumstances, it would seem preferable to couch any general interpretation of the phenomenon of antibody production in biological terms which can be related to general conceptions in other biological fields, rather than to conceal ignorance by a pseudochemical formulation." Burnet treated the Pauling template theory somewhat more charitably, as providing a more impressive physical picture of the antibody molecule, but he questioned the biological basis and biological implications of the Pauling theory.

Like his predecessors, Burnet acknowledged that the information for antibody specificity must be carried by the antigen molecule. His criticisms of the earlier template theories, significantly, questioned not the *chemical* basis for the specificity of the antibody combining site but the *biological* basis for the production of the entire antibody molecule. First, claimed Burnet, direct template theories paid no attention to the modern knowledge of the importance of enzymes in the mechnisms of intracellular metabolism and synthesis. He pointed out, second, that these theories demanded the long-term persistence of antigen throughout the course of antibody formation, an event that Burnet claimed not only had not been formally demonstrated but was probably not even true. Finally, and most significant, Burnet the biologist made his most profound contribution in claiming that "antibody production is a function not only of the cells originally stimulated, *but of their descendants* [my italics]." Here was the key to the problem, which he would utilize so effectively some 18 years later.

Burnet's instructionist theory of antibody formation was very much in line with contemporary biological thought. All proteins (including antibodies) are both broken down and synthesized by special proteinase enzymes. However, in addition to the normal complement of enzymes within a cell, recent work on bacteria had suggested that under special circumstances, "adaptive" enzymes might appear in response to special modifications or requirements of the bacterial organism.[46] From this point of departure, Burnet postulated that, once introduced into the body, antigen would find its way into the cells of the reticuloendothelial system, where contact with local proteinases would result in adaptive modification of the enzymes during the dissolution of the antigen molecule. These newly adapted enzymes would then be able to synthesize a globulin molecule specific for the antigen in question. Moreover, these adaptive enzymes would not only replicate within the antibody-forming cell itself, but the information for antibody specificity that they carried would be perpetuated also within any daughter cells that might result from proliferative activity. Such an expanded population of specifically adapted antibody-forming cells (later called a clone) would account well for the heightened secondary or booster antibody response upon subsequent reexposure to antigen.

In a delightful extension of his theory, Burnet advanced a plausible explanation for the recent observation that when booster injections of antigen are administered, not only is the quantity of antibody increased, but so also is its quality (i.e., its affinity for antigen). Adaptive enzymes, explained Burnet, are not unalterable structures; consequently, over time the adaptive enzymes for any given antibody will slowly deteriorate, thus producing lower-grade specific antibody and ultimately nonspecific "normal" globulin. However, further contact with the same antigen will intensify and make more perfect the adaptation of the enzyme to specific antibody formation, thus resulting in the production of an increasingly higher grade antibody with each booster immunization. Burnet pointed out that it was precisely the ability of his theory to explain the qualitative changes in antibody that accompany prolonged immunization that provided its chief advantage over the earlier template theories.

The Indirect Template Theory of Burnet and Fenner, 1949. The notion that enzymes might be adaptively modified, so popular early in the decade, had begun to lose favor near its close. The formation of protein was now held to be under the master control of an information-laden "genome" of uncertain composition. In a second edition of his book on antibody formation, Burnet, with Frank Fenner, advanced a new indirect template hypothesis.[47] Each antigen, according to this theory, is able to impress the information for its specific determinant upon the (?RNA) genome, against which indirect template antibody specificity might be endowed during protein formation. The new theory continued to stress Burnet's concern with the importance of cellular dynamics in the immune response, since the new genomic copy not only would persist within the cell but also would be reproduced from mother to daughter cells during proliferation. It was these two factors, according to Burnet, that explained the persistence of antibody formation and the accentuated booster response. The genocopy might also deteriorate with time or be sharpened by reexposure to antigen, thus explaining changes in the quality of antibody.

Medawar's early work,[48] demonstrating that tissue homografts are routinely rejected whereas autografts are not, refocused attention on the ability of the immunological apparatus to distinguish between self and not-self. When Ray Owen then showed that nonidentical cattle twins whose circulatory systems were connected *in utero* become antigenic mosaics, unable to respond immunologically to one another's antigens,[49] it became apparent that the distinction between self and not-self was a learned rather than a genetically programmed phenomenon. Burnet and Fenner were the first to recognize the importance of these observations (Burnet would later share the 1960 Nobel prize for this prescience) and the first to insist that an adequate theory of antibody formation must encompass this important biological fact. They therefore suggested that body components acquire "self-markers" at some point in ontogeny, markers whose presence would thenceforth deflect self-components from participation in the immune process.

The Immunocatalysis Theory of Sevag, 1951. I include here, in the interest of completeness, an instruction theory advanced by M. G. Sevag in his book *Immunocatalysis*.[50] Sevag believed that the chemical process of catalysis is important in many aspects of immunology, perhaps nowhere more than in the formation of specific antibodies. He suggested that "the specificity of an antibody molecule is the consequence of specific cellular synthetic processes catalytically modified by an antigen to conform with the configuration of certain active groups of the antigen molecule." Thus, in the production of "normal globulins," the catalytic effect of antigen is to change the configurational pattern of the protein, on the basis of the special structure of the antigenic determinant. There is a certain illogic in this theory. Sevag seems to overextend the accepted definition of catalysis, because catalysts do not make new reactions possible, but merely accelerate preexisting ones.

The Template–Inducer Theory of Schweet and Owen, 1957. It was clear by 1957 that the repository of genetic information lay in DNA. As Schweet and Owen pointed out, information for protein synthesis could no longer be attributed to the *direct* function of other proteins (antigens). They proposed, therefore, a two-phase mechanism of antibody formation.[51] Antigen would first so modify the DNA of the globulin gene as to furnish somatically heritable information for the formation of a new RNA template, producing cells "primed" for specific antibody formation. Antigen would then act further on such cells as an inducer, stimulating the formation of many templates and the exuberant production of antibody. This "biochemical model" of antibody formation not only seemed to accord better with contemporary knowledge but appeared also to furnish a plausible explanation of the difference between primary and booster immunization.

THE IMPLICATIONS OF INSTRUCTION THEORIES

It may be worth pausing for a moment to examine the broader biological implications of the theories that we have examined thus far. When Paul Ehrlich suggested in 1897 that antibodies were natural cell products, the only immunological responses then recognized were to pathogenic organisms and toxic substances. It was thus not unreasonable to suppose that a Darwinian selection pressure had endowed the vertebrate host with the antibody specificities apparently so necessary to its survival. With the expansion of the antibody repertoire to almost unmanageable proportions, including a long list of the unnatural products of the synthetic organic chemist's imagination, a Darwinian explanation no longer seemed possible. In this situation, an instruction theory involving a direct template would be evolutionarily neutral and thus appeared more acceptable. But the indirect template theories, involving the transmission of antigen-induced information from mother to daughter somatic cells, introduced a slightly Lamarckian flavor to the proceedings. The selection theories to which I shall now turn appeared to restore Darwin to favor among immunologists,[52] but simultaneously they posed some of the most interesting and complicated evolutionary problems of all, as I shall point out in Chapter 6.

Selection Theories

The influence of the Second World War on the tempo of scientific discovery cannot be overestimated; in its aftermath new information and new techniques commanded the attention of all biologists. From outside of immunology, perhaps the most significant advances concerned the structure and function of genes. From within immunology, the discoveries of allograft rejection (see ref. 48), of immunological tolerance,[53] and of immunological deficiency diseases[54] heralded a major shift in emphasis from immunochemistry to immunobiology, a field in which selectionist theories of antibody formation would find a more suitable environment. Within the context of the new biology, a plausible theory of antibody formation would now have to address these more biological aspects of the immune response. But even before the biologists led the return to selection theories, one such was advanced by the physicist P. Jordan.

THE QUANTUM-MECHANICAL RESONANCE THEORY OF JORDAN, 1940

Jordan attempted to apply quantum-mechanical arguments to biological systems, most notably to an explanation of the perplexing problem of the reproduction of biologically specific molecules such as enzymes and antibodies. His theory of antibody formation[55] was, in fact, the first of the post-Ehrlich natural selection theories, but it has largely been forgotten. It is presented here in part for completeness, but also to contrast its reception and influence with that of the natural selection theory of Jerne, with which it shared many important features.

Jordan held that injected antigen is first subjected to partial digestion within the host, after which its split-products might combine preferentially with certain naturally occurring molecules, the antibodies. This antigen–antibody complex would then be capable, in special tissues in which the milieu was appropriate, of inducing an autocatalytic reproduction of the antibody moiety. Jordan suggested that quantum-mechanical resonance phenomena would lead to an attraction between molecules containing identical groups and thus to self-reproduction of the antibody molecule. According to this concept, antigen would *select* from a pool of *naturally* occurring antibodies those with which it could specifically interact, and then the antigen would serve as a suitable carrier for the antibody during its autocatalytic phase of reproduction. Jordan even accounted for the Landsteiner observation of graded cross-reactions by suggesting that in many cases the reproductive process might result in daughter molecules whose structure, and therefore specificity, might differ slightly from that of the mother molecule.

Jordan's concept was substantially identical to Ehrlich's, with the substitution of a more "modern" mechanism for the reproduction of the specific antibody molecules. It was even more closely the equivalent of Jerne's natural selection theory, to be discussed next; but it failed completely to attract the attention of biologists. It did, however, come to the attention of Linus Pauling, then promoting his own theory of antibody formation,[41] and he lost no time in attacking the Jordan formulation. The nature and role of intermolecular forces was Pauling's special domain, and he was quick to point out,[56] in Jordan's own quantum-mechanical notation, that resonance attractions were less likely between identical molecules than between complementary molecules, as

Pauling's own theory had suggested. It is of some interest that although Pauling's attack was limited to Jordan's proposed mechanism for the reduplication of antibody molecules, it served also to eclipse the natural selection aspect of the argument.

THE NATURAL SELECTION THEORY OF JERNE, 1955

One of the early observations that led to the concept of a humorally mediated immunity was the existence in "normal" blood and serum of specific antibacterial substances, whose presence could not be accounted for by any known prior exposure to the antigens with which they reacted. These were termed *natural antibodies,* in contradistinction to those acquired after infection or immunization. So long as Ehrlich's side-chain theory of antibody formation was accepted, the presence of spontaneously produced antibodies excited no particular conceptual concern among immunologists. But with the fall into desuetude of Ehrlich's theory and the rise of instructionist theories of antibody formation, natural antibodies could no longer be accounted for, and interest in them waned. With the post-World War II burst of activity in all fields of biology, attention was once again directed to the nature and significance of natural antibodies, thanks in no small measure to a group at the Danish State Serum Institute in Copenhagen, to which Niels Jerne belonged.

In his landmark paper in 1955,[57] Jerne revived the old Ehrlich concept that antibodies of all possible specificities were normally formed by the vertebrate host and delivered in small amounts to the blood. Any antigen that chanced to enter the circulation would then react with those antibodies that were present and specific for the antigenic determinants. Once the antigen–antibody interaction was complete, the role of antigen assigned by Jerne was to carry the antibody to specialized cells capable of reproducing this antibody. When the antigen had fulfilled its task as "selective carrier"[58] of antibody, it had no further role to play, and the internal mechanisms of the antibody-producing cell would then respond somehow to the signal provided by the selected globulins, initiating the synthesis of molecules identical to those introduced, i.e., of specific antibody. In view of the recent demonstration of the importance of ribosomal RNA for the assembly of protein molecules, Jerne suggested that the antibody prototype might initiate the synthesis of a specific RNA, or even modify the structure of a preexisting RNA, upon which further specific antibody molecules might be synthesized.

Jerne's theory appeared, for the moment, to explain satisfactorily most of the biological phenomena associated with the immune response.

The heightened booster response was attributable to the presence of increasing amounts of circulating antibody, thus providing a more efficient stimulus to a greater number of antibody-forming cells than was possible during primary immunization. Similarly, the presence of larger amounts of circulating antibody during the booster response would favor the binding to antigen of higher-affinity antibodies, thus accounting for the increase in the quality of antibodies with repeated immunization. Finally, immunological tolerance was accounted for by postulating that the first natural antibodies produced against self-antigens during embryogenesis would immediately be absorbed by the tissues of the body and thus would be unavailable to serve as stimuli for subsequent autoantibody formation. The demand of an immense number of preexisting antibodies, earlier viewed as the chief objection to Ehrlich's theory, was not even mentioned as a possible drawback to the natural selection theory.

It is curious that although Jerne's theory of antibody formation appears to be the logical equivalent of both Ehrlich's side-chain theory (as Talmage[59] was quick to point out) and Jordan's resonance theory, he referred to neither of them in his paper. All three theories held antibodies to be naturally occurring substances that are selected for by antigens on the basis of their ability to interact specifically. Whereas in the Ehrlich theory this interaction was assumed to occur on the cell surface, signaling antibody formation, in both the Jerne and Jordan formulations the interaction was thought to occur in the blood. In all three theories, the actual antibody formation would then proceed in some sort of intracellular black box, the speculation about mechanisms being governed by the state of knowledge of the day. While future developments would show that the Ehrlich theory was closest to the truth, yet the times were apparently so ripe for this type of biological formulation that it was Jerne's theory that had a seminal influence on further immunological speculation.

It was also pointed out by Talmage that the natural selection theory came close to sharing a critical defect with the earlier instruction theories. By the mid-1950s, it was becoming increasingly evident that the information governing the structure of proteins could flow in only one direction. This constraint was formalized by Francis Crick as the "central dogma" of genetics, which held that information on protein structure flowed from DNA to RNA to protein, and once in the protein, could not escape.[60] Thus, neither antigen nor antibody could carry with it into the cell the information to program the production of specific antibody; it could at best only provide a signal for a preexisting program, a concept that Ehrlich had originally advanced and to which Burnet and others now returned.

The clonal selection theory of antibody formation was first advanced in somewhat vague and general terms by Talmage and Burnet[61] and was then fleshed out in much more specific terms by Burnet,[62] Talmage,[63] and Lederberg.[64] The torch had now clearly passed from the chemists to the biologists.

The opening chapters of Burnet's book, *The Clonal Selection Theory of Acquired Immunity,* point up well the difference in approach between the chemically oriented immunologists, who had dominated the field prior to the 1950s, and the biologically oriented immunologists, who came to the fore during the 1960s. In considering mechanisms of antibody formation, the former group had always placed great emphasis upon two principal characteristics of antibodies: the stereochemical requirement for immunological specificity, and the almost incomprehensibly great size of the antibody specificity repertoire. Burnet, on the other hand, scarcely mentioned these factors. Rather, he placed great emphasis upon such questions as the difference between primary and secondary responses, the phenomena of immunological tolerance and congenital agammaglobulinemia, and the population dynamics of differentiated cells. These factors, he felt, provide the key to the solution of the mechanism of antibody formation, and these factors also must be adequately explained by any suitable theory. The examples he used to illustrate and support his theory came not from structural organic chemistry or chemical physics, but from bacterial genetics, from influenza and myxomatosis virus infections, and from general pathology.

Burnet acknowledged the power of Jerne's suggestion of the presence of preexisting antibodies as the targets of antigen selection, but he found fault with the subsequent steps leading to antibody synthesis. He felt that cells should somehow be more intimately involved in the process—not only single cells but *clones* of cells all devoted to the same function, just as one was accustomed to seeing in any specialized organ of the body or in tumor formation. Burnet therefore suggested, as Ehrlich had before him, that the "natural antibody" should more logically be placed on the surface of a lymphoid cell, phenotypically restricted to one or at most a very few types of specific receptors. The interaction of antigen with these receptors would then trigger (by some mechanism unknown) a signal for cellular differentiation to antibody production, as well as a signal for proliferation to form a clone of daughter cells possessing identical receptors and capable of identical immunological responses. Antigen would thus serve to select and activate specifically the appropriate clonal precursor from a much larger population, thus accounting well for continued antibody formation, for enhanced secondary responses, and for changes in the quality of antibodies. The latter might also benefit from contributions by minor somatic mutations during the course of immunization, yielding closer-fitting antibodies. To explain the usual absence of response to self-antigens and acquired tolerance, Burnet postulated that clonal precursor cells might be especially susceptible to the lethal action of their respective antigens early in ontogeny, an interaction leading to the deletion of those clones that might in the future be embarrassing to the host. Should autoimmune disease develop in later life, it might be accounted for either because the antigen in question had been "sequestered" like lens antigen and not available for clonal deletion or because a somatic mutation might occur, a change leading to the development of a "forbidden clone."

Both Talmage and Lederberg contributed importantly to the elaboration of the clonal selection theory of antibody formation. In addition to expanding on the role of antigen selection and antigen-induced cell differentiation, Talmage alone paid special attention to the question of specificity and the size of the antibody repertoire. He pointed out the important distinction between an antiserum composed of many different specificities and the individual antibodies that it might contain. On the basis of the type of graded cross-reactions so elegantly demonstrated by Landsteiner, Talmage suggested that variable mixtures of a limited number of different antibody specificities may be capable of distinguishing a far greater number of different antigenic determinants, because each combination of cross-reacting antibodies would appear as a distinct specificity. Thus, Talmage made a plausible case for the existence, not of hundreds of thousands or millions of different antibody specificities, but rather something of the order of only 5000 molecular types—not an unreasonable number to have stored in the genome.

Lederberg, on the other hand, specifically addressed some of the genetic implications of the clonal selection theory, contributing to it also the prestige of a Nobel prize-winning molecular geneticist. He claimed that immunological specificity is determined by a unique primary amino acid sequence, the information for which is incorporated in a unique sequence of nucleotides in a "gene for globulin synthesis." To account for antibody diversity, Lederberg suggested the existence in precursor cells of a high rate of spontaneous *and random* mutation of the DNA of the immunoglobulin gene. Such somatic mutation, according to Lederberg, might continue throughout life, rather than being restricted to fetal life as Burnet had suggested. This notion about the somatic generation of antibody diversity would serve as the focus of an extensive subsequent debate between germ-line and somatic theories.[65]

THE MOLECULAR GENETICS THEORY OF SZILARD, 1960

During the 1950s, the famous nuclear physicist Leo Szilard developed a strong interest in the genetic basis of protein formation in general, and of antibody formation in particular. He was for a number of years a familiar figure on the boardwalk at Atlantic City, immediately outside the annual meeting hall of the American Association of Immunologists. He would "hold court" and skillfully and closely cross-examine a selected list of immunological witnesses, whose experiments he had decided were important to the formulation of his concepts. Those immunologists whose data he could not completely extract at the boardwalk sessions were later invited to dinner at his apartment in Washington, where they would be drained dry of useful information. The result of this exercise was a molecular theory of antibody formation, a theory that was based upon the latest information from the new field of molecular genetics and that sought to explain the latest phenomenological observations of the immunologists.[66] As nearly as can be determined, the theory exerted absolutely no influence on the subsequent course of immunological speculation. It is summarized briefly here, not only to complete my review of theories of antibody formation, but also because its attention to detail and its elegance of inner logic cannot fail to excite the interest and even the admiration of the reader.

Szilard postulated that the large variety of enzymes that governed the steps in normal metabolic pathways are encoded by germ-line genes whose duplication and modification result in the formation of proteins that possess similar specific binding sites but lack the catalytic activity of enzymes. These proteins are the antibodies. Immunization was held by Szilard to involve penetration of the antigenic determinant into the cell, where it would combine specifically with the site on a "coupling" enzyme responsible for the formation of a repressor of gene activity. Precipitation of the coupling enzyme would then reduce the rate of repressor formation; consequently, the derepressed antibody gene would engage in the production of large amounts of specific protein. Since the antibody itself could also bind to the repressor, the cell would then be locked in to continue production of the given antibody. The secondary booster antibody response was explained by the existence of an enzyme postulated to inhibit cell division; this inhibiting enzyme possessed many of the properties of serum complement. The injection of new antigen would then lead to intracellular precipitation of immune complexes in those cells already producing antibody, so the enzymatic inhibitor of cell proliferation would be bound to the precipitate, thus freeing the cell for proliferation to daughter cells still restricted to the production of the given antibody.

Szilard attempted to explain the development of immunological tolerance along much the same lines. Now, the presence of excessive amounts of antigen within the cells of the newborn animal might permit it to initiate specific antibody formation but would prevent the cell from locking in on that production, since excess antigen would then precipitate the antibody formed and prevent it from further neutralization of repressor molecules.

Szilard's notions of the basis for antibody formation derived from the contemporary view of the importance of enzyme induction and repression that emerged from the study of bacterial systems. But progress in the field of molecular genetics was so rapid that new approaches had almost superseded the old ones by the time Szilard published his theory; thus, it attracted little attention.

Conclusions

Within a decade of its introduction, the clonal selection theory of antibody formation had won general acceptance for its principal features. The exciting conceptual debate that it engendered—that between germ-line and somatic mutation explanations of the generation of immunological diversity—was resolved, as is so often the case in science, by concessions from both sides.[67] It is well to remember, however, that the theory of clonal selection—indeed the *law* of clonal selection—is based upon two principal concepts advanced 60 years apart: Paul Ehrlich's suggestion that the trigger for the immune response was based upon the interaction of antigen with cell membrane antibody receptors, and Macfarlane Burnet's suggestion that the consequences of the triggering event involve the cellular dynamics of differentiation and proliferation.

In following the course of the history of theories of antibody formation, several interesting aspects of the manner in which a science progresses have been well illustrated. Not long after emerging from its purely bacteriological beginnings, immunology suffered a division into two main traditions or schools of thought: those investigators with a chemical orientation, who dominated the field for almost half a century, and those with a biological orientation, who only became a strong force in the field in the 1960s. Chemically oriented immunologists demanded of a theory of antibody formation primarily that it explain the structural basis of immunological specificity and the overwhelming size of the antibody repertoire, while generally neglecting the more biological aspects of the immune response. Biologically oriented immunologists, on the other hand, paid scant attention to specificity and repertoire size and required only that an acceptable theory of antibody formation explain adequately such aspects of the immune response as the difference between primary and booster immunization, changes in the quality of antibody, and immunological tolerance. For decades, cis- and trans-immunologists spoke different languages and communicated incompletely to one another their views, priorities, and criteria. Only at the very end did it become apparent that a useful theory would have to satisfy the demands of both schools of thought, and indeed the modern synthesis appears to have done this. It has, at the same time, almost completely blurred the boundaries that earlier divided the two camps, although the cis or trans orientation of at least the older generation of investigators can still be discerned.

NOTES AND REFERENCES

1. E. von Behring and S. Kitasato, *Dtsch. Med. Wochenschr.* **16,** 1113 (1980) E. von Behring and E. Wernicke, *Z. Hyg.* **12,** 10, 45 (1892); P. Ehrlich, *Dtsch. Med. Wochenschr.* **17,** 976, 1218 (1891).

2. The details of this important conflict are discussed in Chapter 3.

3. N. K. Jerne, *Cold Spring Harbor Symp. Quant. Biol.* **32,** 591 (1967).

4. See Ernst Mayr's introductory summary of the historical positions of the opposing factions. *In* E. Mayr and W. B. Provine, eds., *The Evolutionary Synthesis: Perspectives on the Unification of Biology,* pp. 1–48. Harvard University Press, Cambridge, Massachusetts, 1980.

5. L. Baldash, *Proc. Am. Philos. Soc.* **112,** 157 (1968); S. C. Brush, *The Temperature of the Earth,* pp. 29–44. Burt Franklin, New York, 1978.

6. There is now reason to believe, however, that prior to its "rediscovery" in 1900 by de Vries, Correns, and Tschermak, Mendel's work had in fact received fairly wide dissemination. See, e.g., R. Olby, *Origins of Mendelism,* 2nd Ed. University of Chicago Press, Chicago, Illinois, 1985.

7. H. Buchner, *Muench. Med. Wochenschr.* **40,** 449, 480, 482 (1893).

8. E. Roux and L. Vaillard, *Ann. Inst. Pasteur, Paris* **7,** 65 (1893).

9. A. Knorr, *Muench. Med. Wochenschr.* **45,** 321, 362 (1898).

10. E. Metchnikoff, *Weyl's Handbuch Hyg.* **9**(1), 48 (1900).

11. E. Hertzfeld and R. Klinger, *Biochem. Z.* **85,** 1 (1918).

12. W. H. Manwaring, *J. Immunol.* 12, 177 (1926).

13. A. L. Locke, E. R. Main, and E. F. Hirsch, *Arch. Pathol.* **2,** 437 (1926). Abstr.

14. G. Ramon, *C. R. Seances Soc. Biol. Ses Fil.* **102,** 287, 379, 381 (1929).

15. See ref. 12. See also W. H. Manwaring, *in The Newer Knowledge of Bacteriology and Immunology* (E. D. Jordan and I. S. Falk, eds.). University of Chicago Press, Chicago, Illinois, 1928.

16. W.H. Manwaring, *J. Immunol.* **19,** 155 (1930); *Science* **72,** 23 (1930).

17. M. Heidelberger and F. E. Kendall, *Science* **72,** 252 (1930).

18. W. W. C. Topley, *J. Pathol. Bacteriol.* **33,** 339 (1930).

19. S. B. Hooker and W. C. Boyd, *J. Immunol.* **21,** 113 (1931).

20. S. B. Hooker and W. C. Boyd, *J. Immunol.* **23,** 465 (1932).

21. E. Berger and H. Erlenmeyer, *Z. Hyg. Infektionskr.* **113,** 79 (1931).

22. M. Marquardt, *Paul Ehrlich.* Schuman, New York, 1957.

23. P. Ehrlich, Die Wertbemessung des Diphtherieheilserums. *Klin. Jahrb.* **60,** 299 (1897). [English translation in *The Collected Papers of Paul Ehrlich,* Vol. 2, pp. 107–125. Pergamon, London, 1956.] The theory was further amplified in Ehrlich's Croonian Lecture to the Royal Society, *Proc. R. Soc. London* **66,** 424 (1900).

24. E. Metchnikoff, *Lectures on the Comparative Pathology of Inflammation.* Kegan, Paul, Trench, Trübner, London, 1893. [Reprinted by Dover, New York, 1968.]

25. C. Weigert, *Verh, Ges. Dtsch. Naturforsch. Aerzte* **68,** 121 (1896).

26. J. Bordet, *Traité de l'immunité dans les maladies infectieuses,* 2nd Ed. Masson, Paris, 1939. In the first edition, Bordet had also called the illustrations "puerile." For a fuller account of the Ehrlich–Bordet debates, see Chapter 5.

27. These studies are well summarized in Karl Landsteiner's book, *The Specificity of Serological Reactions.* Dover, New York, 1962.

28. K. Landsteiner and M. Reich, *Centralbl. Bakteriol.* **39,** 712 (1905).

29. O. Bail and K. Tsuda, *Z. Immunitaetsforsch.* **1,** 546, 772 (1909).

30. The list of attempts to synthesize antibody artificially stretches from Bail to Pauling. Manwaring's collection of such reports (ref. 16), up to 1929, includes 10 items. We know of no efforts in this direction after those of L. Pauling and D. H. Campbell, *Science* **95,** 440 (1942); *J. Exp. Med.* **76,** 211 (1942). A patent (No. 392055) for the production of artificial diphtheria antitoxin was issued in Germany in the late 1920s!

31. O. Bail and H. Rotky, *Z. Immunitaetsforsch.* **17,** 378 (1913).

32. O. Bail, *Z. Immunitaetsforsch.* **21,** 202 (1914).

33. F. H. Thiele and D. Embleton, *Z. Immunitaetsforsch.* **20,** 1 (1914).

34. I. I. Ostromuislensky, *J. Russ. Phys. Chem. Soc.* **47,** 263 (1915); I. I. Ostromuislensky and D. I. Petrov, **47,** 301 (1915). An English abstract of these papers appeared in *Chem. Abstr.* **10,** 214 (1916).

35. W. W. C. Topley, *J. Pathol. Bacteriol.* **33,** 341 (1930).

36. F. Breinl and F. Haurowitz, *Z. Physiol. Chem.* **192,** 45 (1930). See also F. Haurowitz, *Nature (London)* **205,** 847 (1965).

37. S. Mudd, *J. Immunol.* **23,** 423 (1932).

38. J. Alexander, *Protoplasma* **14,** 296 (1931).

39. Haurowitz informs me (personal communication, 1982) that there was little interaction between Bail and the younger members or students in the

department and that Breinl (who had become interested in immunology through Landsteiner's work while at the Rockefeller Institute in 1928 and who invited Haurowitz to join him on his return) in fact worked under the senior virologist, Weil. Haurowitz recalls that even Breinl "considered my chemical aspects of immunology as fantastic" and refused to submit them to the immunology journal.

40. L. Pauling, personal communication, 1984.

41. L. Pauling, *J. Am. Chem. Soc.* **62**, 2643 (1940); *Science* **92**, 77 (1940).

42. It is interesting that the same suggestion had been made earlier by A. Rothen and K. Landsteiner, *Science* **90**, 65 (1939).

43. F. Karush, *Trans. N.Y. Acad. Sci.* **20**, 581 (1958).

44. J. R. Marrack, *The Chemistry of Antigens and Antibodies.* HM Stationery Off., London, 1934.

45. F. M. Burnet, *The Production of Antibodies.* Macmillan, New York, 1941.

46. For a review of the adaptive enzyme story, see J. Monod and M. Cohn, *Adv. Enzymol.* **13**, 67 (1952).

47. F. M. Burnet and F. Fenner, *The Production of Antibodies,* 2nd Ed. Macmillan, New York, 1949.

48. P. B. Medawar, *J. Anat.* **78**, 176 (1944); **79**, 157 (1945); *Harvey Lect.* **52**, 144 (1958).

49. R. D. Owen, *Science* **102**, 400 (1945).

50. M. G. Sevag, *Immunocatalysis,* 2nd Ed. Thomas, Springfield, Illinois, 1951.

51. R. S. Schweet and R. D. Owen, *J. Cell. Comp. Physiol.* **50**, Suppl. 1, 199 (1957).

52. See Alain Bussard's discussion of "Darwinisme et Immunologie." *Bull. Soc. Fr. Philos.* **77**, 1 (1983).

53. R. E. Billingham, L. Brent, and P. B. Medawar, *Nature (London)* **172**, 603 (1953).

54. O. C. Bruton, *Pediatrics* **9**, 722 (1952); O. C. Bruton, L. Apt, D. Gitlin and C. A. Janeway, *Am. J. Dis. Child.* **84**, 632 (1952).

55. P. Jordan, *Z. Immunitaetsforsch.* **97**, 330 (1940).

56. L. Pauling, *Science* **92**, 77 (1940).

57. N. K. Jerne, *Proc. Natl. Acad. Sci. USA* **41**, 849 (1955).

58. Rather than antigen serving as carrier for antibody, the concept of *antibody-as-carrier* was espoused for several decades by Pierre Grabar, *Clin. Immunol. Immunopathol.* **4**, 453 (1975); *Med. Hypotheses* **1**, 172 (1975). Grabar was less interested in *how* antibodies are formed than in *why*. In an approach reminiscent of Metchnikoff and especially of Ehrlich, he viewed the antibody as part of a broader, normal physiological system for the transport and assimilation of both foreign and native substances.

59. D. W. Talmage, *Annu. Rev. Med.* **8**, 239 (1957).

60. F. H. C. Crick, *Symp. Soc. Exp. Biol.* **12**, 138 (1958).

61. F. M. Burnet, *Aust. J. Sci.* **20**, 67 (1957).

62. F. M. Burnet, *The Clonal Selection Theory of Acquired Immunity.* Cambridge University Press, London, 1959.

63. D. W. Talmage, *Science* **129,** 1643 (1959).

64. J. Lederberg, *Science* **129,** 1649 (1959).

65. The somatic theories are best summarized by M. Cohn, *Prog. Immunol.* **2**(2), 261 (1974) and germ-line theories by L. Hood and D. W. Talmage, *Science* **168,** 325 (1970). See also A. J. Cunningham, ed., *The Generation of Immunologic Diversity.* Academic Press, New York, 1976.

66. L. Szilard, *Proc. Natl. Acad. Sci. USA* **46,** 293 (1960).

67. T. J. Kindt and J. D. Capra, *The Antibody Enigma.* Plenum, New York, 1984.

5

The Concept of Immunological Specificity

I N *The Eighth Day of Creation,* Horace Freeland Judson recounts the exciting story of the discovery of the genetic code and of the molecular biology of the storage and retrieval of genetic information.[1] With great insight, he points out that "behind the diversity of discoveries moved a unity, a constant direction of change . . . the development of the concept of biological specificity." In a similar way, the century that has elapsed since Pasteur first established immunology as an experimental science can be viewed as the continuing quest for the meaning and basis of immunological specificity. In the development of immunology, this search appears logically to be divisible into three somewhat overlapping phases. The first centered on the questions of how immunological specificity is expressed, and what its biological implications are. This inquiry involved the study of the major phenomena of immunology—precipitation, agglutination, hemolysis, and the reactions and cross-reactions of immunity and allergy—as well as the pathological, diagnostic, and therapeutic consequences of these phenomena. These were, in general, the principal preoccupations of the bacteriological era of immunology, which saw its peak about the turn of the century, and of the early immunochemical era, which encompassed the decades of the 1920s to 1950s.

The second phase in the development of the discipline addressed the question of how immunological specificity is structurally determined. This inquiry deals with the chemistry and anatomy of the immunoglobulin

molecule, chain sequences, molecular domains, isotypes and idiotypes, as well as the study of the molecular biology of the specific and
nonspecific receptors and factors that initiate or regulate immune
responses. This area was launched in the mid-1950s by the pioneering
work of Porter, Edelman, Putnam, and others[2] on the structure of the
immunoglobulin molecule, but quickly spread from the molecular
immunologists to the cellular immunologists, and soon demanded for
the first time that cis and trans immunologists[3] speak to one another in
mutually comprehensible terms.

Finally, the third phase of investigation has sought to answer the
question of how the information for immunological specificity is carried
and retrieved. Every theory of antibody formation was an attempt to
answer this question, and it finds modern expression in studies of the
molecular biology of the immunoglobulin and immune response genes
and of the nature and function of the receptors on T and B lymphocytes.

The Background to Biological Specificity

The concept of specificity did not appear unheralded when the term was
employed in an immunological context by Pasteur and Koch in the
1880s and by Ehrlich and Metchnikoff in the 1890s. It had, rather, a
long history of usage in many fields of science in one form or another,
and in philosophy as well. Indeed, as early as the sixteenth century, the
physician Hieronymus Mercurialis showed an understanding of that
most basic aspect of immunological specificity when he pointed out,[4] in
criticizing Fracastoro's theory of acquired immunity,[5] that immunity to
smallpox does not protect against measles or leprosy.

MEDICINE AND PHARMACY

The ancient Greek view that disease represents a disturbance of the
humors prevailed in the Western world for about 2000 years and
discouraged the view that individual illnesses might be specific and
subject to differential diagnosis and classification and to specific therapy.
Thus, descriptions of the phenomenon of acquired immunity to plagues
and pestilences from Thucydides down to the Middle Ages carried with
them no implication of specificity, since it was usually not even clear then
or later which of the major infectious diseases was involved in any given
epidemic.[6] Only in the tenth century did the Islamic physician Rhazes
first differentiate between smallpox and measles;[7] and by the sixteenth
century, it was generally understood that diseases such as plague,

smallpox, syphilis, and malaria had more or less specific identities that allowed their differentiation.[8]

In his famous 1546 book *On Contagion,* Fracastoro held that disease "seeds" or "germs" (*seminaria*) had specific affinities for certain targets—some for plants and others for animals. Some germs were held to specifically affect certain animal species and not to affect other species (a primitive notion of natural immunity); and even within a given host, some germs were held to have a specific affinity for certain tissues, organs, or humors. Perhaps even more significant was the contemporary development of the iatrochemical approach to disease, originated by Paracelsus in the early sixteenth century and expanded a century later by van Helmont and many others. Paracelsus helped to replace the lack of specificity of the classical humoralist school by emphasizing the individuality of diseases, their cause by specific agents foreign to the body, and the possibility therefore of specific therapy.[9] This approach has been termed the ontological concept of disease and is essentially the modern one.

Perhaps the greatest impetus to the consideration of diseases as specific entities was provided by Thomas Sydenham in the seventeenth century,[10] as Knud Faber points out in his book *Nosography.*[11] Sydenham's personal emphasis on clinical rather than theoretical medicine and on careful bedside diagnosis convinced him that diseases are specific, subject to uniform laws, and therefore classifiable. This concept led naturally to his later doctrine of specific remedies. On the basis of his knowledge that quinine exerts a specific effect on the ague, "Sydenham entertained no doubt that the Creator had provided specific remedies for the chief diseases."[12] But the notion of therapeutic "specifics" was not new with Sydenham. It has probably always existed in the folklore and even in professional practice, and it persists in sometimes curious form even today. Thus, the physician of the Middle Ages often used ground precious stones as a specific against the plague, mercury was long employed as a specific for syphilis, and pulverized animal horn was and still is employed by many cultures to treat impotence.[13]

Sydenham's approach to medicine exerted a strong influence on his contemporaries, and many of his followers attempted to expand Sydenham's nosological approach, with the idea that diseases could be described and classified in the same way that botanists describe and classify plants. Just as the eighteenth century saw the epitome of botanic taxonomy in the hands of Linnaeus, so did it witness a similar attempt at a grand systematization of disease, most notably by François Boissier de Sauvages. In 1763, Boissier published a *Nosologia*[14] which divided all diseases into 10 classes, these into 40 orders, the orders into genera, and the genera into species—2400 in all! In both botany and medicine, the aim was to distinguish the *specific*. In botany, where structure was easily studied and defined, this approach succeeded; in medicine, where pathological anatomy and pathophysiology were still in their infancy, these classifications proved not very useful.

The eighteenth-century taxonomic excesses in medicine, and the obvious defects of all of the classification systems proposed, induced a reaction in the early nineteenth century to the notion of disease specificity. This response was reinforced by the widely held view of spontaneous generation,[15] in which even microorganisms were not specifically fixed but could develop spontaneously and undergo trans-formations of both form and function. Thus it was that Pasteur experienced great difficulty at the outset in convincing the world of mid-nineteenth-century science of the specificity of action of yeast ferments, of the silkworm parasite, and of the specificity of the agents responsible for the diseases of wine and beer. Pasteur and Koch would later experience the same difficulty when they advanced the germ theory of disease, including as it did the claim that these agents of disease were morphologically specific, were capable of reproduction to type, and were the etiological agents of specific and reproducible diseases. But their notions finally gained broad acceptance, and it was the developments in bacteriology that helped to give true meaning to the term specificity as employed in medicine.

CHEMISTRY

By at least the fifteenth century, the concept of the specificity of action of poisons and of certain drugs was spreading, along with the alchemical understanding that nitric acid, antimony, mercury, sulfur, and many other substances were each able to react in *predictable* fashion with certain other chemicals.[16] Paracelsian iatrochemistry was firmly based on al-chemy and, with overtones of Medieval mysticism, held chemical spe-cificity to be the central issue. Not only did the Paracelsians postulate that every individual physiological action was specific in nature and every disease a distinct entity specific in location, but they also main-tained that the best form of therapy lay in the finding of a chemical able specifically to combat the given disease.

The ability of certain substances to react preferentially with other substances was termed *affinity*. With the discovery that a given chemical might react more strongly with one substance than with another, the late eighteenth and early nineteenth century saw extensive "tables of affin-ity" developed in an attempt to codify the many reactions and cross-reactions observed in the chemistry laboratory.[17] In an age when most sciences were dominated by the popularity of Newtonian mechanics, the speculation of such scientists as Bergman and Berthollet viewed chemical affinity as a force similar in nature to gravity. Only in the nineteenth century did the concept of chemical affinity take on a more significant meaning, with the increasing knowledge of substitution reactions in organic chemistry and with the development of the fields of thermochemistry, electrochemistry, and stereochemistry. All of these trends were crystallized in 1867 in Guldberg and Waage's law of mass action, which showed that the affinity of chemical reactants for one another not only had meaning, but could be quantified.

Developments in biochemistry during the nineteenth century also pointed in the direction of a significant role for affinity and specificity. This notion was nowhere more apparent than in the study of enzymes and of fermentation.[18] In the 1820s Justus Liebig, perhaps the foremost chemist of his day, conceived of disease as the specific consequence of infection by external inanimate ferments and the disease process itself as one of specific fermentation. It was his opposition to this view that preoccupied Pasteur during his early years and perhaps contributed to the transition of his interests from the fermentation of wine and beer to the study of the agents of animal and human disease. As information developed about the multiplicity and mode of action of enzymes, it became quite clear that there exists a remarkable specificity in the interaction of an enzyme with its substrate. This discovery led, in 1892, to the famous metaphor of the noted biochemist Emil Fischer: "To use a picture, I will say that enzyme and glucoside must join one another as lock and key, in order to be able to exert a chemical effect."[19] Fischer's metaphor, as well as the chemical emphasis he gave it, were to exert a profound effect upon Paul Ehrlich and thereby upon the nascent field of immunology.

Thus, by the 1890s, significant progress had been made toward an understanding of the general nature of the specificity of chemical interactions. But problems that persisted in two areas of chemistry would cause great difficulties for immunological theoreticians in the decades to come. The first difficulty involved a lack of understanding of the central difference between the ionic bonds of the electrochemist and what would later be called the covalent bond of the organic chemist. This problem would not be resolved until G. N. Lewis established in 1916 the basis of the strong covalent bond[20] and Linus Pauling showed in 1939 how weak bonds are formed.[21] The second difficulty faced in the 1890s and for some 50 years thereafter involved the difference between chemical and "physical" interactions. Aided in part by the physicist Ernst

Mach and the physical chemist Wolfgang Pauli and attended by a certain degree of mysticism, it was conceived that "colloidal" interactions were all-important in biological systems and involved adsorption processes and reactions with electrolytes that were predominantly nonspecific.[22] Such colloids included proteins, which, at least until the 1930s, were assumed to be nonspecific aggregates of smaller molecules rather than discrete molecular entities themselves.[23]

It was the difference between the *strong* bonds of organic chemistry and the *weak* ionic bonds of electrochemistry that highlighted the conceptual differences between Paul Ehrlich and Svante Arrhenius. Again, Ehrlich's emphasis on firm *chemical* union between antigen and antibody clashed with Jules Bordet's view that the antigen–antibody union represented a weaker, *physical* (colloidal) interaction. The problem of strong versus weak bonds and of chemical versus physical interactions would serve as the leitmotif during the ensuing debates on immunological specificity and its phenomenological consequences.

PHILOSOPHY

Among the philosophical questions that have interested mankind, one has exerted a profound influence in modern times on almost every field of biology. This was the question of whether nature is continuous in all respects or divisible into discrete components and types essentially unrelated to one another. Plato's concept of *essentialism* held that the vast observed variabilities of the world represent complete discontinuities between types (*eidos*), and the Aristotelian classification of animals and plants into separate groups accorded with this notion, as did the later concept of creationism, which maintains that each form of plant or animal life is unique and specific and persists unchanged. In opposition to this view, others saw an overriding continuity in nature and only gradual and quantitative transitions between apparently discrete species of things. Not only did these divergent world views exert a marked effect upon theories of spontaneous generation, on concepts of the fixity of species, and on Darwinian evolution, as Ernst Mayr points out in *The Evolutionary Synthesis*,[24] but they also exerted an interesting influence on immunological thought during the first decades of this century.

The debates over whether nature is seamless or discontinuous persisted throughout the eighteenth and nineteenth centuries. On the one hand was the growing tendency to categorize plants and animals according to the sharply defined differences among them, and on the other was the familiar scholastic expression *natura non facit saltus* and Leibnitz's claim that this was one of his greatest and most highly verified maxims, which he called the law of continuity.[25] Immanuel Kant, in his *Critique of Pure Reason,* suggested that "this logical law of *continuum speciarum . . .* presupposes however a transcendental *lex continui in natura.*"[26] Nature, according to Kant, is herself discontinuous, and only the human mind imposes continuity. In opposition to this, the botanist Karl von Nägeli, like his teacher Mathias Schleiden, held that nature's continuity is real and imposes itself upon the observer. Von Nägeli believed in the continuity of change; he also believed that species differ from one another only by gradual transition and quantitative gradation (*quantitative Abstufung*) rather than by qualitative absolutes. Once again, the "lumpers" and "splitters" were at odds, the former searching for similarities, the latter for differences.

The fascinating implications for immunology of these philosophical differences were pointed out by Mazumdar in her study, *Karl Landsteiner and the Problem of Species, 1838–1968.*[27] In this impressive work, Mazumdar calls attention to the fact that this difference in the approach to nature was responsible for a dispute that covered 130 years and four generations of scientists, of whom the most recent were immunologists. Thus, von Nägeli argued the question of continuity versus discontinuity in botany with the botanist Ferdinand Cohn. In turn, von Nägeli's student Max von Gruber entered into a long-standing dispute in bacteriology, first with Cohn's protegé Robert Koch and then even more violently in immunology with Koch's students Richard Pfeiffer and Paul Ehrlich. Ehrlich next had conceptual differences with Gruber's student Karl Landsteiner. Finally, in the modern era, Landsteiner's student Alexander Wiener engaged in long and bitter controversy in immuno-hematology about the interpretation and nomenclature of the rhesus blood group system, arguing for unity and continuity against the intellectual descendants of the diversity–specificity school, R. A. Fisher and R. R. Race.

This running battle over the period of 130 years may have had its roots in an abstract philosophical difference, but it profoundly influenced the development of modern immunology, as it found expression in concepts of the nature and function of immunological specificity.

Paul Ehrlich: The First Immunochemist

Paul Ehrlich received his medical degree in 1878, for which he presented a thesis on the theory and practice of histological staining.[28] For the next dozen years, most of his work was focused on demonstrations of the usefulness and specificity of chemical stains in histology, hematology, and bacteriology. These studies involved him deeply in problems of

organic synthesis and chemical interaction, and he very early became
aware of the connection between chemical constitution and function and
that such interactions depend upon the presence of specific groups of
atoms. Following the lead of Edward Pflüger, Ehrlich conceived of the
physiological functions of the living cell as dependent upon such specific
atom groups, attached as distinct side chains to the "chemical nucleus" of
the cell. He became interested in the problem of immunity during this
period and undertook experiments in this new field, first privately and
then part-time in Koch's Institute for Infectious Diseases.[29]

Because of Ehrlich's interest in antitoxins and his demonstrated
knowledge of chemistry, he was charged in 1895 to find a solution to
the problem that had vexed workers throughout the world following
von Behring's discovery of diphtheria antitoxin—the measurement and
standardization of both toxin and antitoxin. So elegant was his solution
to this problem that publication of the results gained him almost
instantaneous worldwide recognition and shortly thereafter his own
institute, the Royal Prussian Institute for Experimental Therapy.
Ehrlich's 1897 paper on the measurement of diphtheria antitoxin[30] is of
great historical interest from several points of view. First, it laid the
foundation for the field that would later be known as immunochemistry;
and it pointed the way for 50 years of quantitative studies of the
antigen–antibody interaction. Next, it introduced Ehrlich's concept of
the side-chain receptor theory of antibody formation, which would have
important repercussions on immunological speculation for many decades to come. And finally, it declared to the world that the reactions and
specificity of immunity depend upon the laws of structural chemistry.[31]

THE SIDE-CHAIN THEORY

While the practical applications of preventive vaccines and of antitoxin
serum therapy were being widely exploited, the physiological mechanisms responsible for the functions of immunity were still a mystery. As I
noted in Chapter 1, early theories of acquired immunity pictured the
host as a passive receptacle in which the pathogen itself contributed to its
own demise. Only Elie Metchnikoff, in his theory of cellular immunity,[32] considered that the host might mount an active immunological
defense against infection, but Metchnikoff's phagocytic theory was
widely opposed.[33] The discovery of antibody in 1890 reinforced the
trend toward humoral theories of immunity, and interest in cellular
immunity declined, not to be seriously revived for almost 60 years. After
the work of Emil von Behring and his collaborators,[34] the central
theoretical questions in immunology involved how antibodies are

formed and how they acquire and exercise their specificity. These were the questions that Paul Ehrlich addressed in his famous side–chain theory.

Ehrlich's side-chain theory was not excessively complicated in its initial formulation in 1897. The key postulates were that (1) antibodies are *normal cell products* that serve as cell membrane receptors and that are not "made to order" to fit a given antigen; (2) antibody *specificity* is the consequence of the interaction of chemically defined complementary molecular structures; and (3) the antigen–antibody interaction represents a firm (irreversible) chemical union. Since most of the antibodies recognized at that time were antitoxins,[35] Ehrlich conceived of the antibody molecule as having a single binding site for the haptophore group on the antigen, a site that would simultaneously neutralize the antigen's toxophore group. Very quickly, however, the implications of the newly discovered phenomena of agglutination,[36] the precipitin reaction,[37] and immune hemolysis[38] made new demands upon the side-chain theory, and a complicated set of *ad hoc* hypotheses was required to bring the theory into conformity with the newer facts. Thus, the antitoxin molecule was called by Ehrlich a receptor or "haptine" of the first order, possessing only a binding site for toxic antigens. Receptors of the second order were postulated to contain two different domains, one responsible for interaction with antigen, and a separate portion to account for the secondary biological phenomena of agglutination and precipitation.[39] Ehrlich called this second site the "zymophore" group, believing that agglutination and precipitation were probably the result of some type of enzymatic action. To account for complement-mediated hemolysis and bacteriolysis, Ehrlich postulated the existence of third-order receptors, which possess a site for the binding with antigen (the cytophile group) and a separate site (the complementophile group) to which complement was bound. This complement-fixing antibody, since it contained two receptors, one for antigen and one for complement, Ehrlich termed a *Zwischenkörper* (amboceptor). It is interesting that even this early, Ehrlich conceived of the lytic activity of complement as an enzymatic process, a speculation that would not be confirmed for 60–70 years.[40]

Ehrlich's side-chain theory had a marked effect upon the biological and medical sciences in the decade or two that followed its formulation. This result was due in part to the famous pictures used by Ehrlich and his adherents (Fig. 5.1) to illustrate the structures and their reactions. It is interesting to note that immunologists even today employ the same assortment of geometric shapes to depict different antibody and antigenic specificities. Despite Ehrlich's caution that, "Needless to say, these

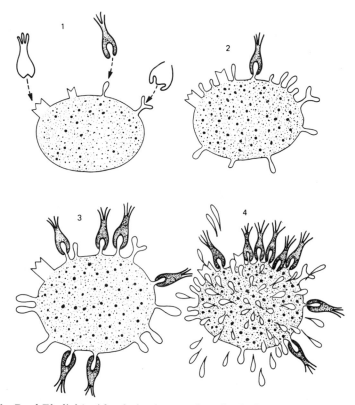

Fig. 5.1. Paul Ehrlich's side-chain theory of antibody formation. (From ref. 41.) Note the use of geometric shapes to indicate different specificities. Antigen selects for the production and release of the appropriate membrane receptors.

diagrams must be regarded as quite apart from all morphologic considerations"[41] they seemed almost to define *and even to be* the molecules and reactions depicted, so that one was almost convinced that one understood the reality from these pictures. These diagrams vexed Jules Bordet, who complained, "By the abuse that it [the Ehrlich theory] has made of quite puerile graphical representations which merely translate the exterior aspect of phenomena without in any way penetrating to their inner meaning, it has extended the deceptive use of explanations that are facile, but illusory."[42] Nevertheless, entire books were devoted to the theory, with chapters on "the side-chain theory in internal medicine," "the side-chain theory in obstetrics and gynecology," and so on.[43] More substantially perhaps, Ehrlich's side-chain theory represented an important contribution to pharmacology and to Ehrlich's new concepts of chemotherapy,[44] to which he devoted most of his activities from the turn of the century until his death in 1915.

THE ANTIGEN—ANTIBODY INTERACTION

It is important to examine more closely Ehrlich's view of toxin—antitoxin and other antigen—antibody interactions, for they not only illustrate his view of the workings of immunological specificity but also introduce for the first time in immunology the equally important concept of affinity.

Ehrlich's studies on diphtheria toxin and antitoxin introduced many now-familiar terms to immunology. Antibody was initially a *receptor* on the cell surface that possessed a configuration specific for antigen. Ehrlich considered the antigen to be a distinct molecular entity, containing a complementary haptophore grouping (Gr. *aptein,* to grasp or fasten) and a second toxophore group responsible for toxicity. He had early recognized that while the toxicity of a preparation of diphtheria toxin might decrease with time, its ability to bind to antibody remained undiminished. He suggested that this represented a deterioration only of the toxophore group, and he named the resulting product a *toxoid*. To explain the discrepancy between L_+ and L_0 values,[45] Ehrlich postulated that the unit of antitoxin had a *valency* of about 200. He suggested further that preparations of diphtheria toxin contained not only toxin and toxoid but also other related substances with different *affinities* for the antibody receptor. Those with the lowest affinity he called toxons, and soon he had introduced a veritable congeries of substances, including α and β modifications of proto-, deutero-, and tritotoxins and toxoids. Ehrlich held that each of these components would react with antibody in sequence, the higher affinity components first and the lower affinity components last. In this manner he sought to explain discrepancies in the titration curve of diphtheria toxin with antibody; he established elaborate charts called "toxin spectra," which purported to show the composition of any preparation in terms of the various high- and low-affinity toxic and nontoxic constituents.[46]

As another example of the extent to which *ad hoc* hypothesis might be carried by Ehrlich and his adherents, I cite the example of the Danysz (or Bordet-Danysz) phenomenon, discovered in 1902.[47] Danysz showed that the degree of neutralization of diphtheria toxin by antitoxin depends upon whether the toxin is added all at once or stepwise. When the addition is made in steps, the supernatant is found to be much more toxic than when the same quantities of toxin and antibody are mixed all at once. By this time, Ehrlich had substantially left immunology to pursue his interest in chemotherapy, but in the Ehrlich tradition von Dungern hypothesized the existence of "epitoxinoids," which were claimed to have even lower affinity for diphtheria antitoxin than did toxon.[48] Von Dungern suggested that the stepwise addition of toxin resulted in the irreversible binding of significant amounts of epitoxinoid, whereas mixing of the toxin and antibody all at once should result in preferential binding and neutralization of the higher-affinity toxin, with the epitoxinoid left substantially unbound.

In his studies on immune hemolysis, Ehrlich and others noted the existence of immunological cross-reactions, such as the ability of rabbit anti-ox erythrocyte antibody to hemolyze goat erythrocytes.[49] Differential absorption studies showed that the goat cells would absorb only the cross-reacting antibody, whereas the homologous ox cells would absorb all hemolysins. Ehrlich explained these results, in the context of his side-chain theory, by assuming that any complex cell must necessarily contain a number of unique antigenic determinants, some of which might be shared among the cells of related species. Thus, immunological specificity was presented as absolute, with cross-reactions resulting only from mixtures of antibodies whose specific antigens happen to be shared by different cells (Fig. 5.2).

The complexity of Ehrlich's formulation of the diphtheria toxin–antitoxin interaction points up the extent to which his fertile imagination was grounded in structural chemistry and concepts of affinity; it was this same commitment, and a willingness to support his theories with extensive *ad hoc* assumptions, that would later carry him into a prolonged debate with Jules Bordet over the mechanism of immune hemolysis and the nature and interactions of complement. But Ehrlich's complex theories aside, one must not lose sight of the important

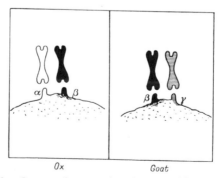

Fig. 5.2. Blood cells of ox and goat, showing specific (α, γ) and common (β) receptors. (From Ehrlich, ref. 49.) Different shadings are used to code for different specificities.

contributions of his work in this area. Apart from advancing for the first time a *practical* method for the standardization of diphtheria toxin and antitoxin, these studies introduced a number of important concepts to immunology. These include the notion that antibody specificity is based upon structural–chemical complementarity of combining sites, the notion of heterogeneity of binding affinity (although in Ehrlich's formulation, heterogeneity was restricted to antigenic variability—the antibody "side chains" reactive with a given antigen were implicitly assumed to be homogeneous), and finally, the observation that antigen–antibody interactions were temperature- and concentration-dependent like any other chemical interaction and were thus amenable to quantitative study.

The Ehrlich–Bordet Debate

Ehrlich maintained that the antigen–antibody bond was the result of a firm and irreversible chemical interaction, with a specificity based on molecular structure. Moreover, Ehrlich held that the receptor on the antibody molecule that fixes complement follows the same rules of specificity and firmness of bonding. This notion forced the conclusion that complement must also be bound firmly by antibody, even in the absence of antigen, since even the side-chain pictures represented the antigen-binding site and the complement-binding site as separate entities on the antibody molecule. Ehrlich and his students, most notably Sachs, also concluded, partly on the basis of experiments but also by strong analogy with the antigen receptor, that just as there were different antigens so were there different complements, each capable of binding specifically to its appropriate receptor on antibody.[50] In both aspects of Ehrlich's side-chain theory, he encountered strong opposition, most notably from the Belgian immunologist Jules Bordet.

The principal difference between the ideas of Ehrlich and Bordet concerned not the existence of immunological specificity but its basis (i.e., the fundamental nature of the antigen–antibody interaction). Ehrlich insisted upon the chemical nature of immunological specificity, which he thought required a firm and irreversible bond. When challenged by data suggesting that antigen–antibody reactions might not proceed to completion or that dissociation was possible—suggested by the diphtheria toxin titration curve and by the Danysz phenomenon— Ehrlich skillfully extended his theory by postulating sufficient new components and sufficient differences in affinity to account for the necessary stoichiometry.

Bordet, on the other hand, approached these problems as a biologist rather than as a chemist. He was convinced from the outset that antigen

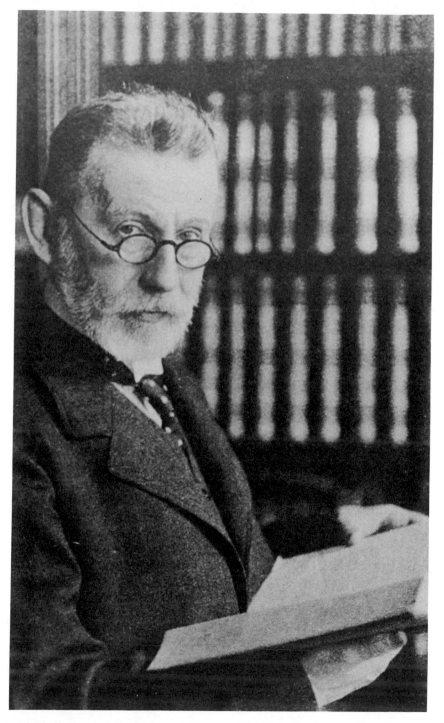

Paul Ehrlich (Courtesy National Library of Medicine)

and antibody might interact in multiple proportions, and that a firm chemical union between them was neither required nor indeed permitted by the pertinent data.[51] Bordet rejected the notion of a chemical interaction between antigen and antibody and suggested instead that the binding was more comparable to the adsorption of dyes. He suggested that the combinations of antibody with antigen are in fact "colloidal" interactions, a term then very popular in many fields and thought to represent an adequate explanation for many different types of phenomena.[52] The large and complex surface area presented by colloids was deemed adequate to encompass almost any sort of adsorptive process. As Bordet claimed, "The affinity of adsorption is sufficiently delicate, graduated, and elective, so that the notion of its participation in antigen–antibody reactions is compatible with that of specificity."[53] Throughout his writings, Bordet repeatedly criticized Ehrlich for his insistence upon chemical notions, and especially for the complexity of his theories. Bordet insisted that he himself was not a theorist and that the ideas that he had advanced were not even worthy to be called theories but rather "merely represent a description of the true state of affairs." He says, however, that

> My predilection for the realities cannot deter me from considering briefly the hypotheses . . . one knows with what luxuriance they have been developed on the fertile ground of immunity, where so much of the unknown still stimulates the imagination and invites audaciously synthetic concepts from the schools desirous of affirming their superiority . . . conceptions that are defended with all of the partisanship that *amour propre* mixed with chauvinism so readily inspire.[54]

If the driving force behind Ehrlich's side-chain theory was the desire to explain immunological specificity and the origin of antibodies, the stimulus to Bordet's more modest speculations was certainly the desire to explain the phenomena of immunity—bacterial agglutination and neutralization, the precipitin reaction, and especially complement-mediated hemolysis. In this approach, the specificity of the primary antigen–antibody interaction seemed less important than the secondary physiological consequences. Bordet apparently did not feel impelled to question closely whether "colloidal interactions" or "physical adsorption processes" were indeed able adequately to explain the striking precision of immunological specificity that was apparent even in those early days. Ehrlich, however, did not hesitate to point out this defect in the "physical" theory of Bordet. It should be noted that this conflict between structural–chemical and physical theories was not restricted to immunology but was then being argued in many fields of biology.[55]

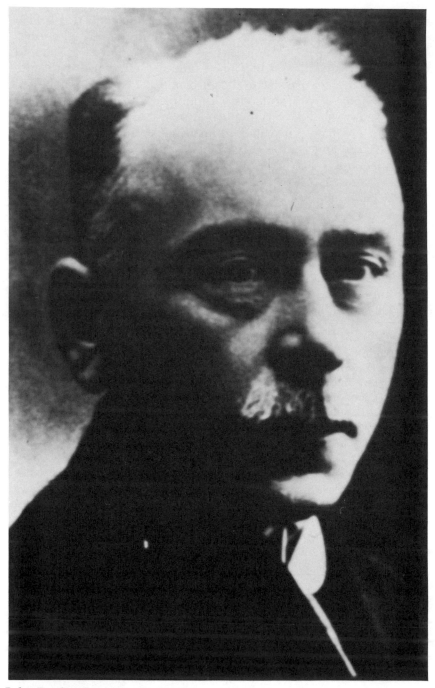

Jules Bordet (Courtesy Institut Pasteur)

The fundamental difference in the approaches of Ehrlich and Bordet is highlighted by their respective responses to the new theory of Arrhenius and Madsen,[56] elaborated in detail by Arrhenius in a book whose title, *Immunochemistry*, named the new field.[57] These authors suggested that antigen reacts with antibody in the same way a weak acid reacts with a weak base, setting up an equilibrium that obeys the law of mass action. Bordet welcomed this new theory, because it showed that the complicated Ehrlich-type theories were not really necessary. However, he maintained that the Arrhenius–Madsen theory could not be correct because it seemed to permit more dissociation of toxin–antitoxin complexes than the data supported. Ehrlich's school, on the other hand, rejected it because it did not adequately explain affinity and specificity.[58]

The second principal dispute between Ehrlich and Bordet centered on the mechanism of complement fixation and immune hemolysis. Ehrlich's chemical concept required two distinctly separate and specific receptors on the antibody molecule, one for antigen and one for complement; and he saw no good reason why complement receptors should not have the range of specificities for different complements that antigen receptors have for different antigens. Thus, for a long time, Ehrlich and his co-workers argued that there was a multiplicity of specific complements in each serum and that the firm complement–antibody interaction could occur independent of the antigen–antibody interaction. Bordet, for his part, was content to have antibody adsorbed onto antigen, an interaction that he suggested would result in a "change of configuration" appropriate for the nonspecific fixation of a single complement.

Even the terminology used by Ehrlich and Bordet typified their different approaches and helped prevent reconciliation. Ehrlich persisted in his use of the German term *Komplement* and referred to hemolytic antibody as the *Zwischenkörper* or *Ambozeptor*, terms suggesting that the function of antibody was to provide a specific link between complement and antigen. Bordet preferred the more French-sounding term *alexine* (actually coined by Buchner) and called antibody *la substance sensibilisatrice*, a phrase implying that the function of the antibody was merely to "sensitize" the antigen-bearing cell so that complement might nonspecifically effect its lysis.

If the major elements of Ehrlich's structural–chemical approach to the antigen–antibody bond (save its irreversibility) were later vindicated, at the expense of Bordet's physical theory, it was Bordet whose general concept of the mode of action of complement was proved correct. From this latter dispute, only Ehrlich's nomenclature survived. But the impressive contributions to immunology of both these scientific giants were subsequently recognized by Nobel prizes. Ehrlich shared his in 1908 with Elie Metchnikoff, and Bordet received this honor in 1919.

The Ehrlich–Gruber Debate

The decade that immediately followed Paul Ehrlich's side-chain theory of antibody formation and definition of the structural–chemical basis for antibody specificity witnessed a flood of new findings that extended the scope of the young field of immunology beyond its original narrow boundaries of protection against bacterial diseases. The discoveries of the precipitin reaction and of hemagglutination quickly demonstrated that antibodies could be raised against a wide variety of nontoxic and even nonbacterial substances. More than this, the phenomenon of complement-mediated immune cytolysis disclosed for the first time that antibodies were not restricted to the destruction of pathogenic bacteria but might engage also in the destruction of other, nonnoxious cell types such as erythrocytes and spermatozoa.[59] The same decade also saw the description of most of the principal phenomena of allergy,[60] including anaphylaxis,[61] the Arthus reaction,[62] and serum sickness.[63] Each of these pathological reactions, as well as the earlier-described Koch reaction in tuberculosis and the tuberculin skin test,[64] were quickly demonstrated to be based upon immunological mechanisms and to obey the general rules of immunological specificity. In yet another direction, these early developments led to the use of antibodies in the new field of serotaxonomy and forensic medicine,[65] in which the interrelationship of animal and plant species was examined in what would be the first of many applications of antibody molecules as molecular probes in other fields of biology.

But one of the important consequences of all of these new discoveries was the growing realization that the repertoire of possible antibodies was very large indeed. Another consequence was the increasing difficulty in establishing the boundaries of immunological specificity itself; certain *in vitro* reactions were found to be highly specific, whereas other reactions might show appreciable cross-reactivity among bacterial species or among different animal sera. It thus became increasingly more difficult to find overwhelming and irrefutable support in the literature for those who argued with Paul Ehrlich for a chemically defined, irreversible binding and a narrow specificity for antibody or for those who argued with Jules Bordet for a physically based, reversible binding and a somewhat broader specificity. But perhaps it might be more appropriate to say that it had become easier to support *either* position, by an appropriate selection from the mass of data that was accumulating. In the event, the controversy continued.

Max von Gruber was, as I have mentioned, descended from a philosophical school of science (Schleiden and von Nägeli) that had long had basic differences with the tradition (Cohn, Koch, and Pfeiffer) to which Paul Ehrlich was heir. For the Ehrlich school, the password had always been discrete specificity–first in botanic classification, then in bacterial action, and currently in the interactions of antigen, antibody, and complement. In the tradition in which Gruber had been reared, the key words were *Kontinuität* and *quantitative Abstufung* (quantitative gradation). A traditional conflict between two differing world views had now shifted its field of battle to the young discipline of immunology.

Ehrlich's controversy with Jules Bordet had always been marked by politeness and respect on both sides. Despite their differences, they continually referred to one another as "distinguished," and Ehrlich even allowed that, while Bordet might be in error, his opposition had served to stimulate much fruitful research that further strengthened the side-chain theory. But Ehrlich's battle with von Gruber was far different—it soon became quite vitriolic, as charges and countercharges appeared month after month in the leading journals. More than once, the dispute was reduced to personal attacks.

When Gruber and Clemens von Pirquet attacked Ehrlich on the question of toxin–antitoxin interactions,[66] Ehrlich responded that "It is all the more remarkable that Gruber should choose the subject of toxins for the main portion of his attack on me, for according to his own admission that is the field which he knows merely from literary studies. Against such critics I am in the unpleasant position of a man who is compelled to discuss colors with the blind."[67] Gruber, in his turn, sent a satirical letter to the *Wiener klinische Wochenschrift* entitled "New Fruits of the Ehrlich Toxin Theory," purportedly addressed to Gruber and signed "Dr. Peter Phantasus, *by God's Grace Chemist.*"[68] It starts, "The Ehrlich side-chain theory has made its triumphant way throughout the world. You, Herr Professor [Gruber], were literally the only one to have called this theory, with astonishing shortsightedness and almost incomprehensible arrogance 'completely worthless, unbridled hypothesis-spinning,' and 'dangerous numbing with words'." Then, in apparent support of the Ehrlich thesis, it employs Ehrlich's approach to prove that distilled water (which also lyses erythrocytes) must contain a whole series of Ehrlich-type toxins, prototoxoids, etc. To this, Ehrlich replied, "I shall now take up Gruber's recent experiments. These were first published in the *Wiener klinische Wochenschrift,* in the form strongly suggestive of the comic supplement of a newspaper."[69] In the introduction to his collected works, Ehrlich takes to task "such authors as Gruber, who have absolutely no personal experience in the main questions, [but] wage a bitter war merely because they have made a few literary studies." And in final exasperation at the Gruber attacks, Ehrlich complains that "In a way, therefore, my position is like that of a chess player who, even though his game is won, is forced by the obstinacy of his opponent to carry on move by move until the final 'mate'."[70]

Gruber's attacks on Ehrlich are extremely interesting, not only because they question the very possibility in Nature of a set of discrete and absolute specificities such as Ehrlich postulated, but also because in the process Gruber raised questions that would continue to vex immunologists for several generations to come. How is it possible to explain even in chemical terms, asked Gruber, the astoundingly large number of different specificities demanded by Ehrlich's theory?[71] Again, Gruber asked how, from the point of view of Darwinian selection, can all of these antibody specificities have evolved to antigens not in the normal environment? For Gruber, the absence of suitable answers to such questions was sufficient cause to reject the Ehrlich hypothesis; and, indeed, these questions may have played a significant role in the fall from favor of Ehrlich's selection theory of antibody formation in the 1920s, and in its replacement by instruction theories that suffered no such defect.

Gruber's central attack, however, was on the key to Ehrlich's theory—specificity—and on its principal implication, the firmness of the antigen–antibody union. Gruber argued against the existence of absolute and discrete specificities for antibodies, which in Ehrlich's hands would not permit extensive serological cross-reactions. For Ehrlich, as for Richard Pfeiffer before him, an antibody could react only with its homologous antigen; any evidence of cross-reactions must imply different antibodies interacting with mixtures of antigens. For Gruber, however, a single antibody could interact, by *graded affinities*, against a number of different antigens. Pfeiffer, in his studies of bacterial agglutination and lysis, and Ehrlich, in his studies of hemolysis, preferred to use weak or diluted antisera whose reactions were narrowly specific. Gruber, on the other hand, always insisted upon "high-grade" antisera, that permitted the study of nonspecific reactions. Each group argued that the other's approach was erroneous.

Throughout the long dispute, few of their differences were resolved, since each spoke a language incomprehensible to the other (see Chapter 8 for a further discussion of the semantic aspects of immunological disputes). The Ehrlich–Bordet disputes are widely remembered in the English-speaking world, thanks in no small measure to the efforts of Bordet's student and translator–popularist, Frederick Gay.[72] The

Ehrlich–Gruber disputes are largely unknown outside Germany and Austria, in part because Gruber had no Gay, but in greatest measure because his work was substantially eclipsed by that of his more famous student Karl Landsteiner, who made the conflict his own.

Karl Landsteiner, The Compleat Immunologist

No single individual contributed so importantly to so many different areas of immunology as did Karl Landsteiner. In a scientific career that spanned almost half a century, he involved himself in almost every significant area of immunology, and on each of them he left his mark.[73] Thus, he founded the field of immunohematology by first describing the ABO system in 1900[74] and followed this up by discovering the M, N, and P erythrocyte isoantigens with Philip Levine in 1926[75] and the Rh antigen system with Alexander Wiener in 1940.[76] He was among the first to produce experimental syphilis in the monkey in 1906,[77] and the first to produce experimental poliomyelitis in the monkey in 1909.[78] In the field of serodiagnosis, Landsteiner (with Donath in 1904) defined the antibody responsible for the first reported autoimmune disease, parox-ysmal cold hemoglobinuria,[79] and later correctly identified the antigen involved in the Wassermann test for syphilis,[80] as well as advancing the first useful serological test for poliomyelitis in 1909.[81] Finally, in collaboration with Merrill Chase, he showed in 1942 that delayed hypersensitivity could only be transferred passively by sensitized leuko-cytes and not by serum antibody,[82] a critical step forward in our understanding of the nature of cellular immunity.

But Landsteiner's most significant work, for the purposes of this discussion of immunological specificity, lay in his studies of the immune response to artificial haptens, which he employed to gain a better understanding of the specificity of serological reactions, as his famous book is entitled.[83] Landsteiner himself apparently considered that the study of hapten–antibody reactions represented his most significant scientific contribution, for when awarded the Nobel prize in medicine in 1930 for his discovery of the blood group antigens, he is reported to have felt that he was recognized for the wrong thing![84]

The Vienna of the 1890s, in which the young Karl Landsteiner took his medical degree and postgraduate training, was both scientifically and intellectually one of Europe's most exciting centers.[85] Like Paul Ehrlich, Landsteiner developed a strong interest in synthetic organic chemistry and spent two years at various laboratories, including that of Emil Fischer in Würzburg. This early training in structural chemistry ulti-mately influenced the direction of Landsteiner's work, but along pathways quite different from those toward which a similar background had pointed Paul Ehrlich. Following additional clinical experience at the University of Vienna, Landsteiner became assistant to Max von Gruber in 1896–97, in the newly established Department of Hygiene. It was here that his interest in serology and immunology was stimulated, and it was here also, from Gruber, that he acquired his basic beliefs about the nature of immunological specificity. Indeed, his first scientific paper in immunology, published in 1897, was on antigen–antibody *cross-reactions*,[86] and this set the tone for his entire life's work in this area.

From the very beginning, in agreement with Gruber, Landsteiner voiced his opposition to Ehrlich's view of a discrete and absolute immunological specificity, and he rejected Ehrlich's structural–chemical approach to the antigen–antibody reaction. In a paper with Jagič in 1903,[87] Ehrlich adopted Jules Bordet's physical (colloid) explanation of the antigen–antibody interaction and claimed that "immune specificity can be seen as in principal the sum of a number of individual, nonspecific reactions." So ardently did Landsteiner espouse the cause of a colloidal interpretation of the antigen–antibody interaction that for a time he, rather than Bordet, was the recognized champion of this viewpoint. However, Landsteiner's commitment to a colloidal interpretation did not survive the decade, and he quietly gave up this "physical" position in favor of a more chemical one, although he never ceased to argue against Ehrlich's absolute specificity and in favor of Gruber's concept of quantitative and almost continuously graded affinities. One who believed otherwise would hardly have devoted his life's work to a study of the cross-reactions of antibodies.

There appeared in 1912 a publication that redirected the course of Landsteiner's future research interests. In this, E. P. Pick published an encyclopedic review of the chemistry of antigens,[88] including an extensive section on the specificity of chemically altered antigens, a door that Obermeyer and Pick had opened with their initial study published in 1906.[89] This paper pointed out that not only were a number of different chemical treatments available, but many of these would also confer new and unique specificities upon proteins, depending only upon the nature and extent of such chemical treatment. Even the normal rules of species specificity might be abrogated. Thus, an antibody raised against a chemically treated egg albumin might now react specifically with horse serum protein treated in a similar manner.

It did not take long for Landsteiner to recognize the power of this new approach; and in 1917 he published two important papers with H. Lampl, an event that marked clearly the course of his future work.[90] In the first of these, he presented data on the cross-reactions of antibodies against a homologous series of acyl-substituted proteins; and in the second study he employed for the first time protein antigens substituted with diazonium compounds. These papers are of singular importance for an understanding both of Landsteiner's future work on immunological specificity and of the contemporary trend of immunological thought. In his work with artificial haptens, Landsteiner saw a powerful tool with which to prove two important immunological points, perhaps best summarized in the following quote from a follow-up paper published with Lampl in 1918:

> We . . . did not think it was possible to explain the workings of normal or immune serum on innumerable cell types by the supposition of innumerable different antibodies and, by analogy, a similar fantastic number of receptors on each cell. We held, like Gruber, that the simpler concept was quite adequate, that an antibody can react with a variety of related but not necessarily identical antigens . . . The specificity of serum reactions appears to be the expression of grades of affinity which reach a maximum in certain combinations—those of antigen and homologous antibody . . . while the Ehrlich theory admits of only a single absolute specificity.[91]

In this quotation, we can almost hear the death knell of Ehrlich's side-chain theory of antibody formation. For if the number of *naturally occurring* antigens was embarrassingly large to be explained on the basis of preexisting antibody side chains, Pick in his review had shown and Landsteiner would soon amply confirm that the number of *synthetic* haptens that might serve as antigenic determinants was immeasurably larger. How could the mammalian host have *prior* knowledge to encompass antibody specificities for such unnatural structures, many of which were not yet even a gleam in the eye of the synthetic organic chemist? I shall show later the direction in which this aspect of Landsteiner's work forced the speculation of chemically oriented immunologists.

The defeat and breakup of the Austro-Hungarian empire following the First World War had serious consequences for Viennese society and for Viennese science.[92] Among those who suffered the effects of this defeat was Landsteiner, who soon lost his position and was pensioned off while still in his early fifties. He had no recourse but to look elsewhere; and after two somewhat insecure years in Holland, he finally received an invitation from Simon Flexner to take up a position at the Rockefeller Institute in New York. Here, his work on antibody cross-reactions with artificial haptens flourished, most notably in collaboration with his colleague James van der Scheer. In much of his work with homologous series of related chemical compounds, he showed repeatedly the nature and extent of the cross-reactions that one might expect from an antibody made against any given member of the chemical series. And yet, despite his continuing emphasis upon *cross*-reactions, it was Landsteiner's work that helped convince the world of the elegance and narrow precision of immunological specificity, in which an antiserum could distinguish clearly among subtle differences in antigenic (haptenic) structure. Landsteiner might argue for graded affinities, but his demonstrations that appropriate antisera could distinguish between optical isomers or between ortho-, meta-, and para-substituted azobenzoates seemed to argue for a sharper specificity.

It is interesting that Landsteiner rarely succumbed to the common practice of contemporary immunologists of drawing Ehrlich-type geometric pictures to designate immunological specificites. (He may have remembered Gruber's distaste of such pictures, and Bordet's comment that these were "quite puerile graphical representations which . . . extended the deceptive use of explanations that are facile, but illusory.") What Landsteiner did publish to display his feelings about the nature of immunological specificity were data of the type illustrated in Table 5.1. It is almost as though Landsteiner saw in the diagonal sweep of + and ± cross-reactions all of the pictorialization that his concept required. For Landsteiner, each of these tables of cross-reactions represented a reconfirmation of his basic belief in how immunological specificity functions. Thus, he could say in the last edition of his famous monograph, *The Specificity of Serological Reactions,* substantially what he had said 25 years earlier:

> The high specificity of many serum reactions led Ehrlich to the view that each antibody is sharply adjusted to one particular structure (receptor), and accordingly that overlapping reactions of antigen must depend upon the presence in each of them of identical substances or chemical groupings . . . From numerous observations on artificial conjugated antigens, however, this notion is seen to be inadmissible, and it is certain that antibodies react most strongly upon the homologous antigen, but also regularly with graded affinity, on chemically related structures. Or, as Haldane wrote regarding an enzyme reaction, "The key does not fit the lock quite perfectly, but exercises a certain strain upon it."[93]

Even though the preceding discussion of Landsteiner's views on the nature of immunological specificity implies a consistency of concept based upon an untroubled consistency in his experimental results, such consistency was true only for Landsteiner's work with the precipitin reaction. Indeed, throughout his career, Landsteiner was beset by a paradox that he was never able fully and satisfactorily to resolve. On the one hand, all of his work on the precipitin reaction with naturally occurring proteins and hapten-substituted antigens suggested extensive

Table 5.1: **Serological Cross Reactions of a Homologous Series of Anilic Acids**

Antigen[a]	Reactions with antisera raised against			
	p-Aminooxanilic	p-Aminosuccinanilic	p-Aminoadipanilic	p-Aminosuberanilic
p-Aminooxanilic (n-0)	+++	0	0	0
p-Aminomalonanilic (n=1)	0	±	0	0
p-Aminosuccinanilic (n=2)	0	+++	+±	+
p-Aminoglutaranilic (n=3)	0	+	++	++
p-Aminoadipanilic (n=4)	0	0	++++	+++
p-Aminopimelanilic (n=5)	0	0	+++	++++
p-Aminosuberanilic (n=6)	0	0	++	++++

Source: After K. Landsteiner and J. van der Scheer, *J. Exp. Med.* **59**, 751 (1934).
[a] The general formula for aminoanilic acids is $NH_2\text{-}C_6H_4\text{-}NH\text{-}CO\text{-}(CH_2)n\text{-}COOH$.

cross-reactions and spectra of graded affinities of antibody for proteins of related species or for haptens of related structure. In contrast, however, all of his work with hemagglutination, starting with the isoagglutinins of the ABO system and later with the M, N, and P antigens and the Rh blood groups, seems to show absolute specificities and few cross-reactions. It was his work on horse–donkey interspecies hybrids[94] that perhaps best pointed up this paradox. Here, even though antibodies against the serum proteins might show extensive cross-reactions between these related species using the precipitin test, agglutinating antibodies could distinguish clearly between the erythrocytes of these closely related species, wherein discrete inherited antigens seemed able to stimulate discrete antibodies more in line with Ehrlich's than with Gruber's concepts.

The lack of accord between the results obtained with agglutination reactions and isoagglutinins and those observed in precipitin tests led Landsteiner and van der Scheer to do a special comparative study.[95] On the basis of this study, they concluded that there must be a difference in the specificities of these two reactions, a conclusion suggesting "an essential difference in the chemical structures which determine the specificity of the two kinds of antigens (precipitinogens and agglutinogens)." This, for Landsteiner, must have been a disappointingly inconclusive result, but it was all that could be said at the time. He attempted to circumvent this inconsistency by pointing out that most of the cell antigens thus far identified (the heterogenetic antigen of Forssman and the pneumococcal polysaccharides of Heidelberger and Avery) were nonprotein haptens. Landsteiner therefore concluded that "there exist two systems of species specificity in the animal kingdom, the specificity of proteins and that of cell haptens. The proteins, it would seem, undergo gradual variation in the course of evolution, while haptens are subject to sudden changes not linked by intermediate stages".[96] Thus, the paradox remained, but did not cause Landsteiner to modify his earlier statement that Ehrlich's view of an antibody sharply adjusted to one particular structure "is seen to be inadmissible."

Specificity and Theories of Antibody Formation

The term *Antikörper*, as it was first coined to describe the agent in the blood that von Behring and Kitasato had shown capable of passively transferring immunity, was originally a noncommittal term. It only implied a recognition that there must exist a discrete entity, or *body*, capable of carrying immunological specificity and thus able to act against (*anti*) the offending toxin. But if a discrete physical entity rather than some vague physiological process were held responsible for acquired immunity, then the nature and manner of formation of such a substance would furnish a valid topic for speculation. While the many theories of antibody formation have been dealt with in detail in Chapter 4, their formulation has been so intimately tied to considerations of antibody specificity (and its corollary, the repertoire size of these specificities) that these theories deserve at least a brief summary in the present context. Indeed, I have already noted that the principal basis for the attack on Ehrlich's theory by Gruber, Bordet, and Landsteiner was precisely their claim that the antigen–antibody interaction was colloidal and thus nonspecific.

At the outset, the protein nature of antibodies was unknown; but even after this was established, no hints were yet available on the nature or mode of production in the body of *any* macromolecules.[97] Before it was appreciated that the repertoire of antibodies was very large, only considerations of immunological specificity drove theoreticians of antibody formation, and it appeared reasonable to Buchner that antigen itself carried the information for specificity, by somehow being incorporated into the antibody molecule in such a manner that it would thenceforth react specifically with other similar antigen molecules.[98] However, such a theory could not long survive the rapidly developing quantitative studies showing that much more antibody was formed than could be accounted for by the amount of antigen injected and that antibody formation, once started, would continue without further administration of antigen.[99]

These objections were dealt with effectively by Paul Ehrlich in 1897, in his side-chain theory of antibody formation. In this prototype of all subsequent natural selection theories, Ehrlich postulated that antibodies are naturally occurring cell products present as receptors on the cell surface, to be selected for specifically by an appropriate antigen. Such an antigen–receptor interaction would then lead to compensatory overproduction of these receptors, which would appear in the blood as circulating antibody. As I have already noted, Ehrlich postulated that the specificity of these antibody receptors was a function of certain stereochemical configurations whose complementarity with structures on the antigen permitted specific interaction. With this theory, Ehrlich dealt simultaneously with the origin of antibodies and with the basis of their specificity. He was, in 1897, untroubled by the problem of the size of the immunological repertoire, since the only antibodies then known were thought to be antitoxins directed against a limited number of human and animal pathogens. Within a very few years, however, the scope of immune reactions was so far extended that it became apparent that the size of the specificity repertoire was almost too great to allow their *natural* occurrence; consequently, the Ehrlich side-chain theory fell into disrepute.

Now specificity *and* repertoire size became the central issues in all theories of antibody formation, an approach reinforced by the changing character of the discipline from about 1910 onward. If the first decades in immunology may be called its Age of Bacteriology, then the period from the 1920s to 1950s may appropriately be termed its Age of Immunochemistry, thanks in part to the stimuli provided by Landsteiner's work on haptens and Heidelberger's work on the pneumococcal polysaccharides and quantitative immunochemistry.[100] Immunology in this period was dominated by chemical approaches and chemical thinking.[101] This hegemony meant inevitably that contemporary theories of antibody formation would have to explain the elegant specificity and extensive specificity repertoire of antibodies; they tended to neglect the more biological aspects of antibody formation, such as its persistence and its ability to undergo anamnestic boosting.

In the main, chemically oriented speculation about the nature of antibody formation sought to explain specificity and its large repertoire by means of instruction theories, wherein the antigen itself somehow transmitted the information for its specificity to a nascent globulin molecule. The most notable of the instruction theories called upon the antigen to act as a template upon which specific antibody might be formed, either by directing the formation of a unique amino acid sequence on the polypeptide chain[102] or by molding a preformed polypeptide chain into an appropriate tertiary configuration in which stereochemical specificity was incorporated.[103] Such direct template theories enjoyed a broad popularity at the time, since they appeared to present the only reasonable explanation for the large number of antibodies that Landsteiner had shown could be formed by the vertebrate host.

In contrast, the developing Age of Immunobiology in the late 1950s and 1960s, arising from observations in fields such as tissue transplantation, immunological tolerance, immunodeficiency diseases, and immunopathology caused a shift toward a more biological direction. The biologists pointed out that "chemical" theories failed to explain how antibody production could persist in the apparent absence of antigen or why a second exposure to antigen should result in an enhanced booster response. Moreover, they provided no explanation for the newer data, which suggested that repeated immunization produces changes in the *quality* of the antibody, in some instances sharpening the specificity and in others considerably broadening the potential for cross-reactions. The

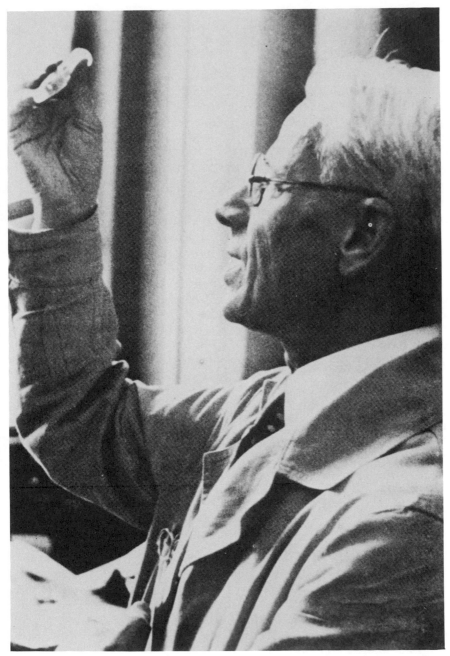
Michael Heidelberger (Courtesy University of Wisconsin Library)

demands upon a theory of antibody formation made by biologists now tended to emphasize exactly these and other biological phenomena, but in the process the structural–chemical aspects of specificity and the repertoire problem were neglected.

This substitution of biological considerations for chemical ones is well illustrated in the several theories that Macfarlane Burnet advanced to explain antibody formation. (Burnet was, at this time, almost unique in bringing a broad background in biology to bear upon questions of theoretical immunology.) In 1941, he proposed an instructionist alternative to the earlier theories,[104] namely, that the function of antigen was to stimulate an adaptive modification of those enzymes necessary for globulin synthesis. As a result of this modification, a unique protein molecule with the required specificity would be formed. But fashions in biology change fairly rapidly, and a decade later the concept of adaptive enzymes was somewhat out of style; now, protein formation was held to be encoded for in a "genome" of uncertain composition. Still impelled by essentially biological considerations, Burnet and Frank Fenner advanced an indirect template hypothesis;[105] in their model each antigen was able to impress the information for its specific determinant upon the (?RNA) genome, against which indirect template a specific antibody might be formed. Not only would this new genocopy persist within the cell, but it would be reproduced from mother to daughter cells during proliferation, thus explaining persisting antibody formation and the heightened booster response.

From the earliest days of the study of immunity, immunologists had been perplexed by finding "natural antibodies" in the serum of normal animals, often present in modest amounts in the absence of overt exposure to the various organisms and toxins with which they reacted. These could hardly be explained by any instruction theory that demanded the presence and even the persistence of antigen. For many decades, the specificity of these natural antibodies was questioned, their provenance mysterious, and their very existence neglected in the main by the proponents of instruction theories of antibody formation. However, in 1955, Niels Jerne focused attention upon these natural antibodies by assigning to them the central role in a "natural selection" theory of antibody formation.[106] Jerne proposed, as had Paul Ehrlich before him, that the host could in fact synthesize small amounts of all possible antibody specificities as part of its normal physiological processes. Jerne suggested that the function of antigen was merely to act as a "selective carrier" of natural antibody, transporting it to appropriate cells somewhere in the body, where it would signal the reproduction of molecules identical to those introduced, i.e., of specific antibody. Jerne's theory appeared to cope quite adequately with most of the biological aspects of antibody formation; it even included an explanation of the newly discovered phenomenon of immunological tolerance. It neglected entirely, however, any discussion of a chemical basis for antibody specificity or any consideration of the size of the antibody repertoire, which had doomed the similar Ehrlich side-chain theory some half-century earlier.

The historic importance of Jerne's theory lies in the fact that it appeared to provide for the first time a biological alternative to the instruction theories of the immunochemists and served as the stimulatory point of departure for biologically oriented theoreticians. The seed that Jerne had planted was not long in germinating, and within three years Burnet, Talmage, and Lederberg had given birth to the clonal selection theory of antibody formation.[107] Central to this concept was Jerne's (and Ehrlich's) postulate that antibodies are natural products; they appear on the cell surface as receptors with which antigen can interact; such interaction signals clonal proliferation of a population of cells phenotypically restricted for the given antibody specificity; and some daughter cells of the clone differentiate into antibody-forming cells while others remain as immunological memory cells, able to participate in an enhanced booster antibody response.

It is probably safe to say that the clonal selection theory took the increasingly biologically oriented world of immunology by storm, save for a few instructionist diehards who were unhappy with its failure to deal adequately with the structural basis of immunological specificity and with the repertoire problem. (Indeed, once the DNA control of antibody structure was accepted, clonal selection theory generated its own repertoire controversy, in a lengthy debate between those who maintained that the entire repertoire was encoded in the germ line and those who argued that immunological diversity was generated by somatic mutation or recombination of a highly restricted number of germ-line genes. I shall discuss this interesting debate more fully in the next Chapter.)

The clonal selection theory appeared to accord well with developments in the new genetics,[108] and especially with Francis Crick's "Central Dogma," which held that information could only pass from nucleic acids to protein and not in the reverse direction,[109] and with the demonstration that the tertiary structure of proteins is under precise genetic control.[110] Moreover, the newer techniques of fluorescent antibody immunohistochemistry[111] and of hemolytic plaque assays,[112] which permitted for the first time the study of single immunocytes in large populations of cells, provided rapid confirmation of the principal aspects of clonal selection theory.

NOTES AND REFERENCE

1. H. F. Judson, *The Eighth Day of Creation*. Simon & Schuster, New York, 1979. This book is the subject of a superb essay review by John T. Edsall [*J. Hist. Biol.* **13,** 141 (1980)], which also emphasizes the importance of the search for biological specificity.

2. The early work in this field is reviewed by R. R. Porter and E. M. Press, *Annu. Rev. Biochem.* **31,** 625 (1962); S. Cohen and C. Milstein, *Adv. Immunol.* **7,** 1 (1962).

3. Niels Jerne, in his typically perceptive discussion of the status of contemporary immunology entitled "Waiting for the End" [*Cold Spring Harbor Symp. Quant. Biol.* **32,** 591 (1967)], first pointed out clearly the schism between trans–immunologists (the molecular immunochemists) and cis–immunologists (the cellular immunobiologists), and their difficulty in communicating with one another.

4. Hieronymus Mercurialis, *De Morbis Puerorum*, Book I, pp. 17–21. Basel, 1584.

5. Girolamo Fracastoro, *De Contagione et Contagiosis Morbis et Eorum Curatione*, 1546 [W. C. Wright translation (with Latin text), Putnam, New York, 1930]. Fracastoro's theory of acquired immunity is discussed in detail in Chapter 1.

6. A. Castiglioni, *A History of Medicine*, p. 243. Knopf, New York, 1947.

7. A. Rhazes, *Treatise on the Small-Pox and Measles* (W. A. Greenhill, trans.). Sydenham Society, London, 1848.

8. Castiglioni, ref. 6, pp. 353 ff; pp. 452 ff.

9. W. Pagel, Paracelsus. *Dict. Sci. Biogr.* **10,** 304–313 (1974). See also Pagel's *Paracelsus. An Introduction to Philosophical Medicine in the Era of the Renaissance.* Karger, Basel, 1958. Pagel also gives a summary of von Helmont's contributions in *Dict. Sci. Biogr.* **6,** 253–259 (1972) and *Bull. Hist. Med.* **30,** 529 (1955).

10. D. G. Bates, Thomas Sydenham. *Dict. Sci. Biogr.* **13,** 213–215 (1976).

11. K. Faber, *Nosography: The Evolution of Clinical Medicine in Modern Times,* 2nd Ed., pp. 1–27. Hoeber, New York, 1930.

12. Faber, ref. 11, p. 16.

13. C. D. Leake, *A Historical Account of Pharmacology to the XX Century.* Thomas, Springfield, Illinois, 1975.

14. François Boissier de Sauvages, *Nosologia Methodica.* 1768.

15. J. Farley, *The Spontaneous Generation Controversy from Descartes to Oparin.* Johns Hopkins University Press, Baltimore, Maryland, 1974.

16. E. von Mayer, *A History of Chemistry* (G. McGowan, trans.). Macmillan, London, 1898. A briefer and more readable account is in H. M. Leicester, *The Historical Background of Chemistry.* Wiley, New York, 1956.

17. von Mayer, ref. 16, pp. 512 ff.

18. J. Fruton, *Molecules and Life: Historical Essays on the Interplay of Chemistry and Biology*, pp. 22–86. Wiley (Interscience), New York, 1972. See also H. M. Leicester, *Development of Biochemical Concepts from Ancient to Modern Times*, pp. 176–188. Harvard University Press, Cambridge, Massachusetts, 1974.

19. E. Fischer, *Ber. Dtsch. Chem. Ges.* **27**, 2992 (1894).

20. G. N. Lewis, The atom and the molecule. *J. Am. Chem. Soc.* **38**, 762 (1916).

21. L. Pauling, *The Nature of the Chemical Bond*, 2nd Ed. Cornell University Press, Ithaca, New York, 1944.

22. J. R. Partington, *A History of Chemistry*, Vol. IV, pp. 729 ff. Macmillan, New York, 1965. See also P. M. H. Mazumdar, *Karl Landsteiner and the Problem of Species, 1838–1968* (thesis), Vol. 2, pp. 379–419. Johns Hopkins Press, Baltimore, Maryland, 1976. Pauli's book of essays [*Physical Chemistry in the Service of Medicine* (M. H. Fischer, trans.). Wiley, New York, 1907] intimately connects the colloidal state with life processes.

23. Fruton, ref. 18, pp. 87–179.

24. E. Mayr and W. B. Provine, eds., *The Evolutionary Synthesis: Perspectives on the Unification of Biology*. Harvard University Press, Cambridge, Massachusetts, 1980.

25. G. W. Leibnitz, Nouveaux essais sur l'entendement. In *Die philosophischen Schriften von Gottfried Wilhelm Leibnitz* (C. J. Gerhardt, ed.), Vol. 5, p. 49. Wiedmann, Berlin, 1882.

26. I. Kant, *Critique of Pure Reason* (N. K. Smith, trans.), pp. 540 ff. Macmillan, New York, 1965.

27. Mazumdar, ref. 22.

28. P. Ehrlich, *The Collected Papers of Paul Ehrlich*, Vol. 1, pp. 65–94. Pergamon, Oxford, 1956.

29. M. Marquardt, *Paul Ehrlich*. Schuman, New York, 1957.

30. P. Ehrlich, Die Wertbemessung des Diphtherieheilserums. *Klin. Jahrb.* **60**, 299 (1897). [English translation in *Collected Papers*, Vol. 2, pp. 107–125.]

31. For recent treatments of Ehrlich's toxin–antitoxin work, see P. M. H. Mazumdar, The antigen–antibody reaction and the physics and chemistry of life. *Bull. Hist. Med.* **48**, 1 (1974). See also L. P. Rubin, *J. Hist. Med.* **35**, 397 (1980).

32. E. Metchnikoff, *Immunity in the Infectious Diseases*, 1905. [Johnson Reprint, New York, 1968.]

33. The battle over the phagocytic theory is detailed in Chapter 3.

34. E. von Behring and S. Kitasato, *Dtsch. Med. Wochenschr.* **16**, 113 (1890). See also E. von Behring and E. Wernicke, *Z. Hyg. Infektionskr.* **12**, 10, 45 (1892).

35. In addition to diphtheria and tetanus antitoxins, Ehrlich himself had shown that antibodies could be formed against the plant toxins ricin and abrin [P. Ehrlich, *Dtsch. Med. Wochenschr.* **17**, 976, 1218 (1890)].

36. M. von Gruber and H. E. Durham, *Muench. Med. Wochenschr.* **43**, 285 (1896).

37. R. Kraus, *Wien. Klin. Wochenschr.* **10**, 736 (1897).

38. J. Bordet, *Ann. Inst. Pasteur, Paris* **12**, 688 (1899).

39. Ehrlich's concept of distinct domains on the antibody molecule would

find striking confirmation three-quarters century later in the work of G. M. Edelman, *Biochemistry* **9**, 3197 (1970).

40. H. J. Müller-Eberhard, *Adv. Immunol.* **8**, 1 (1968).

41. P. Ehrlich, Croonian Lecture—on Immunity . . . *Proc. R. Soc. London* **66**, 424 (1900). This is also the clearest exposition of his side-chain theory.

42. J. Bordet, *Traité de l'immunité dans les maladies infectieuses*, p. 504. Masson, Paris, 1920.

43. See, e.g., L. Aschoff, *Ehrlichs Seitenkettentheorie und ihre Anwendung auf die künstlichen Immunisierungsprozesse.* Fischer, Jena, 1902; P. Römer, *Die Ehrlichsche Seitenkettentheorie und ihre Bedeutung für die medizinischen Wissenschaften.* Hölder, Vienna, 1904.

44. See, e.g., J. Parascandola and R. Jasensky, *Bull. Hist. Med.* **48**, 199 (1974). J. Parascandola's paper on The theoretical basis of Paul Ehrlich's chemotherapy [(*J. Hist. Med.* **36**, 19 (1981)] is especially interesting in this regard.

45. The L$_0$ (*limes* = threshold) dose of toxin would just neutralize 1 unit of antitoxin, whereas the L$_+$ (*limes* death) dose would leave 1 lethal dose free, in the presence of 1 unit of antitoxin. Thus, L$_+$ minus L$_0$ should equal 1 minimum lethal dose (MLD), but in fact might equal 40–60 MLDs or more.

46. P. Ehrlich, *Berl. Klin. Wochenschr.* **40**, 793, 825, 848 (1903). Ehrlich's toxin spectra were elaborated upon by T. Madsen [*Z. Hyg. Infektionskr.* **32**, 214 (1899)], and figured significantly in every comprehensive text on immunology and microbiology for the next 30 years.

47. J. Danysz, *Ann. Inst. Pasteur, Paris* **16**, 331 (1902). Jules Bordet had earlier reported a similar observation on immune hemolysis [*Ann. Inst. Pasteur, Paris* **14**, 257 (1900)].

48. E. von Dungern, *Dtsch. Med. Wochenschr.* **30**, 275, 310 (1904).

49. P. Ehrlich and J. Morgenroth, *Berl. Klin. Wochenschr.* **38**, 569 (1901). [English translation in P. Ehrlich, *Collected Studies in Immunity*, p. 88. Wiley, New York, 1906.]

50. P. Ehrlich and H. Sachs, *Berl. Klin. Wochenschr.* **39**, 297, 335 (1902).

51. Jules Bordet's side of this argument is well summarized in a resumé chapter of his book *Studies in Immunity* [(F. Gay, trans.), pp. 496 ff. Wiley, New York, 1909], and in his famous book *Traité de l'immunité dans les maladies infectieuses* (ref. 42), written while Bordet was isolated in Belgium by the war.

52. Mazumdar (ref. 22) discusses at length the importance attributed at that time to colloidal interactions and the almost mystical role assigned to them in biological processes.

53. Bordet, ref. 42, p. 546.

54. Bordet, ref. 42, pp. vi ff. Bordet's use of the epithet "chauvinism" against his German colleagues is not surprising. I have commented in Chapter 3 on the influences of Franco-German enmity on immunological disputes. See also Rubin, ref. 31.

55. See, e.g., J. Parascandola, *Pharm. Hist.* **16**, 54 (1974); R. E. Kohler, *J. Hist. Biol.* **8**, 275 (1975); Fruton, ref. 18.

56. S. Arrhenius and T. Madsen, Physical chemistry as applied to toxins and

antitoxins. In *Festskrift ved Indvielsen af Statens Serum Institut* (C. J. Salomonson, ed.). Copenhagen, 1902.

57. S. Arrhenius, *Immunochemistry*. Macmillan, New York, 1907.

58. See, e.g., M. Neisser, *Zentralbl. Bakteriol. Parasitenkd.* **36**(1), 671 (1904). Rubin (ref. 31) provides an interesting discussion of the substantive and stylistic differences between Ehrlich and Arrhenius and touches on the broader debate between "physical chemists" and "biologists," an issue that Ehrlich himself addressed in his second Herter Lecture at Johns Hopkins in 1904 (*Collected Papers*, Vol. II, p. 414). In this lecture, curiously, he defended biology from the physical chemist Arrhenius, whereas earlier he had attacked the "biologist" Bordet from a chemical position.

59. See, e.g., the several papers on antitissue antibodies (cytotoxins) in *Ann. Inst. Pasteur, Paris* **14** (1900).

60. An encyclopedic four-volume review of the entire field of allergy, with much historical background, will be found in H. Schadewaldt, *Geschichte der Allergie*. Dustri, Munich-Deisenhofen, 1979.

61. P. Portier and C. Richet, *C. R. Seances Soc. Biol. Ses Fil.* **54**, 170 (1902).

62. M. Arthus, *C. R. Seances Soc. Biol. Ses Fil.* **55**, 817 (1903).

63. C. von Pirquet and B. Schick, *Die Serumkrankheit*. Leipzig, 1905. [English translation: *Serum Sickness*. Williams & Wilkins, Baltimore, Maryland 1951.]

64. R. Koch, *Dtsch. Med. Wochenschr.* **17**, 101 (1891).

65. G. H. F. Nuttall, *Blood Immunity and Blood Relationship*. Cambridge University Press, Cambridge, England, 1904.

66. M. von Gruber and C. von Pirquet, *Muench. Med. Wochenschr.* **50**, 1193 (1903).

67. P. Ehrlich, *Meunch. Med. Wochenschr.* **50**, 2295 (1903). [English translation in Ehrlich's *Collected Studies on Immunity* (C. Bolduan, trans.), pp. 514 ff. Wiley, New York, 1906.]

68. M. von Gruber, *Wien. Klin. Wochenschr.* **16**, 791 (1903).

69. Reference 67, *Collected Studies*, p. 525.

70. Reference 67, *Collected Studies*, p. viii.

71. M. von Gruber, *Muench. Med. Wochenschr.* **48**, 1214 (1901). See also L. Hopf, *Immunität und Immunisierung*, p. 89. Pietzker, Tübingen, 1902. Hans Buchner had also raised this perplexing question earlier [(*Muench. Med. Wochenschr.* **47**, 277 (1900)].

72. J. Bordet, *Studies in Immunity* (F. Gay, trans.). Wiley, New York, 1909.

73. For further information on Landsteiner and his work, see E. Lesky, *The Vienna Medical School in the 19th Century*. Johns Hopkins University Press, Baltimore, Maryland, 1976; P. Speiser, *Dict. Sci. Biogr.* **7**, 622 (1973); Mazumdar, ref. 22; P. M. H. Mazumdar, *J. Hist. Biol.* **8**, 115 (1975); P. Speiser and F. G. Smekal, *Karl Landsteiner: The Discoverer of Blood Groups and a Pioneer in the Field of Immunology* (R. Rickett, trans.). Brüder Hollinek, Vienna, 1975.

74. K. Landsteiner, *Centralbl. Bakteriol. Orig.* **27**, 357 (1900); *Wien. Klin. Wochenschr.* **14**, 1132 (1901).

75. K. Landsteiner and P. Levine, *Proc. Soc. Exp. Biol. Med.* **24**, 600, 941 (1926).

76. K. Landsteiner and A. S. Wiener, *Proc. Soc. Exp. Biol. Med.* **43,** 223 (1940).

77. E. Finger and K. Landsteiner, *Arch. Dermatol. Syph.* **78,** 335 (1906).

78. K. Landsteiner and C. Levaditi, *C. R. Seances Soc. Biol. Ses Fil.* **67,** 592, 789 (1909).

79. J. Donath and K. Landsteiner, *Muench. Med. Wochenschr.* **51,** 1590 (1904).

80. K. Landsteiner, R. Müller, and O. Potzl, *Wien. Klin. Wochenschr.* **20,** 1565 (1907).

81. K. Landsteiner and E. Popper, *Z. Immunitaetsforsch.* **2,** 377 (1909).

82. K. Landsteiner and M. W. Chase, *Proc. Soc. Exp. Biol. Med.* **49,** 688 (1942).

83. K. Landsteiner, *The Specificity of Serological Reactions.* Dover, New York, 1962. [A reprint of the 2nd edition (1945) with a complete bibliography. The original German version, *Die Spezifizität der serologischen Reaktionen,* was published by Springer, Berlin, 1933.]

84. M. W. Chase, personal communication, cited in G. W. Corner, *A History of the Rockefeller Institute,* p. 205. Rockefeller Institute Press, New York, 1964; also in Speiser and Smekal, ref. 73.

85. Lesky, ref. 73.

86. K. Landsteiner, *Wien. Klin. Wochenschr.* **10,** 439 (1897).

87. K. Landsteiner and N. Jagič, *Muench. Med. Wochenschr.* **50,** 764 (1903).

88. E. P. Pick, in *Handbuch der pathogenen Mikroorganismen* (W. Kolle and A. von Wassermann, eds.), 2nd Ed., Vol. 1, pp. 685–868. Fischer, Jena, 1912.

89. F. Obermayer and E. P. Pick, *Wien. Klin. Wochenschr.* **19,** 327 (1906).

90. K. Landsteiner and H. Lampl, *Z. Immunitaetsforsch.* **26,** 258, 293 (1917).

91. K. Landsteiner and H. Lampl, *Biochem. Z.* **86,** 343 (1918).

92. Lesky's book on the Vienna Medical School (ref. 73), while concentrating on its nineteenth century greatness, shows also how it and intellectual Vienna in general declined following the War.

93. Reference 83, p. 266.

94. K. Landsteiner and J. van der Scheer, *Proc. Soc. Exp. Biol. Med.* **21,** 252 (1924); *J. Immunol.* **9,** 213, 221 (1924).

95. K. Landsteiner and J. van der Scheer, *J. Exp. Med.* **40,** 91 (1924).

96. Reference 83, p. 76. See also Landsteiner's presidential address before the American Association of Immunologists [*J. Immunol.* **15,** 589 (1928)].

97. Fruton, ref. 18, pp. 87–179.

98. H. Buchner, *Muench. Med. Wochenschr.* **40,** 449 (1893).

99. See, e.g., E. Roux and L. Vaillard, *Ann. Inst. Pasteur, Paris* **7,** 65 (1893); A. Knorr, *Muench. Med. Wochenschr.* **45,** 321, 362 (1898).

100. Heidelberger's important contributions are perhaps best summarized in the landmark book by his students: E. A. Kabat and M. M. Mayer, *Quantitative Immunochemistry,* 2nd Ed. Thomas, Springfield, Illinois, 1961.

101. The titles of the leading *basic science* books in immunology testify that it was indeed an Age of Immunochemistry. See H. G. Wells, *The Chemical Aspects of Immunity.* Chem. Catalog Co., New York, 1924; J. R. Marrack, *The Chemistry of Antigens and Antibodies.* HM Stationery Off., London, 1934; E. A. Kabat and M. M. Mayer, *Quantitative Immunochemistry* (see ref. 100, 1st Ed., 1949); W. C. Boyd, *Introduction to Immunochemical Specificity.* Wiley (Interscience), New York,

1962; E. A. Kabat, *Structural Concepts in Immunology and Immunochemistry*. Holt, Rinehart & Winston, New York, 1968; D. Pressman and A. Grossberg, *The Structural Basis of Antibody Specificity*. Benjamin, New York, 1968. The leading textbook in the field [W. C. Boyd, *Fundamentals of Immunology*. Wiley (Interscience), New York, 1943] was quite chemically oriented, and was only replaced in 1963 by a text aimed at biologists [J. H. Humphrey and R. G. White, *Immunology for Students of Medicine*. Davis, Philadelphia, Pennsylvania, 1963].

102. F. Breinl and F. Haurowitz, *Z. Physiol. Chem.* **192,** 45 (1930); J. Alexander, *Protoplasma* **14,** 296 (1931); S. Mudd, *J. Immunol.* **23,** 423 (1932).

103. L. Pauling, *J. Am. Chem. Soc.* **62,** 2643 (1940).

104. The biologists' arguments against chemical template theories are best summarized in F. M. Burnet, *The Production of Antibodies*. Macmillan, New York, 1941.

105. F. M. Burnet and F. Fenner, *The Production of Antibodies*, 2nd Ed. Macmillan, New York, 1949.

106. N. K. Jerne, *Proc. Natl. Acad. Sci. USA* **41,** 849 (1955).

107. A clonal selection theory was first hinted at by D. W. Talmadge, *Annu. Rev. Med.* **8,** 239, 247 (1957); outlined by F. M. Burnet, *Aust. J. Sci.* **20,** 67 (1957); fleshed out in detail by F. M. Burnet, *The Clonal Selection Theory of Acquired Immunity*. Cambridge Univ. Press, London, 1959; D. W. Talmadge, *Science* **129,** 1643 (1959); J. Lederberg, *Science* **129,** 1649 (1959).

108. Highly readable accounts may be found in R. Olby, *The Path to the Double Helix*. University of Washington Press, Seattle, 1974; Judson, ref. 1.

109. F. H. Crick, *Symp. Soc. Exp. Biol.* **12,** 138 (1958). See also F. H. Crick, *Nature (London)* **227,** 561 (1970).

110. C. J. Epstein, R. F. Goldberger, and C. B. Anfinsen, *Cold Spring Harbor Symp. Quant. Biol.* **28,** 439 (1963).

111. A. H. Coons, E. H. Leduc, and J. M. Connolly, *J. Exp. Med.* **102,** 49 (1955).

112. N. K. Jerne and A. A. Nordin, *Science* **140,** 405 (1963).

6

Immunological Specificity, Continued

I T WAS evident by the early 1930s that if Paul Ehrlich's biological theory of antibody formation was out of favor, his chemical concept of the basis for antibody specificity was very much in vogue.[1] The very data (primarily Landsteiner's work with synthetic haptens) that had made the antibody repertoire appear too large to be explicable in terms of naturally occurring antibodies almost demanded an immunological specificity based upon a very precise stereochemical complementarity of configuration between antigen and the putative combining site of antibody. Indeed, as I have noted, such a precise structural "fit" between antigen and antibody was explicitly required by most instructionist theories of antibody formation, each of which postulated the existence of some form of template upon which specific configuration might be molded.[2] But the work of Landsteiner on artificial haptens and of Heidelberger and co-workers on polysaccharide antigens accomplished more than this; they signaled to a generation of immunologists that progress in understanding the functions of antibody and the nature of its specificity would only come from chemical approaches to the problem. Nor did biologically oriented immunologists have much to offer at this time in competition with the new trend. Their startling and attractive advances in antitoxic and antibacterial immunity and in novel techniques of serodiagnosis and serotaxonomy and their important contributions to forensic medicine were mostly a generation in the past, and the discovery of immunological tolerance and deficiency diseases, of transplantation immunobiology, and of cellular functions in the immune response would only come with the new biology of a future generation. The occasional development of a new vaccine or the finding of a new blood group thus had little effect upon the growing influence of immunochemistry within the larger field of immunology between about 1920 and 1960.[3]

The introduction of more chemical approaches to immunology—of quantitative methods and studies of the fine structure of antigens and antibodies—had profound implications for the science of immunology. Not only did it reorient the research goals of a generation of scientists, it also led to the production of impressive amounts of "hard" data that altered the very direction of immunological conceptualization. It is typical of the development of a science that in its infancy, conceptual advances are often based primarily upon philosophical viewpoints, given the scarcity and uncertainty of the facts at hand. As the science matures, hypotheses tend to depend less upon the world view of the scientist and more upon the imperatives contained within the growing body of evidence itself. This phenomenon has been no less true of the development of the concept of immunological specificity than in other fields of biology, a source of potential hazard to the chronicler who attempts to trace the history of an idea through the entire time span.

If the earlier period lends itself to more philosophical approaches and furnishes interesting accounts of often vitriolic debates (which the times and the journals then permitted), modern developments tend to make for a drier and more factual presentation. Not only are there more facts to deal with, but the very training and background of the scientist himself becomes an important factor. During the last half of the nineteenth century, the scientist was more likely to have had a classical education that predisposed him to a broad philosophical approach to his discipline, and he could hope to comprehend his own as well as other related disciplines. In the mid-twentieth century, education for a more complex science is often at the expense of the humanities, and the scientist finds it difficult to encompass even his own subspeciality. The gap between C. P. Snow's "Two Cultures" is thus reflected not only in the relationship between science and society, but to a degree also in the "generation gap" that develops within the science itself.

The Structural Basis for Immunological Specificity

By the 1930s, it was known that antibodies were protein in nature, that they belonged to the class of proteins termed globulins, and that antibody activity could be found variously in both the euglobulin and pseudoglobulin classes, as defined by solubility in water and ammonium sulfate solutions. But apart from the knowledge that proteins were composed of chains of apparently randomly arranged amino acids and of indeterminate length, little was known of the protein molecule.[4] A theory had been advanced that the precipitation of antigen and antibody was attained by means of a molecular lattice,[5] a model that implied at least bivalency of the antibody; other than this, the nature of antibody structure and specificity was as little known as that of enzymes. Any approach to the definition of the antibody specific combining site would thus of necessity have to rely upon chemical studies of the antigenic determinants with which they interacted.

APPROACHES TO SPECIFICITY VIA THE ANTIGEN MOLECULE

In his studies of the serological cross-reactions among homologous series of structurally related haptens,[6] Karl Landsteiner provided a powerful tool that permitted the size and shape of the specific site on antibody to be estimated. His demonstration that the precipitation of anti-hapten antibodies by hapten–protein conjugates might be inhibited by free hapten[7] was further seized upon as a means of estimating the thermodynamic characteristics of the antigen–antibody interaction, and these predominantly physicochemical approaches provided a wealth of new, if indirect, information on the structure and function of the specific combining site of antibody.

The Shape of the Specific Antibody Site. The strength of this new approach to the definition of antibody specificity was most forcefully provided by the studies of Linus Pauling and his scientific descendants. By combining quantitative hapten-inhibition studies with the newer knowledge of atomic size and of the orientation of interatomic bonds within and between molecules, Pauling and his students (most notably David Pressman) were able to define precisely, in terms of their van der Waals radii, the configuration of various haptens and therefore by inference the configuration of the "pockets" in the specific antibody site into which they fit. Such studies served also to provide a measure of the varying contributions to the antigen–antibody interaction of ionic interactions, of hydrogen bonding, and of van der Waals forces. These studies are summarized *in extenso* in Pressman and Grossberg's book, *The Structural Basis of Antibody Specificity;*[8] even the difference in size between a chlorine and a bromine atom on a benzene ring influences the binding affinities of haptens, and the influence of the water of hydration of a hapten molecule in solution can be measured.

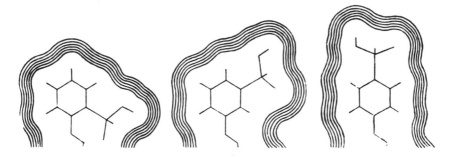

Fig. 6.1. Scale drawing of the antibody cavities specific for *ortho-*, *meta-*, and *para*-azophenylarsonic acid groups. (From Pauling and Pressman, ref. 9.)

As more information became available on the correspondence between the three-dimensional structure of haptens and their ability to combine with specific antibody, molecular diagrams of the type illustrated in Fig. 6.1[9] were drawn and eventually led to the suggestion by Hooker and Boyd and then by Pauling that these structures in fact define a cavity in the globulin molecule into which the hapten might fit more or less tightly,[10] representing thus an interaction of greater or lesser affinity. More careful measurements appeared to show, however, that antibody might not always react with the entire haptenic grouping, especially when the latter attained sizable proportions, an observation that led Pressman to suggest[11] that the cavity in the globulin molecule that determined antibody specificity might sometimes be an invagination, whereas in other instances it might be either a shallow trough or a slit trench, as illustrated in Fig. 6.2.[12]

Antibody Heterogeneity and Thermodynamics. Hapten inhibition studies of immune precipitation quickly confirmed what had long been known—that an immune serum to even a well-defined haptenic grouping was apparently composed of a fairly heterogeneous mixture of antibodies of different affinities. With the revival in the late 1940s by Eisen and Karush of the technique of equilibrium dialysis (involving direct measurements of hapten–antibody interactions free of the complications of secondary phenomena such as precipitation), these observations were elegantly extended and given a firm quantitative basis.[13] Now for the first time it was possible to obtain direct measurements of hapten–antibody interactions and to measure these interactions in absolute rather than relative terms. By assessing the degree of hapten binding at different free hapten concentrations and at different temperatures, measurements could now be made of the free energy of

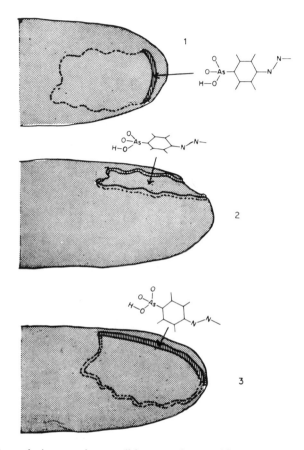

Fig. 6.2. Speculation on the possible ways the specific combining site might be arranged on the antibody molecule. (From Boyd, ref. 12.)

interaction of the hapten and antibody combining site and of the enthalpy and entropy changes associated with these interactions.[14] Only then was the remarkable range of antibody affinities first appreciated: some reacted only weakly with the antigen, with association constants of the order of 10^4 liters/mole, whereas other antibodies might react with their respective haptens with association constants of 10^8 to 10^{10} liters/mole or higher.

Equilibrium dialysis provided two additional types of information about antibodies that were invaluable. From the law of mass action, an appropriate plot of hapten binding data at different initial hapten concentrations should yield a straight-line isotherm. Any deviation of the curve from linearity is a measure of the heterogeneity of affinities in the antibody population measured, and thus it was possible for the first time to obtain a quantitative estimate of the heterogeneity of different antisera and thus of the range of specific affinities present in the mixture.[15] The second advantage of this type of data plot lay in the fact that extrapolation of the curve to the abscissa would give a precise estimate of the valence of the antibody molecule. Immunologists had argued for many years about whether the antibody molecule had only one combining site or many, some suggesting that parsimony of hypothesis did not require more than univalency. Indeed, one prominent immunologist suggested that the single antibody combining site on the globulin molecule was itself so much a miracle that it would be too much to insist upon two such miracles on the same molecule.[16] But equilibrium dialysis settled this question, because it showed that most antibodies were in fact divalent.

The growing notion that a specific antiserum might be composed of a mixture of many different antibodies with greater or lesser "fit," or affinity, for the antigenic structure against which they were formed had a further interesting implication for the concept of immunological specificity. This extension was pointed out most clearly by Talmage in 1959,[17] although in a somewhat different context—that of an attempt to explain away the apparently large size of the immunological repertoire, a subject to which I shall return later. Following an earlier suggestion by Landsteiner,[18] Talmage noted that if indeed the antibody response is degenerate and results in a mixture of antibodies of overlapping specificities and differing affinities for antigen, then such a heterogeneous mixture might appear to react more specifically and to discriminate more finely between related antigenic structures *than would any of its constituent antibodies.* An antigen might fit only partially into the combining site of any particular antibody present in relatively low concentrations but would be well recognized by the totality of all combining sites in a heterogeneous antiserum. By postulating that an antiserum might manifest different specificities depending only upon variations in the relative concentrations of a *limited* number of different specific antibodies, Talmage suggested that the requirement for an unlimited repertoire of antibodies was sharply reduced. In addition, this concept accorded well with the clonal selection theory, which implied the existence of a discrete and discontinuous set of more-or-less specific receptors in the immune response rather than a continuously changing spectrum of affinities such as Landsteiner, and Gruber before him, had suggested.[19]

The Size of the Antibody Combining Site. Numerous studies by Landsteiner and others had shown that a single terminal saccharide, a substituted benzene ring, or even a dipeptide might suffice to determine the specificity of an antibody combining site, and this appeared to set the lower limit on its size. But with the finding that the carrier molecules to which these "immunodominant" groups were attached might influence the antigen–antibody interaction, interest was focused on the maximum size that the antibody combining site might attain. An early and imaginative approach to this question was made by Landsteiner and van der Scheer,[20] who immunized animals with "two-headed haptens," synthesized by attaching symmetrically to a benzene ring two distinctive groupings [such as sym- aminoisophthalylglycine-phenylalanine, or (3-amino, 5-succinylaminobenzoyl)-p-aminophenylarsenic acid]. The antibodies formed against these large structures were invariably specific for one or the other of the two determinants on the molecule and never appeared large enough to encompass both. Using these results, Campbell and Bulman calculated that the specific combining site of an antibody could not be larger than 700 $Å^2$.[21]

A more detailed study of the size of the antibody combining site was made by Kabat.[22] This investigation took advantage of the ability to prepare antibodies against dextran, a molecule composed of long chains of $\alpha 1 \rightarrow 6$-linked glucose units, and of the availability of all of the oligosaccharides of glucose from the disaccharide isomaltose to the heptasaccharide isomaltoheptaose. By testing the ability of the various oligosaccharides to inhibit the precipitation of dextran by antidextran, it was possible to calculate that, whereas simple glucose might contribute about 40% to the total binding energy of the interaction, the addition of further saccharide residues contributed successively less to the interaction, until no further effect could be found beyond isomaltohexaose. These results appeared to set an upper limit on the determinant size of $34 \times 12 \times 7$ Å, if the unlikely assumptions were made that the molecule in solution interacted in its extended form. These findings were substantially confirmed by other investigators employing D-lysine oligopeptides; they found that oligomers beyond a chain length of five or six units made little or no additional contribution to the energy of interaction.[23]

APPROACHES TO SPECIFICITY VIA THE
ANTIBODY MOLECULE

Paul Ehrlich's suggestion in 1897 that immunological specificity is based upon a three-dimensional arrangement of atoms in the antibody molecule that permits a close complementarity to the antigen was a brilliant conceptual leap for his times. Indeed, the verification of his idea would have to wait more than a half-century for the development of appropriate technologies. As I have noted, progress in understanding the protein molecule was almost nonexistent prior to the Second World War, and only indirect information could be obtained about antibodies by studying antigens and haptens. But starting in the late 1930s and for a quarter- century thereafter, a series of technical innovations initiated an explosive burst of progress that permitted the structure of the antibody molecule and the location and nature of its combining sites to be worked out in the finest detail.

The initial steps in defining the antibody molecule were made possible by the development of ultracentrifugation by Svedberg and of electrophoresis by Tiselius, and especially by the subsequent modification of the latter technique to permit immunoelectrophoresis in gels.[24] By allowing antibodies to be separated by weight and by electrical charge, it was established that some antibodies had a molecular weight of about 160,000, whereas others (macroglobulins) had a molecular weight of almost 1 million. Again, some antibodies were found to migrate slowly in an electrical field in the γ region, whereas others migrate in the β- and even α-globulin regions. Most interesting was the observation that differences in biological function (fixation of complement, passage across the placenta, involvement in allergic disorders, etc.) might be correlated with these physical differences. What emerged most forcefully from these early studies was an appreciation of the fact that antibodies, unlike most other serum proteins, constituted a distinctly heterogeneous population of molecules, related in some way to their heterogeneity of specificities and/or to their heterogeneity of biological function.[25]

With the increasing ability to characterize different molecular species and especially with the use of antibody probes with which the *antigenic* character of antibody globulins could be tested, dissection of the immunoglobulin molecule (as it soon came to be known) could be undertaken. Two principal approaches were pursued and strongly complemented each other. The first used the finding that the immunoglobulin molecule can be selectively split by enzymes such as papain and trypsin,[26] and the second used the finding that reductive cleavage of disulfide bonds of the immunoglobulin molecule would lead to a different set of digestion products.[27] Edelman and Poulik[28] then showed that immunoglobulins were composed of two polypeptide chains with molecular weights of 20,000 and about 50,000 [later termed the light (L) and heavy (H) chains]. The chain data and enzyme cleavage results allowed Porter to suggest a structure of the immunoglobulin molecule[29]

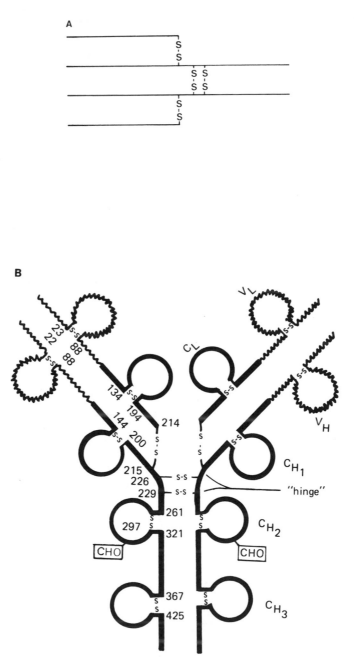

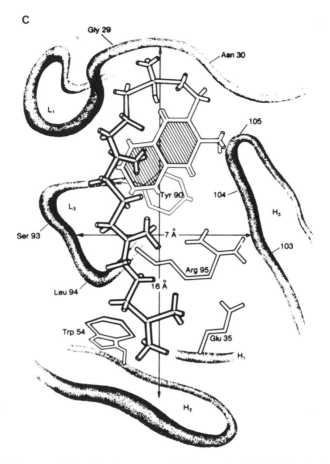

Fig. 6.3. Various models of the immunoglobulin molecule. (A) The 4-chain stick model of Porter in 1963. (From ref. 29.) (B) The heavy- and light-chain domains of Edelman in 1970. (From ref. 30.) (C) The three-dimensional cavity specific for vitamin K, formed of L- and H-chain segments. (From Poljak *et al.*, 1974, ref. 35.)

as illustrated in Fig. 6.3A, and it was now evident that the specific antibody combining site must somehow be formed of portions of both the H and L chains. In addition, it soon became clear that it was a portion of the heavy chain that defined the secondary biological functions of different immunoglobulin classes, a finding that was formalized by Edelman[30] (Fig. 6.3B) in his description of the immunoglobulin molecule as a combination of subunit chains with a set of different functional domains (thus validating Ehrlich's speculation of some 70 years earlier).

All of these structural studies were aided immeasurably by the growing appreciation that the abnormal proteins present in the serum of multiple myeloma patients were fairly homogeneous populations of immunoglobulin molecules[31] and that the Bence-Jones proteins found in the urine of such patients were in fact free immunoglobulin light chains.[32] On the basis of studies of this type, it was finally possible to define a set of immunoglobulin classes (isotypes) and subclasses that depend upon the presence of distinctive heavy chains, each with somewhat different biological properties: immunoglobulin G (IgG), composed of two γ heavy chains and two κ or λ light chains with a molecular formula $H_{\gamma2}L_2$; the pentameric macroglobulin IgM with μ heavy chains; IgA (mono- or dimeric), involved in the secretory immune system, with α heavy chains; IgE, involved in allergic disease, with ϵ heavy chains; and IgD, currently assumed to function as a lymphocyte membrane receptor, utilizing δ heavy chains.

With the increasing ability to split the light and heavy chains of immunoglobulins with a variety of enzymes and with the development of improved techniques to fractionate and establish the amino acid sequences of these fragments, it was finally possible to work out the complete primary structure of an entire immunoglobulin molecule, for which Edelman and Porter shared the Nobel prize in 1972.

The ability to establish the primary amino acid sequence of immunoglobulin molecules did not of itself establish the location or structure of the specific binding site on the molecule, because secondary and tertiary configuration could not be directly inferred from primary structure. But such studies did open the way for a solution to this problem, along two interesting and complementary lines. The first of these derived from the new ability to compare the amino acid sequences of heavy and light chains from antibodies with different specificities and from different species. Not only were there homologies between light and heavy chains and among different segments of both light and heavy chains, a finding suggesting an evolution through gene duplication,[33] but also the amino-terminal segments of both light and heavy chains showed impressive variations in amino acid sequence, especially in certain "hypervariable" regions. The carboxy-terminal portions of these chains, however, were much more constant in composition. A comparison of the sequences of many immunoglobulin chains permitted Wu and Kabat[34] to identify the precise locations of these hypervariable regions and to suggest that these portions of the immunoglobulin chains were most likely to be involved in defining the specific combining site on the antibody molecule. It remained for high-resolution X-ray crystallographic studies to establish the three-dimensional structure of the antibody molecule, to provide a physical picture of the combining site itself, and to confirm that it was in fact a sort of pocket formed by heavy and light chain hypervariable regions, into which the antigen determinant might fit with greater or lesser precision[35] (Fig. 6.3C).

At long last, immunological specificity had been provided with a firm structural basis. But if a unique organization of amino acid sequences with a special spatial configuration were sufficient to determine an antibody binding site, it should also constitute an equally unique *antigenic* determinant on the immunoglobulin molecule; this property was soon confirmed and called an idiotype.[36] It has been possible to obtain antibodies specific for these special structures, whose use has contributed importantly to the analysis of immunologic specificities, and to a clarification of some of the mechanisms that may modulate the immune response.[37]

Specificity in Cellular Immunity

When Elie Metchnikoff introduced the notion of cellular immunity to infection in the 1880s and when he defended and extended his theory over the next 30 years,[38] he identified macrophages (wandering monocytes and sessile histiocytes) and microphages (polymorphonuclear leukocytes) as the mediators of this protection. But Metchnikoff never really addressed in detail the question of the specificity of the phagocytes involved in protective immunity. This omission may have been due in part to his preoccupation with "natural immunity," where discrete specificity was not absolutely demanded. In his first comprehensive review of the subject, he speaks of the "sensitivity" of phagocytes to chemotactic factors released by pathogens and foreign bodies, a sensitivity that leads to enhanced diapedesis and the engulfing and intracellular enzymatic destruction of pathogens. The hallmark of *acquired* immunity, however, is specificity, and Metchnikoff had to concede that immunization might increase the sensitivity of phagocytes (by a mechanism unknown), thus enhancing diapedesis, immigration, and phagocytosis.[39]

When he wrote his famous *Immunity in the Infectious Diseases* in 1901,[40] Metchnikoff was forced to deal with the increasing evidence that not only did the finding of circulating antibody support the opposing theory of humoral immunity, but that these antibodies were themselves highly specific. To counter opposition to this theory, he suggested that these antibodies were in fact merely "stimulins," serving to increase the sensitivity of phagocytes to foreign bacteria. Quoting his student Mesnil, he pointed out that "the effect of the [immune] serum is to stimulate the phagocyte . . . they ingest more quickly, they digest more quickly. The serum is, therefore, a stimulant of the cells charged with the defense of the animal."[41] Elsewhere, Metchnikoff hinted at a specificity of the phagocyte and spoke of the immunized animals as possessing "leukocytes, impressed with a special sensitiveness"[42] but he did not elaborate on this. But even though Metchnikoff generally begged the question of phagocyte specificity in his writings, his theory of cellular immunity based upon phagocytic function imposed on the phagocyte an implicit requirement for specificity; and the "specific phagocyte" would be a recurrent theme in any discussion of cellular immunity for the next 75 years.

For a time, it appeared that the question had been settled by the suggestion that circulating antibody might function as an opsonin (Gr. *opsonein,* to render palatable). According to the opsonic theory, antibodies were thought to coat the pathogen specifically, thus rendering it more susceptible to phagocytic action. This idea was based upon an observation by Denis and Leclef in 1895,[43] who found that the destruction of bacteria by phagocytosis was substantially increased by the addition of specific immune serum. These observations provided the basis for an extensive series of investigations by Wright and Douglas,[44] who sought to mediate the dispute between the cellular and humoral theories of immunity by showing that humoral antibody and phagocytic cells might *collaborate* in combating infectious disease. Indeed, the opsonic theory was broadly accepted for several decades and appeared to explain quite satisfactorily the mechanism of acquired immunity in a number of infectious disease processes. But evidence slowly mounted that certain diseases, most notably tuberculosis, were not so readily explained.

From the very outset, macrophages had been observed to play an important role in the granulomatous inflammation associated with tubercle formation and with the Koch phenomenon and to contribute importantly to the inflammatory infiltrate associated with positive tuberculin tests. However, it soon became clear that there was little or no correlation between circulating levels of anti-tubercle antibodies and immunity to this disease.[45] Moreover, immunity could not be passively transferred with serum antibody. So the intimate collaboration of opsonins and phagocytes in tuberculosis and many other significant diseases appeared questionable, and belief in a "knowledgable" and specific macrophage was revived.

The concept of the immune macrophage was supported by extensive studies by Lurie in the 1930s and 1940s.[46] These studies purported to show with "purified" macrophage preparations that those from immune animals killed or inhibited the growth of tubercle bacilli better than those from normal donors. These findings received additional support from many investigators,[47] although some continued to insist that the protective function of these phagocytic cells was essentially nonspecific in nature.[48] One of the most suggestive observations supporting the notion of the immune macrophage was that of Rich and Lewis,[49] who showed that the normal migration of macrophages from *in vitro* explants of bits of spleen from tuberculous animals could be specifically inhibited by tuberculin.

It was first assumed that the macrophages were directly and specifically killed, an outcome that implied the presence on their surface membrane of receptors specific for the antigen involved. In due course, however, the weight of evidence forced the conclusion that while the macrophage might contribute importantly to cellular immunity and even to antibody formation, its functions were essentially nonspecific. The inhibition of macrophage migration proved to be due to the antigen-induced release of a soluble factor from extremely small numbers of contaminating lymphocytes.[50] The role of the macrophage in antibody formation was ultimately shown to be a nonspecific one, involving the processing and/or presentation of antigen to lymphocytes.[51] But this role was not discovered until after it was suggested that antigen might induce in the macrophage the formation of a specific RNA that could transfer information to antibody-forming lymphocytes,[52] or that, less specifically, an antigen–macrophage RNA complex might serve as a "super antigen" in stimulating lymphocytes to antibody formation.[53]

DELAYED-TYPE HYPERSENSITIVITY

Observations of two sorts helped to slowly define a dichotomy in the phenomenology of immunity and allergy. The first of these were the clinical findings that, whereas the symptoms of local and systemic anaphylaxis, the skin test for allergy, and the hayfever–asthma group of allergies were all characterized by an almost immediate onset following antigenic challenge, the intradermal tuberculin test, the luetin test for syphilis, the lepromin test for leprosy, and the response to vaccination in the sensitized host all required 24 to 48 hours to develop. The former were grouped together under the heading *immediate* hypersensitivities and were acknowledged to be due to the participation of humoral antibodies. The latter, on the other hand, were termed *delayed* hypersensitivities and, since circulating antibody could not be implicated in their pathogenesis, were ascribed to some type of cellular function, or to "cell-bound" antibodies. The appropriateness of this division was made clear when Landsteiner and Chase demonstrated the ability to transfer these hypersensitivities passively with cells and not with serum antibody[54] and when it was recognized that contact dermatitis, allograft rejection, and certain viral and autoallergic diseases somehow belonged to the same category of delayed hypersensitivity cellular responses. With the discovery that certain immunological deficiency diseases might inhibit antibody formation and immediate hypersensitivities while others would impair delayed hypersensitivity and cellular immunity,[55] the stage was set for the establishment of a major division of lymphocytic functions. Thymus-derived cells (T cells) function in cellular immunity, and avian bursal or mammalian bone marrow-derived cells (B cells) are responsible for antibody formation.[56]

The second line of investigation stemmed from the observation that somehow there was a major difference between immunological responses to soluble exotoxins and innocuous antigens and the body's response to infectious agents. This finding led to the early use of such terms as "immunity of infection" and "bacterial allergy." It was not until the late 1920s that Dienes and Schoenheit[57] demonstrated that this type of allergy could be induced even against bland antigens—by injecting them directly into the tubercles of infected animals, a procedure that was considerably simplified by the introduction of complete Freund's adjuvant containing dead mycobacteria. Now delayed-type hypersensitivity could be induced against purified proteins,[58] and it was not long before it was shown that hapten–protein conjugates would serve as well (analogous to Landsteiner's use of artificial antigens for the study of immediate hypersensitivities[59]). The parallelism was not exact, however, for while antibodies raised against a hapten coupled to carrier protein X would interact with the same hapten attached to protein Y, the delayed skin reaction against hapten–protein conjugates did not occur unless the carrier protein employed to elicit the response was the same as that used for sensitization.[60]

Here was a conundrum that taxed the ingenuity of investigators, since it appeared to call for a different order of immunological specificity than that established by the study of serum antibodies. From one direction, Benacerraf and Gell suggested that the specific combining site that mediated delayed hypersensitivity might be larger in physical dimensions than that normally encountered on circulating antibody and would thus encompass both the haptenic determinant and a portion of the adjacent carrier protein molecule.[61] From another direction (and somewhat neglectful of the "carrier effect" while emphasizing the passive transfer experiments), Karush and Eisen suggested that these reactions were due to the participation of very small quantities of very high affinity antibodies, with association constants of the order of 10^{10} or more.[62] But both of these hypotheses were eclipsed by a remarkable series of investigations that showed that in fact *two* different cell types were required for responses to conjugated proteins, one a "helper" cell that recognizes the carrier protein and the other an effector cell that recognizes the haptenic determinant.[63] In delayed hypersensitivity and other forms of cellular immunity, the effector cells proved to be specialized subsets of T lymphocytes, whereas in antibody formation helper T cells were shown to collaborate with effector B cells (both sharing in specificity for antigen) by stimulating the latter to active antibody formation.[64] Evidence was soon forthcoming that antigen-specific T cells might serve other functions as well, such as participating in the feedback suppression of immune responses.[65]

But if lymphocytes are to engage in specific interactions, then they must have on their surface membranes appropriate receptors with the full repertorial range of immunological specificities that immunocyte reactions have been shown capable of distinguishing. For the B lymphocyte, the demonstration of specific surface receptors proved fairly simple, thanks to techniques such as immunofluorescent analysis. These receptors proved to be samples of the antibody specificities for which these cells were programmed, thus providing final vindication of Paul Ehrlich's side-chain theory of 1897 and of Macfarlane Burnet's clonal selection theory 60 years later.

The search for the T cell receptor, however, proved more elusive. As Marrack and Kappler point out in their review of antigen-specific T cell receptors,[66] "Early attempts to isolate these proteins relied heavily on the idea that T cell receptors might be similar, if not identical, to immunoglobulin. In retrospect, although this idea was not unreasonable, it certainly created a good deal of confusion in the field." (It will be remembered that the extremely complicated mechanism for immunoglobulin formation was even then on the horizon; one was loathe at the time to predict that *two* such unique systems had evolved independently, even for so worthy a purpose as the immune response. This suggestion was extremely vulnerable to severe damage by Occam's razor.) In the event, immunofluorescence with anti-immunoglobulin sera usually failed to demonstrate these receptors; and even microchemistry of the surface membrane constituents of T lymphocytes led to very mixed results. Some authors—most notably, Marchalonis and Cone[67]— claimed that the T cell receptor is monomeric IgM, a finding strongly contested by Vitetta and Uhr.[68]

Three findings that appeared in fairly rapid succession indicated that the T cell receptor was indeed not an immunoglobulin. First, it became evident that T and B cell receptors do not recognize the same determinants on a given antigen.[69] Next, it was shown that T and B cells specific for the same antigen often have different cross-reaction patterns with other antigens.[70] Finally, it was shown by several laboratories that immune response genes associated with the major histocompatibility complex affect T cell function, with little *direct* effect upon B cells.[71] A clearer picture of the difference between T and B cell receptors was obtained when Zinkernagel and Doherty showed that, whereas B cells see antigen alone, T cells interact with antigen only in the presence of MHC products.[72] The demonstration that T cells do not contain mRNA for immunoglobulin chains[73] made it evident that a completely different system governs T cell specificity.

I shall not explore *in extenso* the voluminous recent work on the molecular biology of the T cell receptor gene families.[74] It will suffice to indicate that the T cell receptor has been shown to be composed of heterodimeric glycoproteins consisting of an α and a β chain. Each chain, although apparently unrelated to any of the immunoglobulin chains, has both constant and variable regions. Of interest to this discussion is that specificity and a large repertoire are attained just as in the case of Ig molecules—by the rearrangement of numerous gene segments (including multiple V, [D], and J exons). What is especially fascinating is that the T cell receptor shows only modest affinities for the antigen–MHC ligand and that it appears not to interact appreciably with either component alone. (These two features may, in fact, go hand-in-hand, since interaction with and activation by either component might obviate the special functions in the immune response played by T cells.)

TRANSFER FACTOR

No discussion of the basis for and functions of immunological specificity would be complete without mention of the curious substance transfer factor, first described by Lawrence.[75] This material is obtained from the sensitized lymphocytes of certain species following activation with antigen; and it is capable of transferring specific hypersensitivity and immunity to naive recipients. It is, moreover, dialyzable and of relatively low molecular weight (<4000). Transfer factor has been applied clinically with some success in the protection of human immunodeficient patients from a variety of viral and mycotic diseases. Although it has been experimented with for almost 30 years, the precise chemical composition and mode of action of transfer factor remain a mystery. It clearly transfers antigen-specific sensitivity, however, and although unrelated to immunoglobulins, it may be related to the putative T cell receptor discussed earlier. Alternatively, since the specific sensitivity that it transfers is of relatively long duration, the possibility remains open that transfer factor may be an informational single-stranded polynucleotide.

Specific Triggers and Nonspecific Amplifiers

I have thus far treated the phenomena of immunity and allergy that follow upon the interaction of antigen with antibody or antigen with specific lymphocyte as though these complex reactions were entirely specific from start to finish. But progress in sorting out the cellular dynamics and pathophysiology of antibody formation or of delayed and immediate allergic inflammatory responses shows that a number of complicated mechanisms have evolved by which an oft-times exceedingly minor specific immunological trigger may be amplified to a remarkable degree. These depend upon the release of a variety of pharmacological agents whose further function is usually nonspecific in nature.

The first of these nonspecific mediators to be described was complement. Jules Bordet showed originally that complement could effect the hemolysis of erythrocytes that had been sensitized with specific antibody; and he speculated that complement fixation and its consequences were the nonspecific by-products of the antigen–antibody union.[76] The process of complement fixation proved in fact to be nonspecific, and unexpectedly complicated. Thus, complement is composed of a large number of individual components and factors that function in a sequential cascade, with the activation or release of a variety of enzymes that can damage cell membranes and a variety of split-products that may be chemotactic for polymorphonuclear leukocytes or that may exercise physiological effects upon muscle or blood vessels.[77] It is mechanisms of this type, triggered by an initial antigen–antibody interaction, that contribute so importantly to, among others, the inflammatory reaction seen in the Arthus phenomenon and the glomerular damage seen in immune complex disease of the kidney.

Another example of the nonspecific enhancement of a modest immunological interaction occurs in hayfever and asthma-type allergies. Here, exceedingly small amounts of allergen may interact with nanogram quantities of the specialized IgE antibody, but the initial site of interaction on the surface of mast cells leads to their degranulation, with the subsequent release of active pharmacological agents such as histamine and serotonin.[78] These latter substances then incite nonspecific se-quelae, such as dermal wheal and erythema reactions, inflammation of the ocular conjunctiva, and bronchiolar constriction.

Nonspecific mediators and enhancers are no less important in cell-mediated phenomena than they are in those triggered by circulating antibody. It was initially difficult to understand, in passive transfer experiments of delayed hypersensitivity or allograft rejection reactions, why the proportion of *specific* lymphocytes in the inflammatory infiltrate should be so low—often only a fraction of 1% of the lymphocytes present.[79] If these reactions were immunologically specific, as one in fact knew them to be, why then were so many "innocent bystander" cells present at the site? The answer emerged from studies that were stimulated by the phenomenon of antigen-induced inhibition of macro-phage migration, to which I alluded earlier. It was found that the specific interaction of antigen and lymphocyte leads to the release of pharmacologically active substances (lymphokines) able nonspecifically to immobilize (and often activate) macrophages locally (see ref. 50). In time, other agents whose release could be triggered by specific interac-tion with antigen were identified. Some of these act on T cells to attract them to a local site of inflammation and there to stimulate them to mitosis, whereas others appear to act on B cells to induce polyclonal activation and antibody formation.[80] Nor are lymphocytes the only source of nonspecific agents that may contribute to immunogenic reactons. Monocytes may also give rise to such active factors (mono-kines), now often two steps removed from the specific immunological triggering event.[81] Indeed, it is now believed that many other cell types throughout the body, even those unrelated to the immunological apparatus, may be excited by a variety of stimuli (hormones, etc.) to release pharmacologically active agents (cytokines) that act upon lym-phocytes.

It is now clear that without this congeries of nonspecific factors, the workings of protective immunity (and of immunopathology) would be far more modest than those that one sees in actual practice.

Waiting for the End?

For the discipline of immunology, the scientific and even social event of the year 1967 was the International Symposium on Antibodies[82] that convened at Cold Spring Harbor, Long Island, during a sunny week in June. Most of the world's leading immunologists came to discuss their most recent findings, and the proceedings were attended by the electric excitement that characterizes a science in which progress is almost breathtakingly rapid. Indeed, it seemed as though a watershed had been reached or that the divide was at least in sight. All of the important conceptual questions of the past 80 years appeared for the first time to be answerable.

The meeting was opened by Sir Macfarlane Burnet, who declared that a new paradigm now directed the development of hypotheses and the design of experiments in immunology. In less than a decade, the clonal selection theory of antibody formation, based upon genetic control of antibody specificity, had deposed all earlier instruction theories. Moreover, the progress reported during the course of the symposium seemed to foretell the rapid solution of the most pressing problems in immunology. On the molecular level, immunoglobulin chain sequencing had reached the point where the complete structure of the immunoglobulin molecule was in sight, and the genetic basis for the specificity repertoire and the recognition of antigenicity seemed finally to be within reach. Delineation of the steps in antibody biosynthesis appeared well in hand, as did the structure of the antigen-specific lymphocyte receptor. On the cellular level, much information was available on the differentiation pathways of immunocytes and on the collaboration of macrophages. Although T and B lymphocytes had not yet been named, studies of the differences between delayed hypersensitivity and antibody formation and especially the newer information on the role of the thymus and of the avian bursa and the mammalian bone marrow presaged the identification of interacting lymphocyte subsets. One could be justifiably pleased, in June of 1967, that important answers were arriving with impressive rapidity.

The Cold Spring Harbor Symposium was closed with a masterly summary by Niels Jerne, entitled "Waiting for the End." He rightly drew attention to the triumph of the clonal selection theory and implied that cis- (cellular) immunologists, working forward from the first interaction of antigen with cell, and trans- (molecular) immunologists, working backward from the structure of the antibody molecule, were very close to meeting one another somewhere in the middle—at which point all but the minor details would presumably have been settled. As Jerne put it in his final paragraph: "As this younger generation of professionals is pressing rapidly toward the definitive solution of the antibody problem, we older amateurs had perhaps better sit back, waiting for the End."[83]

History suggests, however, that predictions about "definitive solutions" of scientific questions should be made with extreme caution. Thus, for about 2000 years in the case of Aristotle and almost 1500 years in the case of Galen, the Western world appeared to have concluded that little could be added to the natural history writings of the former or to the medical writings of the latter, save perhaps for trivial scholastic disputation.[84] Among the many other examples that might be given, I cite an essay written by the great Rudolf Virchow in 1877, some 18 years after the publication of his landmark book, *Cellular Pathology*.[85] Virchow seemed to imply that it was substantially all over in pathology but the mopping up; he wrote, "What efforts had to be made . . . to assign every phenomenon . . . to its proper place. And yet we seem to have succeeded in bringing firm order out of seeming chaos; the thousands of individual facts have been comprehended in a few well established laws and made easily accessible to the understanding of the younger generation in the new order."[86]

Just a few years later, after almost a century of startling advances in physics, one of the most famous physicists of the day, A. A. Michelson, felt able to come to a similar conclusion about the status of his own field,[87] saying, "it seems probable that most of the grand underlying principles have been firmly established . . . An eminent physicist [he seemed to mean Lord Kelvin] has remarked that the future truths of Physical Science are to be looked for in the sixth place of decimals."[88] Such a view seemed prevalent then in all the sciences. As Price so aptly put it in his *Science since Babylon:* "by about 1890, all natural phenomena had been divided and ruled, and only unimportant problems remained . . . It was obviously reasonable to believe that finality was just around the corner. The only hope for future generations would be to measure each constant of nature to an additional decimal place."[89] This, just a few years before the discovery of X-rays, of radioactivity, and of Einstein's theories produced a new revolution in physics that is still going on.

At the start of this discussion on the development of the concept of immunological specificity, two questions were posed whose history I would attempt to trace: What is the (molecular) basis of immunological specificity? What is its ultimate provenance? It might appear at first sight, from the preceding discussion, that modern immunological science has thoroughly answered both of these questions. Certainly the molecular and even atomic definition of the antibody combining site in terms of unique sequences of amino acids on the heavy and light peptide chains of the immunoglobulin molecule seemed to tell all about *structure* and, thus, about function. Similarly, the identification of a set of germ-line genes for variable and constant regions of heavy and light chains, with an elaborate mechanism provided for the further generation of diversity by somatic mutation, minigene assortment,[90] and variable gene splicing,[91] would appear to answer fully any questions about the *origin* of specific antibodies. Thus, echoing Jerne, one seems to be faced with a "definitive solution of the antibody problem." But in spite of this, at least two conceptual difficulties still persist and demand attention, the one involving the *true* size of the immunological repertoire and the other relating to the mode of evolution of the mechanisms responsible for the generation of diversity. It is difficulties such as these that may announce that investigators are not yet at "the End" in a scientific questions or discipline, rather; they are preparing to cross over into uncharted and hopefully exciting new territory.

The Repertoire Paradox

From the earliest days of immunology, it has been an integral part of the received wisdom that antibody is endowed with a fine specificity for its inducing antigen, a view reinforced by repeated demonstrations of stereochemical molecular complementarity between antigen and antibody and, from outside of immunology, by increasing knowledge of the specificity of enzyme action. The demonstrations by Landsteiner and by Pauling and Pressman of serological cross-reactions among haptens of closely related structure modified this view only slightly, by permitting minor variations in the antibody combining site into which *very closely related* structures might fit with reduced binding energies. However, these same studies with artificial haptens also immeasurably expanded the universe of antigenic structures against which specific antibodies could be formed; and I have noted how the requirement of a large specificity repertoire affected the thinking of immunologists about the mechanism of antibody formation.[92] But does the modern immunogenetic synthesis even now provide sufficient clonal precursors (clonotypes) to encompass the full repertoire requirements of the immunologically active organism? Some investigators think not.

It has always been difficult to arrive at a reasonable estimate of the size of the specificity repertoire of the vertebrate. Some investigators have put the maximum number of *completely different* immunogenic structures as low as 50,000, while the usual number quoted is 10^5 to 10^6. Inman has suggested,[93] on the basis of an analysis of the known natural synthetic structures that have been cataloged, that as many as 10^{16} different antigenic structures may exist, a number appreciably larger than the total number of lymphocytes ($<10^9$) in the immunologically well-studied mouse. There is, however, another approach to the problem.

It has been possible to estimate both the number of different clonotypes that may be produced by a mouse and the precursor cell frequency for each clonotype by employing techniques such as isoelectric focusing, fine specificity analysis, idiotypy, and the transfer of limiting dilutions of clonal precursors to irradiated recipients or to *in vitro* cultures (to allow an actual count of responding clones). These approaches have been extensively reviewed by Sigal and Klinman in their discussion of the B cell clonotype repertoire.[94] With such approaches, it has been estimated that there may be as many as 5000 *different* clonotypes (i.e., specific antibodies of differing primary structure and differing affinity, but reactive nevertheless with the immunizing antigen) for the dinitrophenyl (DNP) or for the 3-iodo-5-nitrobenzoyl (NIP) haptens. It is also estimated that each of these clonotypes is represented by about 10 precursor cells per mouse.[95] With 2 to 3×10^8 B cells in the lymphoid system of a mouse, there could be only about 6000 *different* antigenic determinants against which the adult mouse might be capable of responding. This figure accords well with the finding that about 1 in 5000 B cells in the mouse is specific for DNP and between 1 in 7000 and 1 in 15,000 B cells is specific for NIP.[96] Thus, even though the total clonotype repertoire of the mouse may be quite large ($\sim 10^7$), the degeneracy of the immune response appears to allow an almost embarrassingly restricted coverage of the universe of potential stimuli.[97]

This paradox is further pointed up by observations in other areas. Whereas man with his 10^{13} lymphocytes might have little difficulty in expressing a suitably broad specificity repertoire, smaller vertebrate species such as the mammalian shrew at 1 to 2 gm or certain species of fish at less than 100 mg of adult weight (with proportionately fewer lymphocytes) might experience greater difficulties. Yet these small animals appear to cope very well and to survive attack by their respective pathogens with little sign of immunological impairment. Indeed, du Pasquier has shown that the tadpole with about 10^6 lymphocytes (and perhaps one-third as many B cells) can form an adequate immune response against a variety of antigens.[98]

The dilemma posed by these data has been countered by the suggestion that the antibody combining site may not be as tightly restricted to a small antigenic determinant as had earlier been supposed. The hypothesis has been advanced that the combining region on antibody might be "polyfunctional," in that it might be large enough to permit the binding of two or more quite disparate molecular structures.[99] Thus, an immune response to antigenic determinant A might involve several clonotypes, one binding determinants A and B, another binding determinants A and C, etc. The resulting immune serum would *appear* to have anti-A specificity, because other specificities would be at very low concentration. On such a basis, the universe of different antigens could be dealt with. There is even some direct indication in the literature that such a general multispecificity of the antibody combining site may exist. Some monoclonal myeloma proteins are able to bind unrelated haptens such as ε-DNP lysine (with an affinity constant of 10^5 L/mol) and 2-methyl-1,4- naphthoquinone (menadione) with an affinity constant of 2×10^4 L/mol, and neither of these may represent the "best fit" hapten.[100] Similarly, a myeloma protein that reacts with three unrelated structures (dinitrophenyl, 5-acetouracil, and purines) has been found;[101] and the homogeneous human immunoglobulin Wag has been shown to bind both ε-DNP lysine and an Fc fragment of IgG.[102] Finally, in another biological system whose specificity appears to have a basis similar to that of antibodies, enzymes that bind a number of structurally unrelated compounds to their binding sites have been found.[103]

A theory of receptor site multispecificity was first advanced by Talmage[104] in an attempt to show that a heterogeneous immune serum might show a greater specificity for antigen than any of its constituent antibodies. This suggestion has been taken up and extended by Inman and by Richards *et al.* as "the only reasonable solution" to the continuing repertoire paradox.

The Evolutionary Paradox

During the decade-long debate on the genetic basis of immunological diversity, one of the most telling arguments employed by the proponents of a paucigene model expanded by somatic variation[105] against those who espoused the idea that all specificities were encoded in the germ line[106] focused on the problem of Darwinian evolution. How, they asked, could the gene pool be maintained when any given organism was likely to employ such a small proportion of its specificity repertoire during its lifetime and when so many of the specificities that it did employ were against antigens that posed little threat to survival? In the absence of positive selective pressures, it would not take long for such unused or "unimportant" genes to lose their identity. But even though modern molecular biology has "split the difference" between somaticists and germ liners, by showing an endowment of several hundred V_H and V_L genes and an elaborate mechanism for the further generation of immunological diversity,[107] the evolutionary question still remains with us.

There are, in fact, three different questions to be asked about the evolution of the specificity repertoire in immunology: (1) How has the complicated overall mechanism evolved, a mechanism including multiple V_L and V_H genes and an elaborate mechanism for the somatic expansion of their specificity potential and for their splicing to J_L, J_H,

D_H, and the constant region sequences of DNA, and even for intracodon recombination? (2) What is the nature of the specificities encoded for by the germ-line genes, that Darwinian selective pressures might function to maintain their integrity? (3) How can speciation of these *linear sets* of immunoglobulin genes be explained? Scientists are still far from understanding the answers to *any* of these questions; and the questions may not even have been phrased correctly.

EVOLUTION OF THE IMMUNOGLOBULIN MECHANISM

Immunology is not unique in presenting the problem of the Darwinian evolution of complex biological systems, often involving multiple independent constituents acting in sequence to produce a complicated physiological result. As Ernst Mayr points out, the self-reproduction of complex biological systems that are based upon the trials and errors of several thousand million years of evolution is what distinguishes the biological from the physical sciences.[108]

In tracing the evolution of a complex biological system, it may not always be necessary to posit a step-by-step *forward* development from the first reactant. Thus, the complicated vertebrate blood clotting system, involving multiple factors and cofactors, proenzymes and enzymes acting in sequence, might have started in evolution at the end result— the selective advantage of a fairly simple clotting protein in metazoan invertebrates (*Limulus*, for example)—and then evolved elaborate and more efficient mechanisms by working *backward* to what are now considered to be the initiating factors in clotting. Again, the complicated cascade reactions seen in the complement system, involving a dozen or more components acting sequentially and along at least two different pathways,[109] might have started somewhere in the middle, perhaps with the physiologically important activities associated with the third or fifth components of complement. In this instance, one can conceive of evolution working in both directions: backward, to select the earlier components that render the production of chemotactic factors and anaphylotoxins more efficient, and forward, to extend the utility range of the complement system to additional biological functions.

In defining the molecular evolution of the immunoglobulins, one is impressed by the amino acid sequence homology between the variable and constant regions of the light chains, among the different domains on the heavy chains, and among the light and heavy chains themselves,[110] a homology suggesting an evolution through gene duplication.[111] But what is the molecular starting point for such an evolution? Here, one is impressed by the sequence homology of immunoglobulins with β_2-microglobulin.[112] The immunoglobulin Urpeptide (and its immediate evolutionary descendants) may well have functioned as cell-membrane recognition or adhesion molecules, whose selective value in the differentiation and maintenance of integrity of *all* multicellular organisms is well recognized.[113]

But what can be said of the complicated genetic mechanisms that, starting from a limited number of germ line V regions, permit the individual to generate so extensive a clonotype repertoire of immunological specificities? Ohno has addressed this question in a most imaginative way, pointing out that the answer to this question may be as applicable to the functional diversity of the nervous system and human intelligence as it is to immunity.[114] By analogy with the Greek myth of the Titan brothers, foresighted Prometheus and hindsighted Epimetheus, he suggests that there may be in fact two types of evolution—an Epimethean process based upon *past* adaptations (corresponding to classic Darwinian principles) and a Promethean process that may prepare the organism advantageously for *future* adaptations. Given that the generation time of viral and bacterial pathogens is several orders of magnitude less than that of vertebrate hosts, Ohno suggests that Epimethean natural selection might not afford adequate time to catch up with the rapid adaptive changes that parasites may manifest, and thus there may be much selective advantage in the development of a new evolutionary mechanism based upon Promethean principles. It is understandably difficult to evaluate this stimulating suggestion, although it must be pointed out that invertebrates, apparently devoid of any semblance of the molecular immune system of vertebrates, seem to cope well in this pathogen-ridden world.

WHAT IS ENCODED BY GERM-LINE V REGION GENES?

Whatever may be the basis for the further somatic expansion of the immunological repertoire, it appears necessary to invoke Darwinian selective forces for the maintenance intact of the set of variable region genes with which vertebrates are endowed in the germ line. But the single gene does not, as I have noted, define a specificity—this is a function of the V_H and V_L combination. Fortunately, selection acts not upon the genotype but upon the phenotype; so even though an individual would presumably be deselected should he suffer functional loss of a single V region gene whose light or heavy chain product was critically important for survival, the population would survive.

What, then, are the germ-line specificity phenotypes? Jerne, impressed by the large number of T cells that show specificity for alloantigens shared within a species,[115] proposed that the germ-line V genes code for receptor specificities that recognize the full range of the species' polymorphic histocompatibility units.[116] He cites the importance in the ontogeny even of invertebrates of cell-to-cell recognition, to enable differentiation and histogenesis to take place; and he suggests that the parallel evolution of a set of histocompatibility units and V gene combinations may mediate these important interactions. Pointing to the tremendous lymphocyte proliferation in the thymus (and bursa of Fabricius), Jerne suggests that these organs may in fact function as mutant-breeding sites, where the immunological repertoire is somatically expanded by stepwise mutational deviations from the histocompatibility-determinant starting point.

On the other hand, Cohn *et al.* have pointed out that alloaggression and allospecificities appear to be significant only with respect to the T cell repertoire and seem not so prominent in the B cell repertoire. They support this view by noting also that whereas B cells appear to recognize only antigen, T cells usually recognize the combination antigen-and-self [i.e., gene products encoded in the major histocompatibility complex (see ref. 72)]. Thus, while willing to concede that the specificity of the germ line T cell repertoire *may* be for alloantigens, they insist that the specificity of the germ line B cell repertoire must be devoted to the important infectious pathogens, to assure their selective survival.[117] (The differences between B and T cell repertoires, with respect to their structural basis as well as their repertorial compass, does not as yet support any conclusion along these lines.)

THE PROBLEM OF SPECIATION

In dealing with the evolution of single genes, it is easy to understand that mutations which do not impair the physiological function of the gene product may introduce species-specific DNA sequences or a polymorphism associated with the presence in a population of multiple alleles at a single locus.[118] But if one considers the effect of speciation on tandemly arranged sets of genes of related function, such as those of the immunoglobulin system, then the acquisition of shared species characteristics by *all* members of such gene families becomes more difficult to explain. In considering the evolution of immunoglobulin chains, the question of speciation may be posed at two different levels.

The first problem is to explain how species-specific substitutions, including allotypes, on the constant regions of the immunoglobulin chains or on the framework regions of the variable portions of these chains can be achieved simultaneously by tandemly arranged gene families during the evolution of a species. While a number of allotypic markers in species such as rabbit and man appear confined to one or another of the heavy chain isotypes, and thus to a single gene, some allotypic markers appear to be shared by multiple genes (e.g., the several V_H allotypes of the rabbit and the light chain INV marker in the human.) In addition, other nonpolymorphic species marker sequences appear to exist elsewhere in immunoglobulin chains.[119]

It may not be necessary, however, to postulate some novel genetic mechanism that would ensure that speciation be accompanied from the outset by an abrupt *and concerted* shift of species markers by all members of a given gene family. Edelman and Gally originally proposed a mechanism for the conservation of homology among the members of immunoglobulin gene families. They called this mechanism "democratic gene conversion;"[120] and Baltimore has recently revived it.[121] Edelman and Gally suggested that gene conversion (the transfer of DNA sequence information from gene to gene) may have played the most significant role in immunoglobulin evolution, by ensuring the uniform acquisition (or, rather, the uniform spread) of species markers along the linear array of a given family of immunoglobulin genes.

The problem of speciation becomes more difficult, however, when we consider the evolution of the set of germ-line V region genes—if, in fact, the specificities for which they code are species-related. Assuming, with Jerne, that the germ-line V region genes of T cells encode for receptor specificities that recognize species-specific histocompatibility alloantigens, speciation would require a concerted redirection of the entire family of V genes to include now a new library of allospecificities. Such a genetic shift would appear to impose a greater conceptual problem than does the suggestion that the germ-line V genes encode for the antigens carried by the major pathogens, for, in addition to the obvious selective value that such immunity would confer, the susceptibility of related species to similar sets of pathogens would obviate the requirements for a major shift in V gene-coded specificities.

Conclusions

I have attempted, in these chapters on the development of the concept of immunological specificity, to trace the history of one of the most central ideas in immunology (and, indeed, in biology in general). The result must be viewed as preliminary and incomplete and as an invitation to others to add, to amend, and even to disprove. Nevertheless, several interesting conclusions that may be drawn reveal much about the workings of immunology in particular, and perhaps science in general.

First, the roots of any important scientific concept (such as that of immunological specificity) do not grow in isolation; they draw nourishment from many other disciplines. Similarly, the growth of an important concept within a given discipline will have far-reaching implications and fruits for other fields of science. Second, one notes that the manner in which immunology is currently practiced has changed markedly from that of the end of the last century. The quantum leaps forward in funding, in numbers of scientists, and in masses of crucial data have not been without a certain cost—the substantial reduction in elegant *personal style* that characterized so many of our scientific forebears and that makes so interesting and even enjoyable the reading of their reports. Finally, one sees again and again how much philosophical bases and disciplinary upbringing determine a scientist's approach, the questions asked, and the type of answers he or she will accept. Throughout much of immunology's history, as Jerne put it so well,[122] cis- and trans-immunologists hardly spoke to one another. Or rather, a cis-immunologist sometimes spoke to a trans-immunologist, but the latter rarely answered! Fortunately, one of the attributes of scientific progress is a merging of these disparate languages and eventual mutual comprehension.

NOTES AND REFERENCES

1. P. Ehrlich, Croonian Lecture—On Immunity. *Proc. R. Soc. London* **66,** 424 (1900).

2. See Chapters 4 and 5.

3. That this was indeed the Age of Immunochemistry is discussed in Chapter 5, ref. 101, and in Appendix A1.

4. J. Fruton, *Molecules and Life: Historical Essays on the Interplay of Chemistry and Biology.* Wiley (Interscience), New York, 1972.

5. J. R. Marrack, *The Chemistry of Antigens and Antibodies.* HM Stationery Off., London, 1934.

6. K. Landsteiner, *The Specificity of Serological Reactions.* Dover, New York, 1962.

7. K. Landsteiner, *Biochem. Z.* **104,** 280 (1920).

8. D. Pressman and A. Grossberg, *The Structural Basis of Antibody Specificity.* Benjamin, New York, 1968.

9. L. Pauling and D. Pressman. *J. Am. Chem. Soc.* **67,** 1003 (1945).

10. S. B. Hooker and W. C. Boyd, *J. Immunol.* **42,** 419 (1941); L. Pauling and H. A. Itano, eds., *Molecular Structure and Biological Specificity.* American Inst. of Biological Sciences, Washington, D.C., 1957.

11. D. Pressman, in *Molecular Structure and Biological Specificity* (L. Pauling and

H. A. Itano, eds.). American Inst. of Biological Sciences, Washington, D.C., 1957.

12. These factors are reviewed by W. C. Boyd, *Introduction to Immunochemical Specificity*. Interscience, New York, 1962.

13. H. N. Eisen and F. Karush, *J. Am. Chem. Soc.* **71**, 363 (1949). A forerunner of this technique had first been employed by J. R. Marrack and F. C. Smith, *J.Exp.Pathol.* **13**, 394 (1932).

14. F. Karush, *Adv. Immunol.* **2**, 1 (1962).

15. See, e. g., L. Pauling, D. Pressman, and A. Grossberg, *J. Am. Chem. Soc.* **66**, 784 (1944); F. Karush and M. Sonnenberg, *J. Am. Chem. Soc.* **71**, 1369 (1949); F. Karush, *J. Am. Chem. Soc.* **78**, 5519 (1956).

16. The author recalls having heard this comment at a meeting, perhaps 20–25 years ago, and believes it was made by Felix Haurowitz. Prof. Haurowitz (personal communication, 1982), while not remembering it specifically, allows that he could well have made it.

17. D. W. Talmage, *Science* **149**, 1643 (1959).

18. K. Landsteiner, *Wien. Klin. Wochenschr.* **22**, 1623 (1909).

19. The philosophical background to the dispute about continuity or discontinuity in nature and its implications for immunology are discussed in Chapter 5. See also P. M. H. Mazumdar, *Karl Landsteiner and the Problem of Species 1838–1968* (thesis). Johns Hopkins Press, Baltimore, Maryland, 1976.

20. K. Landsteiner and J. van der Scheer, *J. Exp. Med.* **67**, 709 (1938).

21. D. H. Campbell and N. Bulman, *Fortschr. Chem. Org. Naturstoffe* **9**, 443 (1952).

22. E. A. Kabat, *J. Immunol.* **77**, 377 (1956). See also E. A. Kabat, *J. Immunol.* **97**, 1 (1966); E. A. Kabat, *Structural Concepts in Immunology and Immunochemistry*. Holt, Rinehart & Winston, New York, 1968.

23. R. Arnon, M. Sela, A. Yaron, and H. A. Silber, *Biochemistry* **4**, 948 (1965); H. van Vunakis, J. Kaplan, H. Lehrer, and L. Levine, *Immunochemistry* **3**, 393 (1966).

24. P. Grabar and C. A. Williams, Jr., *Biochim. Biophys. Acta* **10**, 193 (1953); **17**, 65 (1955). See also P. Grabar and P. Burtin, *Immunoelectrophoretic Analysis*. Elsevier, Amsterdam, 1964. Also critical for the development of immunoelectrophoresis and of great importance in its own right was the introduction of immunoprecipitation in gels by J. Oudin, *Ann. Inst. Pasteur, Paris* **75**, 30 (1948); A. Ouchterlony, *Acta Pathol. Microbiol. Scand.* **26**, 509 (1949).

25. J. L. Fahey, *Adv. Immunol.* **2**, 41 (1962).

26. R. R. Porter, *Biochem. J.* **46**, 479 (1950); M. Fried and F. W. Putnam, *Fed. Proc.* **18**, 230 (1959); A. Nisonoff, F. C. Wissler, and D. L. Woernley, *Biochem. Biophys. Res. Commun.* **1**, 318 (1959). As early as the mid-1930s, I. A. Parfentiev had obtained patents on the pepsin cleavage of diphtheria antitoxin without altering its antibody activity [U.S. Patents 2,065,196 (1936); 2,123,198 (1938)].

27. G. M. Edelman, *J. Am. Chem. Soc.* **81**, 3155 (1959); F. Franěk, *Biochem. Biophys. Res. Commun.* **4**, 28 (1961).

28. G. M. Edelman and M. D. Poulik, *J. Exp. Med.* **113**, 861 (1961).

29. R. R. Porter, *Br. Med. Bull.* **19,** 197 (1963).

30. G. M. Edelman, *Biochemistry* **9,** 3197 (1970).

31. R. J. Slater, S. M. Ward, and H. G. Kunkel, *Harvey Lect.* **59,** 219 (1965).

32. G. M. Edelman and J. A. Gally, *J. Exp. Med.* **116,** 207 (1962). See also F. W. Putnam and S. Hardy, *J. Biol. Chem.* **212,** 261 (1955).

33. R. L. Hill, H. E. Lebowitz, R. E. Fellows, and R. Delaney, in *Gamma Globulin Structure and Control of Biosynthesis* (J. Killander, ed.). Almqvist & Wiksells, Stockholm, 1967; H. M. Grey, *Adv. Immunol.* **10,** 51 (1969); L. Hood, J. H. Campbell, and S. C. R. Elgin, *Annu. Rev. Genet.* **9,** 305 (1975). For a more general discussion of the gene duplication mechanism, see S. Ohno, *Evolution by Gene Duplication.* Springer, New York, 1970.

34. T. T. Wu and E. A. Kabat, *J. Exp. Med.* **132,** 211 (1970). The reader should be aware that much of the progress in understanding the relationship between Ig structure and function, Ig evolution, and even the clarification of genetic mechanisms involved has depended upon comparisons of the amino acid sequences of Ig chains and thus upon such tabulations as those of E.A. Kabat, T. T. Wu, and H. Bilofsky, *Variable Regions of Immunoglobulin Chains. Tabulations and Analyses of Amino Acid Sequences, Medical Computer Systems.* Bolt, Baranek, & Newman, Cambridge, Massachusetts, 1976; *Sequences of Immunoglobulin Chains. Tabulation and Analysis of Amino Acid Sequences of Precursors, V-regions, C-regions, J-chain, and β₂ Microglobulins,* Publ. 80-2008. U.S. Dept. of Health, Education and Welfare, Bethesda, Maryland, 1980; M. O. Dayhoff, ed., *Atlas of Protein Sequence and Structure* (multiple volumes and supplements). Nat. Biomed. Res. Found., Washington, D.C.

35. R. J. Poljak, L. M. Amzel, H. P. Avey, B. L. Chen, R. P. Phizackerley, and F.Saul, *Proc. Natl. Acad. Sci. USA* **70,** 3305 (1973); **71,** 1427 (1974).

36. H. G. Kunkel, M. Mannik, and R. C. Williams, *Science* **140,** 1218 (1963); J. Oudin and M. Michel, *C. R. Hebd. Seances Acad. Sci.* **257,** 805 (1963). The early history of idiotypes and anti-idiotypes is discussed in Chapter 10.

37. N. K. Jerne, *Ann. Immunol.* (*Paris*) **125C,** 373 (1974); A. Nisonoff and M. I. Green, *Prog. Immunol.* **4,** 57 (1980). The contribution of idiotypes and anti-idiotypic antibodies to the definition of immunological specificity, the study of repertoire size, and the functions of what Jerne called *immune networks* of immonoregulation is one of the most active fields of immunology today, and its full implications cannot yet be assessed. For a hint of its breadth, see *International Conference on Immune Networks.* N.Y. Acad. Sci., New York, 1983.

38. See Chapter 3.

39. E. Metchnikoff, *Lectures on the Comparative Pathology of Inflammation.* Keegan, Paul, Trench, Trübner, London, 1893. [Reprinted by Dover, New York, 1968, pp. 154 ff.]

40. E. Metchnikoff, *L'Immunité dans les maladies infectieuses.* Masson, Paris, 1901. [English translation: Macmillan, New York, 1905; reprinted by Johnson Reprint, New York, 1968.]

41. Reference 40 (Engl. trans.), pp. 270–274.

42. Reference 40 (Engl. trans.), p. 306.

43. J. Denis and J. Leclef, *Cellule* **11,** 177 (1895). The observation was soon

confirmed by F. Mennes, Z. Hyg. Infektionskr. **25**, 413, 1897; W. B. Leishman, Br. Med. J. **1**, 73 (1902).

44. A. E. Wright and S. R. Douglas, Proc. R. Soc. London, Ser. B **72**, 364 (1903); **73**, 136 (1904); A. E. Wright, Studies on Immunization and Their Application to the Treatment of Bacterial Infection. Constable, London, 1909.

45. The best summary of the early work on tuberculosis and on the relationship of immunity and allergy to its pathogenesis is still that of A. R. Rich, The Pathogenesis of Tuberculosis, 2nd Ed., Thomas, Springfield, Illinois, 1951; see also Chapter 9.

46. M. B. Lurie, J. Exp. Med. **57**, 181 (1933); **75**, 247 (1942).

47. S. S. Elberg and K. Faunce, Jr., J. Bacteriol. **73**, 211 (1957); S. S. Elberg, Bacteriol. Rev. **24**, 67 (1960); E. Suter, J. Exp. Med. **97**, 235 (1953).

48. G. B. Mackaness, Am. Rev. Tuberc. **69**, 495 (1954). For more general reviews, see D. Rowley, Adv. Immunol. **2**, 241 (1962); E. Suter and H. Ramseier, Adv. Immunol. **4**, 117 (1964); D. S. Nelson, Macrophages and Immunity. North-Holland Publ., Amsterdam, 1969.

49. A. R. Rich and M. R. Lewis, Bull. Johns Hopkins Hosp. **50**, 115 (1932). These authors thought that antigen killed the macrophages, but see B. H. Waksman and M. Matoltsy, J. Immunol. **81**, 220 (1958).

50. B. R. Bloom and B. Bennett, Science **153**, 80 (1966); J. R. David, Proc. Natl. Acad. Sci. USA **56**, 72 (1966).

51. G. Möller, ed., Role of macrophages in the immune response. Immunol. Rev. **40**, (1978); E. R. Unanue and A. S. Rosenthal, eds., Macrophage Regulation of Immunity. Academic Press, New York, 1980.

52. M. Fishman and F. L. Adler, J. Exp. Med. **117**, 595 (1963); J. Fong, D. Chin, and S. S. Elberg, J. Exp. Med. **118**, 371 (1963).

53. B. A. Askonas and J. M. Rhodes, Nature (London) **205**, 470 (1965). See also O. J. Plescia and W. Braun, eds., Nucleic Acids in Immunology. Springer, New York, 1968.

54. K. Landsteiner and M. W. Chase, Proc. Soc. Exp. Biol. Med. **49**, 688 (1942).

55. D. Bergsma, Immunologic Deficiency Diseases in Man. The National Foundation, New York, 1968.

56. J. F. A. P. Miller and G. F. Mitchell, Transplant. Rev. **1**, 3 (1969); A. J. S. Davies, Transplant. Rev. **1**, 43 (1969); H. N. Claman and E. A. Chaperon, Transplant. Rev. **1**, 92 (1969).

57. L. Dienes and E. W. Schoenheit, Am. Rev. Tuberc. **20**, 92 (1929).

58. See, esp. J. Uhr, S. B. Salvin, and A. M. Pappenheimer, Jr., J. Exp. Med. **105**, 11 (1957); S. B. Salvin, J. Exp. Med. **107**, 109 (1958).

59. K. Landsteiner, Proc. K. Ned. Akad. Wet. **31**, 54 (1922); J. Exp. Med. **39**, 631 (1924); K. Landsteiner and J. van der Scheer, J. Exp. Med. **57**, 633 (1933).

60. B. Benacerraf and P. G. H. Gell, Immunology **2**, 53 (1959); B. Benacerraf and B. B. Levine J. Exp. Med. **115**, 1023 (1962).

61. B. Benacerraf and P. G. H. Gell, Immunology **2**, 219 (1959).

62. F. Karush and H. N. Eisen, Science **136**, 1032 (1962).

63. N. A. Mitchison, in Immunological Tolerance (M. Landy and W. Braun, eds.), p. 149. Academic Press, New York, 1969.

64. H. N. Claman, E. A. Chaperon, and R. F. Triplett, *Proc. Soc. Exp. Biol. Med.* **122,** 1167 (1966); G. F. Mitchell and J. F. A. P. Miller, *J. Exp. Med.* **128,** 801, 821 (1968).

65. R. K. Gershon, *Contemp. Top. Immunol.* **3,** 1 (1974); T. Tada and K. Okumura, *Adv. Immunol.* **28,** 1 (1979).

66. P. Marrack and J. Kappler, *Adv. Immunol.* **38,** 1 (1986).

67. J. J. Marchalonis, J. L. Atwell, and R. E. Cone, *Nature (London)* **235,** 240 (1972); M. Feldmann and G. J. V. Nossal, *Transplant. Rev.* **13,** 3 (1972); R. E. Cone and J. J. Marchalonis, *Biochem. J.* **140,** 345 (1974).

68. E. S. Vitetta, C. Bianco, V. Nussenzweig, and J. W. Uhr, *J. Exp. Med.* **136,** 81 (1972); E. S. Vitetta, J. W. Uhr, and E. A. Boyse, *Proc. Natl. Acad. Sci. USA* **70,** 834 (1973); J. W. Uhr, in *Genetic Control of Immune Responsiveness* (M. Landy and H. O. McDevitt, eds.), p. 228. Academic Press, New York, 1972.

69. C. R. Parish, *J. Exp. Med.* **134,** 21 (1971); V. Schirrmacher and H. Wigzell, *J. Exp. Med.* **136,** 1616 (1972).

70. M. Hoffmann and J. W. Kappler, *J. Immunol.* **106,** 261 (1972); J. H. L. Playfair, *Nature (London) New Biol.* **235,** 115 (1972).

71. D. H. Katz, T. Hamaoka, M. E. Dorf, P. E. Maurer, and B. Benacerraf, *J.Exp. Med.* **138,** 734 (1973); J. L. Press and H. O. McDevitt, *J. Exp. Med.* **146,** 1815 (1977).

72. R. M. Zinkernagel and P. C. Doherty, *J. Exp. Med.* **141,** 1427 (1975); *Adv. Immunol.* **27,** 51 (1979).

73. M. Kronenberg *et al., J. Exp. Med.* **152,** 1745 (1980); **158,** 210 (1983).

74. See, e.g., ref. 66. See also T. A. Waldmann, *Adv. Immunol.* **40,** 247 (1987). A feeling for the rapidity of progress in this field may be obtained by comparing the foregoing reviews with that of Tada and Okumura, ref. 65.

75. H. S. Lawrence, *J. Clin. Invest.* **33,** 951 (1954); *Harvey Lect.* **68,** 239 (1974). See also M. S. Ascher, A. A. Gottlieb, and C. H. Kirkpatrick, eds., *Transfer Factor: Basic Properties and Clinical Applications.* Academic Press, New York, 1976.

76. J. Bordet, *Ann. Inst. Pasteur, Paris,* **12,** 688 (1899). See also Chapter 5.

77. L. M. Lichtenstein *et al., Immunology* **16,** 327 (1969). See also H. J. Müller-Eberhard and R. D. Schreiber, *Adv. Immunol.* **29,** 1 (1980).

78. M. Plaut and L. M. Lichtenstein, in *Allergy: Principles and Practice* (E. Middleton, E. Ellis, and C. E. Reed, eds.), pp. 115–138. Mosby, St. Louis, Missouri, 1978.

79. R. T. McCluskey, B. Benacerraf, and J. W. McCluskey, *J. Immunol.* **90,** 466 (1963); R. A. Prendergast, *J. Exp. Med.* **119,** 377 (1964).

80. S. Cohn, E. Pick, and J. J. Oppenheim, eds., *Biology of Lymphokines.* Academic Press, New York, 1979.

81. R. E. Rocklin, K. Bendtzen, and D. Greineder, *Adv. Immunol.* **29,** 55 (1980).

82. Antibodies. *Cold Spring Harbor Symp. Quant. Biol.,* Vol. 32 (1967).

83. N. K. Jerne, in ref. 82, p. 601.

84. A. Castiglioni, *A History of Medicine,* 2nd Ed., p. 221. Knopf, New York, 1947; H. M. Leicester, *Development of Biochemical Concepts from Ancient to Modern Times,* Chap. 2 and 7. Harvard University Press, Cambridge, Massachusetts, 1974.

85. R. Virchow, *Die Cellularpathologie in ihrer Begründung auf physiologische und pathologische Gewebelehre*, Hirschwald, Berlin, 1858. [English edition: *Cellular Pathology*. Dover, New York, 1971.]

86. R. Virchow, Standpoints in scientific medicine. In *Disease, Life, and Man: Selected Essays by Rudolf Virchow* (L. J. Rather, ed.), p. 143. Stanford University Press, Stanford, California, 1958. Virchow had written an essay with the same title 30 years earlier (also in Rather, ed., p. 26), in which he had outlined many of the outstanding problems in pathology, whose solution had presumably been attained by the cellular approach.

87. See L. Badash's discussion, The completeness of nineteenth century science. *Isis* **63**, 48 (1972).

88. A. A. Michelson, *Univ. Chicago Q. Calendar* **3**, (Aug.), 15 (1894).

89. J. D. de S. Price, *Science since Babylon*, p. 37. Yale University Press, New Haven, Connecticut, 1961.

90. Following their definition of the V_L and V_H chains as being composed of three hypervariable (complementarity determining) regions isolated by four framework regions, the imaginative suggestion was made by Kabat and co-workers [E. A. Kabat, T. T. Wu, and H. Bilofsky, *Proc. Natl. Acad. Sci. USA* **75**, 2429 (1978); *J. Exp. Med.* **149**, 1299 (1979)] that these seven DNA sequences might represent independently assorting germ-line "minigenes," whose variable assemblage would provide for V_L and V_H diversity. However, subsequent DNA sequence data have shown that, whereas framework and hypervariable regions are not independent, there are in fact true minigenes that contribute to variability of the third "hypervariable region." These minigenes include a set of five J minigenes for light chains and two or more D and four J minigenes for heavy chains, with special mechanisms for splicing these to one or the other of the V_L or V_H and C_L or C_H segments. The minigenes contributing to the variability of the third hypervariable region are reviewed in detail in ref. 91; see also E. A. Kabat, *Pharmacol. Rev.* **34**, 23 (1982). The important contributions of Susumu Tonegawa to these developments are summarized in the report of his Nobel prize award, *Science* **238**, 484 (1987).

91. M. Potter, *Adv. Immunol.* **25**, 141 (1977); P. Leder, E. E. Max, and J. G. Seidman, *Prog. Immunol.* **4**, 34 (1980).

92. The role of repertoire size in the decline of Ehrlich's side-chain theory and in the stimulation of instructionist theories is discussed in Chapter 4.

93. J. K. Inman, in *Theoretical Immunology* (G. I. Bell, A. S. Perelson, and G. H. Pimbly, Jr., eds.), p. 243. Dekker, New York, 1978.

94. N. H. Sigal and N. R. Klinman, *Adv. Immunol.* **26**, 255 (1978).

95. H. W. Kreth and A. R. Williamson, *Eur. J. Immunol.* **3**, 141 (1973); J. R. L. Pink and B. Askonas, *Eur. J. Immunol.* **4**, 426 (1974). See also G. Köhler, *Eur. J. Immuno.* **6**, 340 (1976)

96. N. R. Klinman, *J. Exp. Med.* **136**, 241 (1972); J. L. Press and N. R. Klinman, *Eur. J. Immunol.* **4**, 155 (1974); G. J. V. Nossal, J. W. Stocker, B. Pike, and J. W. Goding, *Cold Spring Harbor Symp. Quant. Biol.* **41**, 237 (1977).

97. The degeneracy of the immune response is perhaps best pointed up by the reports of J. Sharon, E. A. Kabat, and S. L. Morrison, [*Mol. Immunol.* **18**, 831 (1981); **19**, 375, 389 (1982)] on 12 hybridomas to $\alpha 1 \rightarrow 6$ dextran, no two of

which are identical with respect to idiotypic specificity, binding affinity, or moiety of the antigenic determinant with which they interact.

98. L. Du Pasquier, *Curr. Top. Microbiol. Immunol.* **61**, 37 (1973). See also H. N. Eisen, *Progress in Immunology,* p. 243. Academic Press, New York, 1971.

99. See ref. 14. See also F. F. Richards and W. H. Konigsberg, *Immunochemistry* **10**, 545 (1973); F. F. Richards, W. H. Konigsberg, R. W. Rosenstein, and J. M. Varga, *Science* **187**, 130 (1975); J. A. Berzofsky and A. N. Schechter, *Mol. Immunol.* **18**, 751 (1981).

100. H. N. Eisen, M. C. Michaelides, B. J. Underdown, E. P. Schulenberg, and E. S. Simms, *Fed. Proc.* **29**, 78 (1970).

101. D. Schubert, A. Jobe, and M. Cohn, *Nature (London)* **200**, 882 (1968).

102. H. Metzger, *Proc. Natl. Acad. Sci. USA* **57**, 1470 (1967); N. S. Otchin and H. Metzger, *J. Biol. Chem.* **246**, 7051 (1971).

103. A. N. Glazer, *Proc. Natl. Acad. Sci. USA* **65**, 1057 (1970).

104. Reference 17.

105. See, e.g., M. Cohn, *Prog. Immunol.* **2**(2), 261 (1974).

106. W. J. Dreyer and J. C. Bennett, *Proc. Natl. Acad. Sci. USA* **54**, 864 (1965); L. Hood and D. W. Talmage, *Science* **168**, 325 (1970). See also A. J. Cunningham, ed., *The Generation of Antibody Diversity.* Academic Press, New York, 1976.

107. M. Potter, *Adv. Immunol.* **25**, 141 (1977); P. Leder, E. E. Max, and J. G. Seidman, *Prog. Immunol.* **4**, 34 (1980); E. A. Kabat, *Pharmacol. Rev.* **34**, 23 (1982).

108. E. Mayr, *The Growth of Biological Thought.* Harvard University Press, Cambridge, Massachusetts, 1982.

109. D. T. Fearon, *Crit. Rev. Immunol.* **1**, 1 (1979); H. J. Müller-Eberhard and R. D. Schreiber, *Adv. Immunol.* **29**, 1 (1980).

110. Kabat *et al.,* ref. 34; Dayhoff, ref. 34.

111. R. L. Hill, H. E. Lebowitz, R. E. Fellows, and R. Delaney, in *Gamma Globulin Structure and Control of Biosynthesis* (J. Killander, ed.). Almqvist & Wiksells, Stockholm, 1967; H. M. Grey, *Adv. Immunol.* **10**, 51 (1969); L. Hood, J. H. Campbell, and S. C. R. Elgin, *Annu. Rev. Genet.* **9**, 305 (1975). For a more general discussion of the gene duplication mechanism, see S. Ohno, *Evolution by Gene Duplication.* Springer, New York, 1970.

112. P. A. Peterson, B. A. Cunningham, I. Berggard, and G. M. Edelman, *Proc. Natl. Acad. Sci. USA* **69**, 1697 (1972); M. D. Poulik, *Prog. Clin. Biol. Res.* **5**, 155 (1976).

113. D. H. Katz. *Adv. Immunol.* **29**, 137 (1980). A possible evolutionary precursor of the vertebrate major histocompatibility complex is discussed by V. L. Scofield, J. M. Schlumpberger, L. A. West, and I. L. Weissman, *Nature (London)* **295**, 499 (1982). Edelman and co-workers suggest that Igs may derive from primitive cell adhesion molecules; see B. A. Cunningham *et al., Science* **236**, 799 (1987); G. M. Edelman, CAMS and Igs: Cell adhesion and the evolutionary origins of immunity. *Immunol. Rev.* **100**, 11 (1987).

114. S.Ohno, *Perspect. Biol. Med.* **19**, 527 (1976); *Prog. Immunol.* **4**, 577 (1980). See also M. Cohn, R. Langman, and W. Geckeler *Prog. Immunol.* **4**, 153 (1980).

115. M. Simonsen, *Acta Pathol. Microbiol. Scand.* **40,** 480 (1967); D. B. Wilson and P. C. Nowell, *J. Exp. Med.* **131,** 391 (1970).

116. N. K. Jerne, *Eur. J. Immunol.* **1,** 1 (1971).

117. The suggestion has also been made [L. Thomas in *Cellular and Humoral Aspects of Hypersensitivity States* (H. S. Lawrence, ed.). Hoeber, New York, 1959] that the evolutionary significance of the vertebrate immunological apparatus is not so much to protect against *exo*genous pathogens as to mount a surveillance against *endo*genous tumor formation. This proposal was explored at length in R. T. Smith and M. Landy, eds., *Immune Surveillance.* Academic Press, New York, 1970; and in *Transplant. Rev.* **28** (1976).

118. Among the many remarkable genetic mechanisms associated with the immune response, we have thus far not mentioned yet another that is important to an understanding of immunological specificity. The utilization of immuno-globulin genes is characterized also by allelic exclusion, which permits only one (paternal or maternal) chromosomal allele to be transcribed within a given cell. Whatever the molecular basis for this phenomenon [see Leder *et al., Prog. Immunol.* **4,** 34 (1980)], without it most antibodies might be *heteroligating* and inefficient, with two different specificities on a single Ig molecule.

119. R. Mage, *Contemp. Top. Mol. Immunol.* **8,** 89 (1981). See also *Ann. Immunol.* *(Paris)* **130C,** (1979).

120. G. M. Edelman and J. A. Gally, in *The Neurosciences: Second Study Program* (F. O. Schmitt, ed.), p. 962. Rockefeller University Press, New York, 1971.

121. D. Baltimore, *Cell (Cambridge, Mass.)* **24,** 592 (1981). See also R. Egel, *Nature (London)* **290,** 191 (1981).

122. N. K. Jerne, in ref. 82, p. 591.

7

Horror Autotoxicus: The Concept of Autoimmunity

*It would be exceedingly dysteleologic, if in
this situation self-poisons, autotoxins, were
formed.*
—Paul Ehrlich

WHEN PAUL Ehrlich speculated in 1901 about
whether an individual is able to produce toxic autoantibodies and about the implications of such antibodies for disease,[1] it
might almost have appeared that he was making one of those alogical
conceptual leaps into the unknown that occasionally accelerate the
normally slow pace of science. A closer examination of contemporary
ideas, however, reveals that this new concept was the eminently logical
result of the convergence of three historically important trends:[2] the
two-thousand-year-old tradition of Greek humoral medicine; the
century-old developments in the new (but not yet so-named) pathophysiology; and more recent developments in the new sciences of bacteriology and immunology. If the implacably logical Ehrlich (see Chapter 10)
was at all out of step with his times, it was with the concept of *horror
autotoxicus* itself.

The teachings of Hippocrates and Galen held that disease results from
dysfunctions of the four humors, usually instigated by external (and
often demonic) factors.[3] While not then expressed in such modern
terms, it is apparent that normal bodily functions might be disturbed,
leading to quantitative changes in the humors (too much or too little) or
to qualitative changes (a "sharp" humor), with resulting disease. With
the advent of a more scientific medicine, these ancient concepts were
translated in the nineteenth century by John Brown and François
Broussais into a new physiological concept of health and disease, in

which disease was defined as a disturbance of normal (and now presumably identifiable) physiological processes.[4] Claude Bernard's famous 1865 book, *Introduction to the Study of Experimental Medicine,* became the classic exposition of this new pathophysiology,[5] which held that disease is essentially a *functio laesa,* i.e., one of the patient's inherent bodily processes in a state of disorder.

It was this pervasive nineteenth-century view of the close relationship of the normal and the pathological, strongly supported by August Compte's positivist philosophy of biology,[6] that lent support to the notion that just as altered normal bodily functions might cause disease, so they might be recruited to fight disease as well. Thus, Elie Metchnikoff was able to invoke the normal digestive functions of phagocytes in his cellular theory of immunity to infectious diseases, and Paul Ehrlich proposed that antibodies are normal cell receptors with *preassigned* functions in the bodily economy.

The next step in this conceptual progression came from the young field of bacteriology. With the triumph of the germ theory of disease, thanks to Pasteur and Koch, it was held initially that bacterial toxins (rather than the organisms acting directly) were the major offenders, a view reinforced by the identification of diphtheria and tetanus toxins. Not only were such toxins elaborated directly by pathogenic organisms, but they might also result from the action of even saprophytic bacteria on normal bodily elements, leading to the formation of a variety of noxious ptomaines and so-called toxalbumins. This notion led Charles Jacques Bouchard to advance a theory of autointoxication in 1886.[7] He proposed that toxic products arising most usually in the intestinal tract from otherwise normal digestive processes (or occasionally interstitially from the action of cellular metabolism) could produce a variety of different diseases. It is remarkable how popular the notion of autointoxication became in the 25 years prior to the First World War. Hundreds of papers were written on the implications of autointoxication for one or another disease process or organ system, and extensive reviews were published on the implication of autointoxication for medical specialties such as ophthalmology, pediatrics, and internal medicine.[8] To cite but a single case, autointoxication from colonic stasis was deemed so important that great numbers of surgical procedures for colon bypass or colectomy were performed for indications ranging from lassitude to epilepsy![9] Even Metchnikoff developed a fascination for the intestinal tract and its imperfections, for the treatment of which he advocated yogurt. Indeed, he was instrumental in popularizing yogurt in the Western world.[10]

It was thus at almost the height of general interest in so-called autointoxication and after it had been shown, primarily at the Institut Pasteur in Paris, that toxic antibodies (cytotoxins) could be formed against a variety of cells in the body[11] that Paul Ehrlich considered the question of autotoxic antibodies. Given the prevailing views, it is not surprising that he would speculate on the possibilities that antibodies against self might account for yet another kind of autointoxication. What is surprising is that he should conclude, in the face of a general contemporary belief in so many other forms of autointoxication (of which he should have been aware), that the production of toxic autoantibodies was "dysteleologic in the extreme."[12] Why postulate an immunological *horror autotoxicus* in quite absolute terms when no such horror appeared to exist in other physiological processes?

The Real Meaning of *Horror Autotoxicus*

As I noted in Chapter 4, Ehrlich's side-chain theory of antibody formation viewed the antibody, not as a unique attribute of the immune apparatus, but as part of a larger physiological system of cell receptors. While some of these receptors might function as antibodies to neutralize bacterial toxins, others served to promote drug action, to assimilate the nutrients required by cells, or even to aid in the breakdown and elimination of both foreign bacteria and native effete cells. When Bordet showed that anti-erythrocyte antibodies could mediate immune hemolysis[13] and cytotoxic antibodies against a variety of other cell types were demonstrated, it was but a simple and logical step to imagine that *self*-produced hemolytic antibodies might assist in the normal destruction of worn-out erythrocytes. But an intensive search for such hemolytic autoantibodies carried out by injecting animals with their own blood and that of other members of their species led only to the formation of isoantibodies, and never to autoantibodies. It was only then that Ehrlich concluded that either autoantibody formation does not occur because the appropriate receptors do not exist in the individual or, more probably, that they may be formed but are inhibited in their toxic action. As Ehrlich put it:

> the organism possesses certain contrivances by means of which the immunity reaction, so easily produced by all kinds of cells, is prevented from acting against the organism's own elements and so giving rise to autotoxins . . . so that we might be justified in speaking of a "horror autotoxicus" of the organism. These contrivances are naturally of the highest importance for the individual.[14]

Here is the true meaning of Ehrlich's *horror autotoxicus*, as Dietlinde Goltz makes abundantly clear in her treatise on this subject.[15] Ehrlich's dictum of *horror autotoxicus* makes no claim that autoantibodies may not be formed; it only suggests that *they are somehow prevented from acting.* As Goltz pointed out, several generations of immunologists have misunderstood Ehrlich, to the detriment of progress in the science of autoimmune diseases. An interesting case in point is that of Ernest Witebsky, a "second generation Ehrlichite" (by way of Ehrlich's student and Witebsky's teacher Hans Sachs). When Witebsky and his students discovered thyroid autoantibodies in experimental thyroiditis animals in the early 1950s, Witebsky (as a fervent adherent of the Ehrlich theories) refused for some time even to believe his own data.[16] He actually withheld publication of the results for over three years, while the experiments were repeated and reexamined to find the error that had produced data in such apparent contravention of Ehrlich's rule.[17]

One can be fairly certain that Ehrlich did not intend with the phrase *horror autotoxicus* to prohibit all autoantibody formation. When Serge Metalnikoff in Metchnikoff's laboratory produced autoantispermatozoa,[18] Ehrlich did not object to the antibodies themselves but argued that they were not autocytotoxins "within our meaning," since they did not function to destroy spermatozoa in their normal *in vivo* location.[19] But how then did Ehrlich picture the putative "regulatory contrivances" that would inhibit the development of autoimmune diseases? For a while, when it seemed that autoanti-antibodies (what would later be called anti-idiotypes) were produced with great facility, Ehrlich (along with Besredka in Paris) conceived of a steady-state immunoregulation provided by the balanced production of autoantibodies and their neutralizing anti-antibodies. (This fascinating interlude, a long-forgotten forerunner of modern theories of idiotype–anti-idiotype network immunoregulation, will be discussed in greater detail in Chapter 10). But belief in the existence of autoanti-antibodies was short lived in the early twentieth century, and the search for the theoretical basis of such regulatory mechanisms was left to a later generation of immunologists.

The Classical Period of Autoimmunity Research

Despite the teleological appeal of Ehrlich's *horror autotoxicus,* the first decade of the twentieth century witnessed an ever-increasing willingness to speculate that autoantibodies might contribute to the pathogenesis of certain diseases. This movement was especially notable among investigators such as Landsteiner in Vienna and Weil in Prague who did not accept Ehrlich's teachings as gospel, but it was detectable even among the faithful. It appears to have been based primarily upon observations made in two different experimental areas, each of which contributed

importantly to the intellectual environment that favored such speculation.

The first set of observations, as previously noted, involved the
demonstration that hetero- and even isoantibodies (cytotoxins) could be
obtained against almost any organ or cell type one chose to inject into the
experimental animal. Many investigators turned to this diverting pas-
time during the next decade, and few were the tissue types that were not
put to this test, as was witnessed by the many reviews that were published
on this subject.[20] To many, it seemed but a short step from an
isoantibody to an autoantibody, and even though Metalnikov's autoantispermatozoa were only cytotoxic *in vitro* and did not cause obvious
disease in the experimental subject, they appeared to point in the same
direction.

The second and perhaps even more significant contribution to this
speculative environment came with the succession of discoveries that
antibodies (or something remarkably similar) could in fact produce
disease. In 1902, Portier and Richet discovered anaphylaxis;[21] in 1903,
Arthus discovered the phenomenon named after him;[22] and in 1906,
von Pirquet and Schick described and analyzed serum sickness.[23] Even
though there was a general disinclination to identify these reactions with
the same mechanisms that produced protective antitoxins and antibacterial immunity—hence the special term *allergy*, or altered reactivity—
yet there was more than a hint that the mechanisms that protected from
a disease and those that led to a disease were somehow interrelated.
Anaphylaxis became thenceforth a sort of passkey to the study of disease
causation, especially among clinicians interested in explaining the pathogenesis of their particular subspecialty group of interesting diseases.[24]
Where exogenous factors that might serve as inciting antigens were not
immediately apparent, it was only a short step to the conclusion that
endogenous antigens and "autoanaphylactic responses" might hold
the key.

PAROXYSMAL COLD HEMOGLOBINURIA (PKH)

The details of the discovery by Julius Donath and Karl Landsteiner[25] in
1904 of the mechanism responsible for this rare hemolytic disease will be
covered more fully in the next chapter, since it illustrates other important sociological and linguistic aspects of immunological science. Suffice
it to say here, in the context of autoimmunity, that these authors may be
credited with the discovery of the first human disease based upon an
autoimmune pathogenesis. In carefully controlled experiments, they
showed that there exists in the blood of PKH patients an autoantibody of

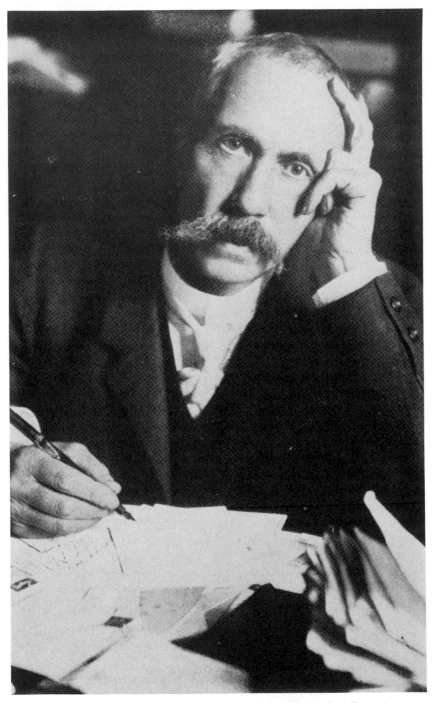

Charles Richet (Courtesy University of Wisconsin Library)

a special type, one that combines with its specific antigen on the surface of the patient's own erythrocytes only in the cold. Rewarming of the erythrocyte–antibody complex is required before complement is able to participate, to effect the immune hemolysis of the now-sensitizied cell. All of the clinical symptoms were explicable in terms of these autoimmune events: the "cold" because of the special characteristics of this peculiar antibody; the "paroxysmal" because it occurred suddenly after exposure of the patient's extremities to the cold; and the "hemoglobinuria" as a consequence of the sudden release of so much hemoglobin following intravascular hemolysis. Here was a useful precedent for an autoimmune disease, which even Ehrlich and his followers could not gainsay, despite its incompatibility with the rule of *horror autotoxicus*. This finding in PKH would ease the way for later speculations on the autoimmune nature of other disease entities.

THE WASSERMANN ANTIBODY

Not long after Bordet and Gengou showed that *any* antigen–antibody interaction could be measured by the nonspecific uptake of complement,[26] it occurred to numerous investigators that here was a useful method for the detection either of antigen with a known antibody[27] or of specific antibody with the appropriate antigen. Wassermann and Bruck,[28] and Citron[29] independently, showed that bacterial extracts could be successfully substituted for whole bacteria in these reactions, and it was demonstrated that complement fixation could be applied to the serodiagnosis of tuberculosis, using various tuberculin preparations as antigen. The recent isolation of *Spirochaeta pallida*[30] had stimulated numerous studies on experimental syphilis, and Wassermann and his colleagues quickly realized that here was an important serodiagnostic application of the complement fixation test. But since the spirochete could not be cultured, Wassermann, Neisser, and Bruck[31] utilized extracts of the organs of syphilitic humans as antigen and showed that the sera of syphilitic monkeys would yield positive results. Shortly thereafter the same authors, with Schucht[32] (and, independently, Detré[32]) extended this method to the diagnosis of syphilis in human beings. These and many other investigations very quickly showed that syphilis might be more-or-less reliably diagnosed by testing the blood and even the cerebrospinal fluid of infected individuals.

The history of the Wassermann reaction, including its acceptance by the scientific community, was the object of a very detailed study by the Polish serologist Ludwik Fleck in his 1935 book, *Genesis and Development of a Scientific Fact*.[34] Fleck's thesis, which has attracted much recent

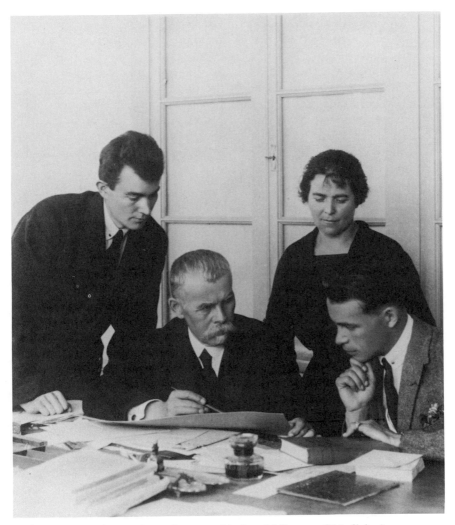

Maurice Arthus (Courtesy National Library of Medicine)

attention from sociologists and epistemologists of science,[35] was that the directions of research are generally determined by the body of contemporary views held by a *Denkkollektiv,* that group of intellectual leaders in the field whose views establish what Thomas Kuhn would later call the reigning paradigm. Furthermore, even a scientific "fact," according to Fleck, does not actually become one until it is accepted by and integrated within the normative science of the day. [In an interesting aside on scientific revisionism, Fleck called attention to a lecture by Wassermann in 1920, in which the latter claimed sole title to the discovery of the "Wassermann" reaction (called by the French the Bordet–Wassermann reaction) and egregiously revised the history of its development. These claims were quickly challenged by Wassermann's former student Carl Bruck and by Wassermann's long-time opponent from Prague, E. Weil; and there ensued a series of exchanges among the three that was both vituperative and *ad hominem*[36]].

Many investigators were attracted by the new serodiagnostic test for syphilis, and the next few years saw many modifications and improvements that rendered the test both more specific and more sensitive. But the most curious new observation revealed that extracts of syphilis-infected organs were not actually required for positive results—extracts of *normal* organs would function as combining antigen just as well.[37] This finding was extremely perplexing, since all previous experience indicated that only *specific* antigen could interact with antibody to fix complement and yield a positive diagnostic test. If the antigen in these extracts was not of spirochetal origin, then what was it, and why should it have stimulated antibody formation in the syphilitic individual?

It was not long before Weil and Braun offered a possible explanation, entirely consistent with earlier speculations on the broad biological functions of antibody. Infection with *Treponema pallidum* induces tissue breakdown in the affected organs, claimed these authors, and the antibodies circulating in syphilitic patients are in fact autoantibodies specific for the breakdown products! This explanation would account also, they held, for the "false positive" cross-reactions seen in diseases such as malaria and leprosy, where analogous tissue breakdown also occurred. Indeed, they claimed that such autoantibodies would exacerbate the disease:

> When the very tissue destruction which follows the first infection has led to antibody formation, so it will during the further course of its formation be generally directed not only against the material formed from damaged cells, but also against [normal] human cell substances . . . thus these autoantibodies attack the cells to liberate antigen, which is able to evoke further autoantibody formation. Should the newly formed protein possess

toxicity for the organism, then will the antibody contribute to enhance this toxicity.[38]

In an interesting extension of this provocative speculation, Weil and Braun also considered the possibility that paresis, one of the more prominent symptoms of tertiary syphilis, might be attributed to the same pathogenetic process. Should the infection spread to the brain and there cause analogous cell breakdown, then autoantibodies to neuroantigens might further attack and destroy the normal cells of the brain, thus accounting for the progression of the neurological complications of syphilis. But even as they advanced 'this hypothesis, they cautiously suggested that it might be better to reject it as too hypothetical, "because specificity has not yet been demonstrated."[39]

Now, 80 years later, an acceptable explanation for the presence of these serodiagnostic antibodies in syphilis (which have been shown to differ from those that react specifically with known treponemal antigens) is still awaited. The antigen active in complement fixation tests for syphilis was quickly shown to be a lipid and later was purified and named cardiolipin, but the origin of the antibodies from syphilitic patients with which it reacts is still a mystery. Modern science has not gone much further in this respect than Weil in 1907, who concluded that "the facts seem rather to speak to the view that the complement-binding material [antibody] is the consequence and not the cause of [the disease]."

AUTOIMMUNITY TO LENS PROTEINS

In his contribution to the festschrift in 1903 honoring the sixtieth birthday of Robert Koch, Paul Uhlenhuth opened up a new chapter in immunological research by demonstrating the organ specificity of the proteins of the lens of the eye.[40] This was the first clear demonstration, not only that unique antigens might exist within a single organ and nowhere else in the body, but also that these antigens might be shared from species to species. Here was a finding whose implications would fascinate both clinicians interested in ocular diseases as well as generations of immunopathologists searching for the underlying basis of autoimmune disease. Over the next few years, Uhlenhuth's report was confirmed in a number of different laboratories and extended in several provocative directions. First, Kraus and co-workers[41] showed that these organ-specific lens antigens can induce both active and passive anaphylaxis in experimental animals, a finding quickly confirmed by Andrejew.[42] Then Uhlenhuth and Haendel[43] showed that a guinea pig could be rendered sensitive to its *own* lens protein and sent into anaphylactic shock with the protein from any other lens. But these authors made no further comment on the possible clinical significance of this phenomenon, although the ophthalmologist P. Römer had earlier speculated that the pathogenesis of senile cataract formation might possibly involve the production of autocytotoxins.[44] It remained for the ophthalmologist F. F. Krusius to perform the critical experiment relating lens anaphylaxis to an actual ocular disease, by showing that the experimental rupture of the lens capsule in a *normal* guinea pig could not only actively sensitize the animal but also function as the antigenic challenge of the "anaphylactic" state, with resulting ocular disease.[45] All of these data were reevaluated, and their implications considered in a lengthy review of the field by Römer and Gebb in 1912. In a separate section "on the question of the formation of autoanaphylactic antibodies by means of lens proteins," these authors asked whether autologous lens can actually be characterized as *foreign* in the guinea pig, or "whether the 'law of immunity research,' which Ehrlich has popularly termed horror autotoxicus, does not rather apply to the lens."[46]

The first part of this question is an interesting one. Here, as early as 1912, is a preview of what would later be called the "sequestered antigen" theory. If indeed the body cannot respond immunologically to "self," then *ipso facto* such antigens as do stimulate the immune response must be foreign, i.e., somehow sequestered from the immunological apparatus of the host. But Römer and Gebb did not yet misunderstand Ehrlich's rule of horror autotoxicus as future investigators would, as is made clear by the way that they interpreted Ehrlich's law. In a further elaboration of this understanding, they state that "we shall by no means assert that the homologous [read autologous] lens protein fails in all circumstances with respect to the formation of these anaphylactic autoantibodies. We are rather convinced that the regulatory mechanism of the organism can and will refuse to serve under special conditions. And the investigation of these situations will further promote our understanding of pathological states."[47]

This statement clearly advances Ehrlich's original proposition by a significant step forward. Ehrlich was willing to permit the formation of autoantibodies, but he invoked an immunoregulatory process to inhibit their deleterious reactions. Now, in the light of these more recent experiments, Römer and Gebb can conceive of a *failure* of these regulatory mechanisms, with consequent autoimmune disease.[48]

SYMPATHETIC OPHTHALMIA

Sympathetic ophthalmia is a blinding disease that has long fascinated ophthalmologists, because of its curious sequence of clinical events.

Sometimes long after a penetrating injury to the eye, that eye may suddenly become inflamed, a response accompanied by a spontaneous involvement of the contralateral eye. It has variously been speculated that bacteria, fungi, and viruses (depending upon the current vogue) might provide the etiological triggers for these events. When, after the turn of the century, anaphylaxis captured the attention of medical researchers, it was quickly called upon to help to explain sympathetic ophthalmia as well.

It was the Italian Santucci who in 1907 first drew attention to the fact that sympathetic ophthalmia might be due to the formation of cytotoxins (autoantibodies) following resorption of damaged ocular tissue in the first eye, which could then attack and cause disease in the hitherto normal fellow eye.[49] This conjecture was accompanied by experiments showing that injection of emulsified ocular tissues into rabbits and guinea pigs would produce endophthalmitis. Scarcely had this thesis begun to attract attention when a counterclaim for priority was submitted from Russia under the title "Hypothesis of the Autocytotoxic Origin of Eye Diseases."[50] In this, S. Golowin complained that no one in the West appeared to be aware of the fact that as early as 1904 he had published his theory in a Russian journal.[51] "Soon after the appearance of the work of Bordet and others, it occurred to me to propose a new hypothesis for the still enigmatic pathogenesis of sympathetic ophthalmia, with the help of the doctrines of cytotoxins." He suggested that lesions of the ciliary body lead to the release of antigens and to the formation of autocytotoxins, which circulate and act specifically on the iris and ciliary epithelium of the fellow eye to cause inflammatory disease. Golowin named these autoantibodies *cyclotoxins.*

Now enters the ophthalmologist Elschnig from Prague (later to become perhaps the foremost academic ophthalmologist of his day). Elschnig soon became the leading exponent of an autoimmune pathogenesis of sympathetic ophthalmia; and he published a series of papers on this subject.[52] In the first of these, while acknowledging Golowin and Santucci, he implied that it was rather "the idea of Professor Weil on the origin of sympathetic ophthalmia that calls absolutely for further studies." Weil, one of the most active workers in immunology during that period, apparently served as Elschnig's immunological mentor in these studies, and together they formulated the hypothesis that as a result of the resorption of antigen in the damaged uveal tissue, there develops a hypersensitivity (one of the earliest uses of this term) in the organism, and especially in the homologous organ, the second eye. This response leads to a heightened ability to react, so that the slightest disturbance in the sensitized second eye leads to inflammation with serious consequences. Elschnig performed numerous experiments in animals to test this theory, and eventually he identified the pigment so abundantly present in the pigment epithelial cells of the iris and ciliary body as the antigenic culprit.

GENERAL OBSERVATIONS ON THIS PERIOD

The preceding examples, while they might soon fade from the view of mainstream immunology, permit one to draw some interesting conclusions about the immunological practices and the immunological beliefs extant in the decades preceding the First World War. First, it was clearly a Golden Age of immunological and immunopathological research, during which time the groundwork was laid for many later immunological subspeciality areas. Second, it is clear that Ehrlich's theories held great sway (especially outside France) and that the concept of *horror autotoxicus* was not misunderstood then, as it would be later. Finally, the concepts of anaphylaxis and cytotoxins were extremely attractive to experimental pathologists and were in the forefront of the candidates nominated to explain the pathogenesis of almost any disease then poorly understood.

The Dark Ages of Autoimmunity Research

I have noted how the 15 years immediately preceding the First World War witnessed an expansion of the young field of immunology into many interesting and fruitful areas of research. There was, at the same time, a flurry of interest in anaphylaxis and related mechanisms of disease and a no less intense interest in the production and possible functions of autoantibodies. "Basic" scientists were interested then as now in what autoantibodies might tell them about the processes underlying the immune response, while clinicians were interested in their implications for disease pathogenesis. But interest in autoantibodies and autoimmune diseases very rapidly slowed and then ceased within the mainstream of immunology, not to be resumed for another 40 years or so. Of course, not *all* activity in these areas was everywhere terminated, and all previous knowledge was not lost. Just as during the Dark Ages in Europe, this period saw that some institutions continued their scholarly pursuits, and here and there isolated individuals appeared to revive and to extend past knowledge. The study of anaphylaxis and related phenomena passed, in the main, into the hands of clinical allergists (see Chapter 9); clinical ophthalmologists maintained an interest in the pathogenesis of sympathetic ophthalmia and of endophthalmitis phacoanaphylactica; and the occasional experimental pathologist or immunochemist might publish a sporadic study on autoimmune encephalitis, on the meaning of the Wassermann antibody, or on the autoantigens of the thyroid. It was evident, however, that the earlier continuity and interconnections of immunological and biomedical thought had substantially waned between the two World Wars. What was accomplished in the immunological study of disease during this period received little consistent attention from immunological leaders interested in other problems.

How can one account for this 40-year-long hiatus? The disruptions that accompanied and followed the 1914–1918 war surely contributed substantially to the lapse. Defeated Germany, formerly the leader in the field, went into eclipse in the biomedical sciences. Paul Ehrlich died in 1915, and no one took his place to maintain the tradition. In Austria, conditions were just as bad; Karl Landsteiner lost his position and was forced to emigrate to the United States to carry on his work. Even in victorious France, immunology went into decline. With the death of Metchnikoff in 1916, even the Pasteur Institute seemed to give up its long and glorious tradition of leadership in theoretical and experimental immunology. The war had caused the center of gravity of scientific research to shift from Europe to America, although even there little attention was paid to fundamental biomedical studies in immunology.

It is of interest that the slowdown in immunological activity between the two World Wars was not part of a more general phenomenon suffered by *all* biomedical research fields. Significant advances continued to be made in endocrinology and other physiological pursuits, in genetics, and in virology. In biochemistry, the 1920s and 1930s were the halcyon years of nutrition and vitamin research. Even within immunology, immunochemistry continued its productive course, in the hands of Landsteiner, Heidelberger, Marrack, Pauling, Boyd, and many others. Here perhaps is one of the important clues to the decline of interest in autoimmunity. During its first 30 years, immunology had primarily been the domain of biologically and medically oriented individuals who were interested in its implications for disease prevention and disease causation. With the exhaustion of the search for vaccines against the most important pathogens, and especially with the decline of the phagocytic theory of immunity at the hand of the more readily available and manipulable circulating antibody, biologists were replaced by chemists at the leading edge of immunological research (see Chapter 3). These investigators focused their attention on the molecule rather than on the whole organism. They were more interested in the size, shape, and structure of the antibody than in its possible role in the pathogenesis of disease. Thus, the conceptual foundations of the new *Denkkollectiv* were markedly different from those of the old one, and the guidelines for research and for conceptual advance that accompanied this change were markedly different. This shift is well illustrated not only by the types of study deemed worthy of pursuit and worthy of publication in journals of immunology but also by how immunological phenomena were being interpreted. As I noted in Chapter 4, this was the era of instructionist theories of antibody formation—theories that Macfarlane Burnet would later criticize as being too chemically oriented and too neglectful of biological phenomenon and biological realities.

It is no wonder, then, that interest in autoimmune diseases waned during the period between the wars. This may be best appreciated by an examination of Table 7.1, in which are listed for each organ or disease entity the date of the last significant contribution during the "classical"

Table 7.1: **The Dark Ages of Autoimmunity**

Disease/System	Last "classical" contribution	First "modern" contribution
Hemolytic disease	1909	1945: Coombs et al.[a]
Sperm and testicular	1900	1951: Voisin[b]
Encephalomyelitis	1905	1947: Kabat et al.[c]
Sympathetic ophthalmia	1912	1953: Collins[d]
Phacoanaphylaxis	1911	1963: Halbert and Manski[e]
Thyroid	1910	1955: Witebsky and Rose; Roitt et al.[f]
Wassermann antibody	1909	—
Platelet disease	—	1949: Ackroyd[g]

[a] R. R. A. Coombs, A. E. Mourant, and R. R. Race, *Br. J. Exp. Pathol.* **26,** 255 (1945). For an early history of the antiglobulin test, see R. R. A. Coombs, *Am. J. Clin. Pathol.* **53,** 131 (1970). It is interesting that Moreschi in 1908 had described the same phenomenon as the Coombs antiglobulin test [C. Moreschi, *Zentralbl. Bakteriol.* **46,** 51 (1908)], a finding forgotten in the interval. I might have listed here the work of Dameshek and Schwartz in 1938,[53] although they only hinted at *auto*hemolysins. But they were heard at the time only by fellow hematologists. The antiglobulin "Coombs test" is perhaps a better landmark, even though it involved at first only the detection of Rh *iso*antibodies in erythroblastosis fetalis. Its use very quickly showed autoantibodies in acquired hemolytic anemias, an observation of which the immunological community was now fully aware.
[b] G. Voisin, A. Delaunay, and M. Barber, *Ann. Inst. Pasteur, Paris* **81,** 48 (1951). Important contributions to this field were also made by J. Freund, M. M. Lipton, and G. E. Thompson, *J. Exp. Med.* **97,** 711 (1953).
[c] E. A. Kabat, A. Wolfe, and A. E. Bezer, *J. Exp. Med.* **85,** 117 (1947); **89,** 395 (1949).
[d] R. C. Collins, *Am. J. Ophthalmol.* **36** (Part II), 150 (1953).
[e] S. P. Halbert and W. Manski, *Prog. Allergy* **7,** 107 (1963).
[f] E. Witebsky and N. R. Rose, *J. Immunol.* **76,** 408 (1955); I. M. Roitt, D. Doniach, P. N. Campbell, and R. Vaughan-Hudson, *Lancet* **ii,** 820 (1956).
[g] J. F. Ackroyd, *Clin. Sci.* **8,** 269 (1949).

period, and of the first significant contribution during the "modern" era. For those systems for which both starting and ending dates are available, the average interlude is 44 years! This is a long period in a field whose total life span to the time of this writing numbers scarcely more than 100 years.

As might be expected, interest in autoimmune disease was not completely extinguished during the interim. The ophthalmologists Verhoeff and Lemoine examined clinical cases of lens-induced ocular inflammation and coined the term phacoanaphylactic endophthalmitis in 1922;[54] and other ophthalmologists extended the study of retinal pigment as the autoantigen responsible for sympathetic ophthalmia.[55] In 1933 the experimental pathologist Rivers created the model of experimental allergic encephalomyelitis[56] that would later be exploited so productively by other workers. In the 1920s also, the immunologist Ludvig Hektoen and co-workers did careful studies on the autoantigenicity of thyroid antigens.[57] These latter investigators, however, were not interested in disease; rather, they utilized thyroid proteins to study species interrelationships by means of antigenic cross-reactions, in the tradition of Nuttall (see ref. 27). One of the more unique curiosities of the time was the attempt to utilize autoimmunity for beneficial purposes. A number of efforts were made to utilize sperm antigens in antifertility vaccines,[58] a subject that has recently been revitalized.[59]

Such sporadic investigations as occurred during this interbellum period were, as I have mentioned, out of touch with most contemporary immunological activity. They went substantially unremarked, if they were even seen, by the immunological leaders of the day. The same situation appears to have been true of the early stirrings of activity in experimental immunopathology, by investigators such as Louis Dienes, Jones and Mote, Simon and Rackemann, and Arnold Rich, as noted in Chapters 3 and 9. It required the biological sea-change in concept that followed the Second World War to attract interest once again in the biological and medical aspects of immunology and thus in the autoimmune diseases, i.e., the establishment of a new *Denkkollektiv* and a new paradigm.

The Modern Period of Autoimmunity Research

CONCEPTUAL PROGRESS

In the years immediately following World War II, biological phenomena and biological reasoning penetrated the field of immunology with ever-increasing effect. This synthesis was stimulated by Medawar's work on the immunology of skin graft rejection,[60] by reports of immunological deficiency diseases,[61] by new sources of funding for biomedical research, and, equally important, by the entry into immunology of a new generation of young scientists with few ties to the old dogma. Here was a biomedical renaissance in which autoimmunity research participated. One of the key observations that stimulated thought in the latter field was that of Ray Owen on chimerism in cattle twins.[62] This author showed that dizygotic calves whose circulatory systems were connected *in utero* would show after birth not only mixtures of their erythrocyte blood types but also an inability to respond immunologically to each other's antigens. This new biological fact about immunology would demand consideration in any future concept of antibody formation and focus attention on the ability *and inability* of these mechanisms to react to self. In addition, three other events made it easier for investigators to work with and to think about autoantibodies and autoimmunity. These were (1) the Coombs test, which helped to detect such antibodies; (2) the introduction of Freund's adjuvants,[63] which substantially simplified their production; and (3) Byron Waksman's review of 1959,[64] which helped to give focus and direction to these studies. Waksman's call to arms was especially significant at the time, in that it focused attention on the role of delayed hypersensitivity mechanisms in these autoimmune phenomena, and on the importance of a careful interpretation of accompanying cytological and histopathological changes.

Immunological Tolerance. Whereas Burnet's 1941 book,[65] *The Production of Antibodies,* made no mention at all of autoimmunity or autoantibodies, this gap was rectified in his 1949 revision of the book with Frank Fenner.[66] They took note of Owen's observations; and even in the context of an instructionist theory of antibody formation (see Chapter 4), they proposed an explanation for how the immunological apparatus might distinguish between "self" and "not self." (Medawar's earlier work on graft rejection and Landsteiner's blood group story had already drawn attention to the antigenic differences among individuals of the same species.) According to Burnet and Fenner, there was established on every cell during fetal or neonatal life a set of "self markers," subsequent recognition of which would inhibit an active immune response. Any antigen present during this maturational process (such as the foreign erythrocytes of Owen's calves) would be marked "self" and thus be exempt from future autoantigenicity. These events occur even in nature, with implications for congenital infections, as Burnet and Fenner pointed out. They cited the observations of Traub during the 1930s on lymphocytic choriomeningitis (LCM) virus infection of mice;[67] fetal infection from the mother appeared to render the animal incapable of mounting an immune response to the viral antigens after birth as a result of "the development of a tolerance to the foreign microorganism during embryonic life,"[68] possibly the first use of this term in an immunological context. (Perhaps the LCM story itself should have provided the trigger for speculations on immunological tolerance during the 1930s, but the observation was apparently premature and, even if known to immunologists, would have been difficult to assimilate within the chemically oriented paradigm of the times.)

Once Burnet had called attention to them, the implications of Owen's observations were considered so important that they figured significantly in every subsequent theory of antibody formation. But it was Burnet himself who fully developed the concept of self and non-self and of immunological tolerance in his clonal selection theory of antibody formation.[69] If the potential for antibody formation is preformed in clonal precursor cells (especially if generated by somatic mutations[70]), then Burnet insisted that this process must be a random one. A mechanism should therefore exist to delete those anti-self clones that would threaten the integrity of the body. This result could be accomplished by a mechanism of "clonal deletion," in which antigen present during embryonic life would somehow cause the destruction of such dangerous self-reactive clones. Here was a thesis with obvious experimental implications, and it was quickly put to the test and validated by Billingham, Brent, and Medawar[71] (for which Burnet and Medawar shared the Nobel prize in 1960).

It may be well to recall at this point that somewhat analogous observations had been made earlier on the immune response to polysaccharide antigens. In this case, *adult* animals had been rendered immunologically unresponsive by the adminstration of large doses of these antigens,[72] while modest dosages would lead to satisfactory levels of antibody formation. The explanation proposed was that the excess antigen had somehow "clogged" the apparatus, preventing its function. The phenomenon was termed immunological paralysis, and while it appears to be related to the difficulty with which certain polysaccharides are metabolized (and thus to their long-term persistence), the phenomenon has yet to be satisfactorily explained.

The phenomenon of acquired immunological tolerance attracted much attention and experimental confirmation during the 1950s, not only at the hands of Billingham, Brent, and Medawar working with mice, but also by Milan Hašek's group in Prague, who worked with parabiotic chick embryos[73] and later by Weigle, who studied tolerance induced in neonatal rabbits.[74] The ability to induce tolerance with fairly large doses of antigen *in utero* and even during the neonatal period was abundantly confirmed, although tolerance was found in general not to be absolute but to depend upon the persistence of antigen. This finding implied not that the attainment of tolerance is a single and irreversible event, but that the state of unresponsiveness has to be actively maintained. Another indication that immunological tolerance is not absolute and qualitative but quantitatively variable came from studies (especially in the transplantation field) showing that various degrees of *partial* tolerance might exist.[75] Indeed, partial or "incomplete" tolerance to self-antigens may be the rule rather than the exception, since low levels of circulating antibody to a variety of tissue autoantigens is a fairly common finding in otherwise normal individuals.

Yet another observation that modified the view of how tolerance is induced came with the realization that the mammalian fetus may show a wide range of immunological competencies even fairly early in gestation in some species,[76] and that the induction of tolerance may require *prior* immunological competence to respond to the antigen in question, rather than taking place during an immunological "null" state. All of these new facts suggested that tolerance is not a negative state but a positive and even dynamically equilibrated regulatory mechanism.

The unraveling of the mechanism of induction of acquired immunological tolerance was further complicated by the finding that extremely *low* doses of antigen administered repeatedly to an experimental animal might also induce the unresponsiveness, even in the adult animal.[77] Here was yet another clue that tolerance may not be based upon some form of antigenic cytotoxicity directed against clonal precursors, to induce a "gap" in the immunological repertoire. (Such gaps have been experimentally produced, however, in the "immunological suicide" experiments of Ada and Byrt[78] and of Humphrey.[79] The injection of highly radioactive antigen into naive animals causes a radiation-induced death of specific clonal precursors; and the animal is incapable thereafter of mounting an antibody response against the antigenic determinants involved.) Still another observation that argued against clonal deletion was the finding that tolerance to a given antigenic determinant might be "broken" by the administration of related, cross-reactive antigens.[80]

A new era in the interpretation of the basis of immunological tolerance was ushered in by the finding that the cellular contributions to the immune response were divided among a variety of lymphocyte subsets, each with well-defined and highly specialized functions. B cells, originating in the bone marrow (and in avians, regulated by the bursa of Fabricius), are responsible for active antibody formation and provide the plasma cells, whose function Astrid Fagraeus had originally pointed out[81] and Albert Coons' fluorescent antibody immunohistochemical techniques had confirmed.[82] These cells, however, cannot act alone. They require the active intervention of macrophages to process and efficiently present the antigen to the immunocyte,[83] and of T cells (which undergo functional maturation of the thymus). Such "helper" T cells apparently interact first with antigen, to somehow provide the trigger for B cell activation.[84] The importance of the T cell receptor in recognizing self antigens was further emphasized by the finding that these cells, so important in defense against viral infections, act by responding not to virus alone but to viral antigen only when presented in the context of a self antigen (a Class II component of the major histocompatibility complex).[85]

All of these observations on the induction *and breakage* of immunological tolerance, coupled with numerous reports on clinical and experimental examples of autoimmunity (to be detailed later), forced even the doubters to concede the reality of autoimmunity. But it did more; it forced acceptance of the fact that all antibody formation, all immunological tolerance, and the presence or absence of pathological autoimmunity are the result of a complicated system of *immunoregulatory mechanisms.* Thus, Ehrlich's conjecture that *horror autotoxicus* means regulatory control of unwanted reactions against self was apparently now validated. While the microeconomics of the regulation of the cells active in the immune response would soon be assigned to a congeries of chemical signals (lymphokines, monokines, etc.), two new theories would compete to provide an explanation for the macroeconomics of immunoregulation. In an interesting replay of the old cellularist–humoralist debate in immunology (described in Chapter 3), one of these theories would be predominantly cellular in its interpretation and the other predominantly molecular. Both would attempt to explain why autoimmune disease exists at all and why it is not more common.

The Basis of Immunoregulation. The finding that B lymphocytes require the assistance of T lymphocytes in their antibody response to antigenic stimulus opened up a new avenue of research. Different subsets of T lymphocyte lineage would soon be described, each with its own distinctive set of surface membrane markers,[86] including helper cells, cytotoxic cells, and others. Many of these cell types appeared to function in the up-regulation of the immune response, but Gershon and Kondo[87] soon showed that some lymphocytes might contribute to down-regulation. These they called suppressor T cells. And, like helper T cells, these lymphocytes can be passively transferred and perform their functions in naive recipients. Indeed, Gershon and Kondo showed that the information for down-regulation of the immune response might even pass from cell to cell, and they spoke of an "infectious immunosuppression."[88] Since most of these immunoregulatory cells appeared to be antigen-specific, here was an elegant hypothesis to explain how the immune response might be modulated. Depending upon their numbers and specificities, the intercommunication of these regulatory cell types among themselves and with primary immunocyte responders would decide whether the response to a given stimulus would be high or low. In terms of autoimmunity, a "normal" balance of helpers and suppressors would hold in check the ever-present threat of embarrassing responses to self, whereas an imbalance among the cells of the regulatory system might lead to serious autoimmune disease.

An alternative theory of immunoregulation arose at about the same time, from a different direction. It was discovered that the binding site on an antibody possesses a highly distinctive three-dimensional structure (the idiotype) that might itself act as an antigenic determinant to stimulate the formation not only of heteroantibodies in another species but even of autoantibodies within the same host. With the realization that the anti-idiotype would possess a structure similar to that of the antigenic determinant (since both could interact with the same antibody combining site), and that nothing prevented the development of a cascade of anti-antibodies, anti-anti-antibodies, etc., Niels Jerne put forth a theory of immunoregulation based upon purely molecular considerations. This was his idiotype–anti-idiotype network theory,[89] in which the various levels of autoanti-idiotypes could interact with and inhibit the previous levels, thus establishing an immunoregulatory balance that would determine the extent of an immune response. (The details of this network theory will be examined more fully in Chapter 10.)

Phenomenological and Technical Progress

It is not my purpose here to provide a detailed description of each of the many diseases and syndromes that have been added to the ever-lengthening list of proved or probable autoimmune conditions. The bibliography of such findings has become too massive for this, and many useful summaries are available.[90] I hope, rather, in what follows to provide the reader with a feel for the explosion of interest and activity that has taken place in this area since the Second World War, to indicate some of the more important observations that helped to stimulate this interest, and to touch upon some of the newer directions taken by laboratory and clinical research in the autoimmune diseases.

SINGLE-ORGAN AUTOIMMUNE DISEASE

When the conceptual dam that had blocked acceptance of the fact of autoimmune disease was broken in the late 1940s and early 1950s by clinical data from the hemolytic anemias and by laboratory data from tolerance studies, there followed a flood of new findings and new experimental models. Autoimmune orchitis with aspermatogenesis was shown to be a reality,[91] as were "allergic" encephalomyelitis,[92] sympathetic ophthalmia,[93] and phacoanaphylaxis.[94] To these were added autoimmune thyroiditis,[95] adrenalitis,[96] pemphigus vulgaris[97] bullous pemphigoid,[98] and numerous others. Particularly worthy of note is the fact that the pathogenesis of some of these diseases such as the hemolytic anemias, thrombocytopenias, and pemphigoid involves uniquely the participation of circulating antibodies and presumably of complement. On the other hand, there is a group of autoimmune diseases that, while they may be accompanied by the formation of circulating antibodies, seem to require cell-mediated immune mechanisms to effect the tissue destruction seen. Among these are diseases such as allergic encephalomyelitis and autoimmune thyroid disease, in which passive transfer of the disease state to naive recipients is possible only with sensitized lymphoid cells, and not with specific antibodies.

There is another group of antibody-mediated autoimmune diseases whose elucidation promises to lend an added dimension to the concept of autoimmunity. These conditions involve the formation of autoantibodies directed at certain of the surface receptors of cells so important to their proper physiological function.[99] The role of such receptors in cell nutrition and toxicity reactions had been stressed by Paul Ehrlich; and even before him Newport Langley had suggested in 1878[100] that the opposing actions of atropine and pilocarpine or of nicotine and curare involved the competition of the two drugs for the same "receptive substance." It is now known that all biological signals mediated by hormones, neurotransmitters, and other small molecules operate by attaching to specific cell receptors. Should an autoantibody be formed against the receptor itself to compete for the site with the active molecule, then normal function may be inhibited, with resulting disease. Recent evidence suggests that this is in fact what may underlie Graves disease, involving autoantibody to the receptor for thyroid-simulating hormone (TSH);[101] myasthenia gravis, in which autoantibody to the acetylcholine receptor at the neuromuscular endplate interferes with the electrical transmissions governing muscular responses;[102] and insulin-resistant diabetes, where autoantibodies against the insulin receptors in various tissues interfere with glucose metabolism.[103] These interesting studies open new pathways to the diagnosis and therapy of a number of important human diseases.

MULTIPLE-SYSTEM AUTOIMMUNE DISEASE

There are a number of diseases of probable autoimmune pathogenesis that target not a single organ but multiple organs or organ systems throughout the body. Among these are systemic lupus erythematosus (SLE), rheumatoid arthritis, and Sjögren's syndrome. While each of these may be not so much a single disease as a group of related processes, each is characterized by a fairly well defined immunopathology. In the case of SLE, most of the symptoms can be ascribed to the presence of antinuclear autoantibodies, which account not only for the LE cell phenomenon but also for the immune complexes that cause the damage in susceptible target organs (e.g., at the dermal–epidermal junction, a reaction yielding erythematous skin rashes, or in the glomeruli, causing lupus nephritis).[104] In rheumatoid arthritis, the autoantibodies are anti-type II collagen and anti-immunoglobulins, which form immune complexes whose presence in synovial linings activates complement to induce the effusion characteristic of rheumatoid synovitis.[105] Sjögren's syndrome differs from the previous two conditions in that, while autoantibodies and hypergammaglobulinemia may be present, the lesions of the lacrimal, salivary, and other exocrine glands appear rather to be due to the effects of immunocyte (and macrophage) activation.[106]

One of the more interesting consequences of the study of these autoimmune diseases was the growing realization of the importance of genetic constitution, a finding confirmed by the strong predilection of certain inbred strains of laboratory animals (e.g., the NZB, MRL, and RCS strains of mice and the BUF and BB/W strains of rats) to develop a variety of autoimmune diseases.[107] Among these genetic influences are certain predispositions for disease, located within the major histocompatibility gene complex (MHC) at loci that code for the formation of the principal human leukocyte antigens.[108] Yet another group of immunological dysregulations appears to depend upon a set of immune-response genes at another location within the MHC.[109] These factors will be discussed at greater length in Chapter 11.

TECHNOLOGICAL ADVANCES

To the extent that most autoimmune diseases represent undesirable active responses to self antigens, it follows that they should be amenable to immunosuppressive therapy with the variety of chemotherapeutic agents that have emerged, primarily from developments in cancer chemotherapy. But other more elegant and more specific approaches to both diagnosis and therapy are in the process of development. The newer techniques of molecular biology have made available monoclonal antibodies and RNA–DNA molecular probes to identify and even to reproduce the antigenic epitopes that are the targets of the autoimmune response. This technical development offers the possibility that genetically engineered antigens may be employed therapeutically to down-regulate these dangerous responses. Alternatively, where a receptor-specific autoantibody can be identified as the cause of a disease, its (temporary) alleviation may be obtained (as in myasthenia gravis) by removing the antibody by means of plasmapheresis[110] or perhaps, eventually, specific immunosorbents.

Conclusions

With the possible exception of a Lamarckian period of interest in instructionist theories of antibody formation, most of the important conceptual threads that run through the fabric of immunology have been strongly influenced by Darwinian precepts. In his clonal selection theory of antibody formation, Macfarlane Burnet acknowledged his strong debt to Darwin, and Darwinism has more recently contributed importantly and positively to the development of theories about the evolution of the immunoglobulin apparatus and the molecular biology of its genetic underpinnings.[111] It will be obvious from the above account of the early history of autoimmunity that Darwinism exerted its influence here also, although perhaps not always with positive effect. Both Metchnikoff with his phagocytic theory and Ehrlich with his antibody theory made obeisances to Darwin, each claiming that the mechanisms he proposed were part of a larger biological system whose evolution brought with it improvements in the organism's ability to nourish itself and, incidently, to protect itself from infection. But Metchnikoff was always willing to concede that the advantages of such an evolution might be accompanied by certain disadvantages. Thus, he recognized that cellular inflammation might produce local tissue damage as well as overall benefit, and he accorded a role to the phagocyte in such deleterious aging processes as the graying of the hair, the wrinkling of the skin, and the deterioration with age of the brain and other organs. Ehrlich, for his part, seeemed to have been unwilling to concede a down-side to the Darwinian evolution of the receptor antibodies that he had proposed. His concept of *horror autotoxicus* was in fact his denial that some other biological price might be exacted for the benefits that antibodies endow upon the individual organism. It was exactly this denial, strongly reinforced by the triumph of Ehrlich's humoralist views over the cellularist notions of Metchnikoff, that made it so difficult for immunological theoreticians to accept the reality of autoimmunity for over 50 years. In spite of the Donath–Landsteiner finding of an autoantibody in paroxysmal cold hemoglobinuria and in spite of increasing evidence from clinical subspecialties of the existence of autoimmune diseases, the teleological appeal of *horror autotoxicus* (= no autoantibody) made the acceptance of the reality of autoimmune disease difficult, if not impossible. To force such an acceptance would require a conjunction of events that many different scientific disciplines eventually experience: the accumulation of a large number of observations not explicable in terms of the current dogma, and a major change in the direction of thought in the field that would allow the previously unthinkable now to be thought. In the immunology of the 1950s and 1960s, the former was represented by the many new clinical and experimental models of autoimmune disease (and of immunopathological responses in general) then being reported, while the latter reflected the shift of immunology from a chemical to a more biological discipline.

NOTES AND REFERENCES

1. P. Ehrlich, *Verh. 73 Ges. Dtsch. Naturforsch. Aerzte* (1901). [Reprinted in *The Collected Papers of Paul Ehrlich*, Vol. 2, p. 298. Pergamon, New York, 1957.]

2. Among the few discussions of the history of autoimmunity in the literature are J. M. Cruse, D. Whitcomb, and R. E. Lewis, Jr., *Concepts Immunopathol.* **1**, 32 (1985); D. Goltz, *Horror Autotoxicus. Ein Beitrag zur Geschichte und Theorie der Autoimmunpathologie im Spiegel eines vielzitierten Begriffes.* Thesis, Münster, 1980; A.-M. Moulin, Histoire du Système Immunitaire: Immunologie et Médicine (1880–1980). Thesis, University of Lyon, 1987; A. Eyquem, Arch. Inst. Pasteur, Tunis 58, 281 (1981).

3. H. E. Sigerist, *A History of Medicine*, Vol. II. Oxford University Press, New York, 1961.

4. See O. Temkin, Health and disease. In *Dictionary of the History of Ideas* (P. P. Wiener, ed.), Vol. 2, pp. 395–407. Scribner's, New York (4 vols., 1974). See also G. Canguilhem, *On the Normal and the Pathological*. Reidel, Boston, Massachusetts, 1978.

5. C. Bernard, *Introduction to the Study of Experimental Medicine* (H. C. Greene, trans.). Macmillan, New York, 1927.

6. I. A. M. F. X. Compte, *Cours de Philosophie Positive,* Vol. 3. Paris (6 vols., 1830–1842).

7. C. J. Bouchard, *Union Med.* Apr. 10, 577 (1886); *Lectures on Autointoxication* (T. Oliver, trans.). Davis, Philadelphia, Pennsylvania, 1894.

8. See, e.g., T. Paczkowski, *Die Autointoxication als Grundlage zu Erkrankung.* E. Demme, Leipzig, 1900; V. Jahn, Die gastrointestinalen Autointoxikationspsychosen des späten 19 Jahrhunderts. *Zuercher Medizingesch. Abh.* **111** (1975).

9. J. L. Smith, *Ann. Intern. Med.* **96,** 365 (1982).

10. See, e.g., E. Metchnikoff, *The Prolongation of Life* [English trans. by P. C. Mitchell of *Essais Optimistes.* Putnam, New York, 1908].

11. See, esp. vol. 14 (1900) of *Ann. Inst. Pasteur, Paris* for individual reports and a broad review by Bordet on *cytotoxines.*

12. Reference 1, *Collected Papers,* p. 315.

13. J. Bordet, *Ann. Inst. Pasteur, Paris* **12,** 688 (1899). Perhaps Ehrlich was aware that Rudolf Virchow, the greatest pathologist of his day and a believer in pathology as altered physiology, speculated that such alterations resulted from "insufficiency of the regulatory apparatuses" [R. Virchow, Lecture "Über die heutige Stellung der Pathologie," Naturforscherversammlung in Innsbruck, 1869. In K. Sudhoff, *Rudolf Virchow und die deutschen Naturforscherversammlungen,* p. 93. Akad. Verlagsges., Leipzig, 1922.

14. P. Ehrlich and J. Morgenroth, *Berl. Klin. Wochenschr.* **28,** 251 (1901). [Reprinted in English translation in Ref. 1, *Collected Papers,* p. 253.]

15. Goltz, ref. 2.

16. N. R. Rose, personal communication, 1986. As late as 1954, even while sitting on his own thyroid autoantibody data, Witebsky could say (at the Ehrlich centennial celebration) "The validity of the law [*sic*] of *horror autotoxicus* certainly should be evident to everyone interested in the field of blood transfusion and blood disease. Autoantibodies—namely, antibodies directed against the receptors of the same individual—are not formed." [E. Witebsky, Ehrlich's side-chain theory in the light of present immunology. *Ann. N.Y. Acad. Sci.* **59,** 168 (1954).] Even in the face of positive Coombs tests in cases of acquired hemolytic anemias, Witebsky suggested in 1952 [*Proc. Int. Congr., 4th, Int. Soc. Hematol., Mar del Plata, Argent., 1952,* p. 295. Grune & Stratton, New York, 1954] that the immunologist "should keep an open mind . . . toward the theory of autosensitization . . . it might be well to seek additional causes" for acquired hemolytic anemia of the adult.

17. By the time that Witebsky accepted the implications of these data and they were finally published [E. Witebsky and N. R. Rose, *J. Immunol.* **76,** 408 (1955); N. R. Rose and E. Witebsky, *J. Immunol.* **76,** 417 (1956)], Roitt *et al.* [*Lancet* **ii,** 820 (1956)] had made similar findings in human Hashimoto's disease, and priority of discovery is now adjudged to be shared equally.

18. S. Metalnikoff, *Ann. Inst. Pasteur, Paris* **14,** 577 (1900).

19. P. Ehrlich and J. Morgenroth, *Berl. Klin. Wochenschr.* **38,** 251 (1901), p. 255 footnote.

20. E. Metchnikoff, Sur les cytotoxines. *Ann. Inst. Pasteur, Paris* **14**, 369–377 (1900); H. Sachs, in *Handbuch der Technik und Methodik der Immunitätsforschung*, Vol. 2, p. 186. Fischer, Jena, 1909.

21. P. Portier and C. Richet, *C. R. Seances Soc. Biol. Ses Fil.* **54**, 170 (1902).

22. M. Arthus, *C. R. Seances Soc. Biol. Ses Fil.* **55**, 817 (1903).

23. C. von Pirquet and B. Schick, *Die Serumkrankheit*. Deuticke, Vienna, 1906. [English translation: *Serum Sickness*. Williams & Wilkins, Baltimore, Maryland, 1951.]

24. See, e.g., A. von Szily, *Die Anaphylaxie in der Augenheilkunde*. Enke, Stuttgart, 1914.

25. J. Donath and K. Landsteiner, *Muench. Med. Wochenschr.* **51**, 1590 (1904). Other instances of autoimmune hemolytic anemias were reported a few years later by A. Chauffard and J. Troisier, *Sem. Med. (Paris)* **28**, 345 (1908); **29**, 601 (1909).

26. J. Bordet and O. Gengou, *Ann. Inst. Pasteur, Paris* **15**, 289 (1901).

27. See especially the extensive studies by Nuttall on comparative analyses of antigens from different species [G. H. F. Nuttall, *Blood Immunity and Blood Relationships*. Cambridge University Press, Cambridge, 1904]. It is of interest that von Wassermann's original intent in his serological studies was the detection of *antigen* and not of antibody.

28. A. von Wassermann and C. Bruck, *Dtsch. Med. Wochenschr.* **32**, 449 (1906).

29. J. Citron, *Zentralbl. Bakteriol.* **41**, 230 (1906).

30. F. Schaudinn and E. Hoffmann, *Arb. ReichsgesundhAmt.* **22**, 527 (1905).

31. A. von Wassermann, A. Neisser, and C. Bruck, *Dtsch. Med. Wochenschr.* **32**, 745 (1906).

32. A. von Wassermann, A. Neisser, C. Bruck, and A. Schucht, *Z. Hyg.* **55**, 451 (1906).

33. L. Detré, *Wien. Klin. Wochenschr.* **19**, 619 (1906).

34. Ludwik Fleck, *Entstehung und Entwicklung einer wissentschaftlichen Tatsache. Einführung in die Lehre vom Denkstil und Denkkollektiv*. Benno Schwabe, Basel 1935. [English translation: *Genesis and Development of a Scientific Fact*. University of Chicago Press, Chicago, Illinois, 1979.]

35. See, e.g., Thomas Kuhn's acknowledgment of Fleck's influence in the introduction to his book *The Structure of Scientific Revolutions*. University of Chicago Press, Chicago, Illinois, 1980. See also R. S. Cohen and T. Schnelle, eds., *Cognition and Fact: Materials on Ludwik Fleck*. Reidel, Boston, Massachusetts, 1986.

36. See the numerous broadsides fired by Wassermann, Bruck, and Weil, in *Berl. Klin. Wochenschr.* **58** (1921).

37. This observation was reported almost simultaneously from many laboratories, including A. Marie and C. Levaditi, *Ann. Inst. Pasteur, Paris* **21**, 138 (1907); F. Plaut, *Muench. Med Wochenschr.* **44**, 1458 (1907); L. Michaelis, *Berl. Klin. Wochenschr.* **44**, 1103 (1907); E. Weil and H. Braun, *Wien. Klin. Wochenschr.* **20**, 527 (1907).

38. E. Weil and H. Braun, *Wien. Klin. Wochenschr.* **22**, 372 (1909).

39. Reference 38, p. 374.

40. P. Uhlenhuth, in *Festschrift zum 60 Geburtstag von Robert Koch.* Fischer, Jena, 1903.

41. R. Kraus, R. Doerr, and M. Sohma, *Wien. Klin. Wochenschr.* **21,** 1084 (1908).

42. P. Andrejew, *Arb. Kais. Gesundheitsamt* **30,** 450 (1908).

43. P. Uhlenhuth and Haendel, *Z. Immunitäetsforsch* **4,** 761 (1910).

44. P. Römer and H. Gebb, *Albrecht von Graefes Arch. Ophthalmol.* **60,** 175 (1905).

45. F. F. Krusius, *Arch. Augenheilkd.* **67,** 6 (1910).

46. P. Römer and H. Gebb, *Albrecht von Graefes Arch. Ophthalmol.* **81,** 367, 387 (1912).

47. Reference 46, p. 393.

48. Not only does Römer's use of Ehrlich's concepts and even phrases testify to their popularity at that time, but it will be recalled that it was this same Römer who in 1904 wrote a 403-page treatise on *The Ehrlich Side-Chain Theory and Its Meaning for Medical Science.* Hölder, Vienna, 1904.

49. Santucci, *Riv. Ital. Ottal. Roma* **2,** 213 (1906) [abstracted in *Z. Augenheilkd.* **17,** 297 (1907)].

50. S. Golowin, *Klin. Monatsbl. Augenheilkd.* **47,** 150 (1909).

51. S. Golowin, *Russky Vratch.* May 29, No. 22 (1904).

52. A. Elschnig, *Albrecht von Graefes Arch. Ophthalmol.* **75,** 459 (1910); **76,** 509 (1910).

53. W. Dameshek and S. O. Schwartz, *N. Engl. J. Med.* **218,** 75 (1938); *Am. J. Med. Sci.* **196,** 769 (1938).

54. F. H. Verhoeff and A. N. Lemoine, *Proc. Int. Congr. Ophthalmol., Washington, D.C.* p. 234 (1922).

55. A. C. Woods, *Allergy and Immunity in Ophthalmology.* Johns Hopkins University Press, Baltimore, Maryland, 1933.

56. T. M. Rivers, F. F. Schwentker, and G. P. Berry, *J. Exp. Med.* **58,** 39 (1933); T. M. Rivers and F. F. Schwentker, *J. Exp. Med.* **61,** 689 (1935).

57. L. Hektoen and K. Schulhof, *Proc. Natl. Acad. Sci. USA* **11,** 481 (1925); L. Hektoen, H. Fox, and K. Schulhof, *J. Infect. Dis.* **40,** 641 (1927).

58. Reviewed by S. Katsh, *Am. J. Obstet. Gynecol.* **77,** 946 (1959).

59. D. J. Anderson and N. J. Alexander, *Fertil. Steril.* **40,** 557 (1983).

60. P. B. Medawar, *J. Anat.* **78,** 176 (1944); **79,** 157 (1945).

61. O. C. Bruton, *Pediatrics* **9,** 722 (1952).

62. R. D. Owen, *Science* **102,** 400 (1945).

63. J. Freund and K. McDermott, *Proc. Soc. Exp. Biol. Med.* **49,** 548 (1942); J. Freund, *Am. J. Clin. Pathol.* **21,** 645 (1951).

64. B. H. Waksman, Experimental Allergic Encephalomyelitis and the "Autoallergic" Diseases. *Int. Arch. Allergy Appl. Immunol.* **14,** Suppl. (1959). See also B. H. Waksman, *Medicine (Baltimore)* **41,** 93 (1962).

65. F. M. Burnet, *The Production of Antibodies.* Macmillan, New York, 1941.

66. F. M. Burnet and F. Fenner, *The Production of Antibodies,* 2nd Ed. Macmillan, New York, 1949.

67. E. Traub, *J. Exp. Med.* **64,** 183 (1936); **68,** 229 (1938); **69,** 801 (1939).

68. Reference 66, p. 104.

69. F. M. Burnet, *The Clonal Selection Theory of Antibody Formation.* Cambridge University Press, London, 1959. An earlier version appeared in *Aust. J. Sci.* **20,** 67 (1957).

70. J. Lederberg, *Science* **129,** 1649 (1959).

71. R. E. Billingham, L. Brent, and P. B. Medawar, *Nature (London)* **172,** 603 (1953).

72. L. D. Felton and B. Ottinger, *J. Bacteriol.* **43,** 94 (1942). For later work on this problem, see R. T. Smith, *Adv. Immunol.* **1,** 67 (1961). See also A. Coutinho and G. Möller, *Adv. Immunol.* **21,** 114 (1975).

73. M. Hašek, A. Lengerová, and T. Hraba, *Adv. Immunol.* **1,** 1 (1961).

74. W. O. Weigle, *Adv. Immunol.* **16,** 61 (1973).

75. For a discussion of the theoretical and practical implications of partial tolerance, see G. J. V. Nossal, *Annu. Rev. Immunol.* **1,** 33 (1983).

76. J. Šterzl and A. M. Silverstein, *Adv. Immunol.* **6,** 337 (1967); J. B. Solomon, *Foetal and Neonatal Immunology.* North-Holland Publ., Amsterdam, 1971.

77. N. A. Mitchison, *Proc. R. Soc. Med.* **161,** 275 (1964).

78. G. L. Ada and P. Byrt, *Nature (London)* **222,** 1291 (1969); G. L. Ada *et al.* in *Developmental Aspects of Antibody Formation and Structure* (J. Šterzl and I. Říha, eds.), Vol. 2, p. 503. Academic Press, New York, 1970.

79. J. H. Humphrey and H. U. Keller, in Šterzl and Říha, eds., ref. 78, p. 485.

80. W. O. Weigle, *J. Exp. Med.* **114,** 111 (1961).

81. A. Fagraeus, *Acta Med. Scand., Suppl. No.* 204 (1948).

82. A. H. Coons, E. H. Leduc, and J. M. Connally, *J. Exp. Med.* **102,** 49 (1955).

83. E. R. Unanue, *Adv. Immunol.* **15,** 95 (1972). See also E. R. Unanue and A. S. Rosenthal, eds., *Macrophage Regulation of Immunity.* Academic Press, New York, 1980.

84. H. N. Claman, E. A. Chaperon, and R. R. Triplett, *Proc. Soc. Exp. Biol. Med.* **122,** 1167 (1966); G. F. Mitchell and J. F. A. P. Miller, *J. Exp. Med.* **128,** 801, 821 (1968); N. A. Mitchison, *Eur. J. Immunol.* **1,** 18 (1971).

85. R. M. Zinkernagel and P. C. Dougherty, *Adv. Immunol.* **27,** 52 (1979).

86. I. F. C. McKenzie and T. Potter, *Adv. Immunol.* **27,** 179 (1979).

87. R. K. Gershon and K. Kondo, *Immunology* **18,** 723 (1970).

88. R. K. Gershon and K. Kondo, *Immunology* **21,** 903 (1972).

89. N. K. Jerne, *Ann. Immunol. (Paris)* **125C,** 373 (1974); *Harvey Lect.* **70,** 93 (1974).

90. I. R. Mackay and F. M. Burnet, *Autoimmune Diseases.* Thomas, Springfield, Illinois, 1963; N. R. Rose and I. R. Mackay, eds., *The Autoimmune Diseases.* Academic Press, New York, 1985; R. S. Schwartz and N. R. Rose, Autoimmunity: Experimental and Clinical Aspects. *Ann. N.Y. Acad. Sci.* **475** (1986).

91. Voisin *et al.*, Table 7.1. See also K. S. K. Tung and A. C. Menge, in Rose and Mackay, eds., ref. 90, p. 537.

92. Kabat *et al.*, Table 7.1. See also B. G. W. Arnason, in Rose and Mackay, eds., ref. 90, p. 400.

93. Collins, Table 7.1. See also J.-P. Faure, Autoimmunity and the Retina. *Curr. Top. Eye Res.* **2,** 215 (1980).

94. G. E. Marrack, R. L. Font, and F. P. Alepa, *Ophthalmic Res.* **8,** 117 (1976); **9,** 162 (1977).

95. See ref. 17. See also P. E. Bigazzi and N. R. Rose, in Rose and Mackay, eds., ref. 90, p. 161.

96. J. Anderson, R. Goudie, K. Gray, and G. Timbury, *Lancet* **1,** 1123 (1957); R. Blizzard and M. Kyle, *J. Clin. Invest.* **42,** 1653 (1963).

97. E. H. Beutner and R. E. Jordon, *Proc. Soc. Exp. Biol. Med.* **117,** 505 (1965); L. A. Diaz *et al.,* in Rose and Mackay, eds., ref. 90, p. 443.

98. R. E. Jordon, E. H. Beutner, E. Witebsky, G. Blumenthal, W. L. Hale, and W. F. Lever, *J. Am. Med. Assoc.* **200,** 751 (1967).

99. L. C. Harrison, in Rose and Mackay, eds., ref. 90, p. 617.

100. J. N. Langley, *J. Physiol. (London)* **1,** 339 (1878).

101. S. W. Manley, A. Knight, and D. D. Adams, *Springer Semin. Immunopathol.* **5,** 413 (1982); T. F. Davies and E. De Bernardo, in *Autoimmune Endocrine Disease* (T. F. Davies, ed.), p. 127. Wiley, New York, 1983.

102. J. A. Simpson, *Scott. Med. J.* **5,** 419 (1960); W. L. Nastuk, O. J. Plescia, and K. E. Osserman, *Proc. Soc. Exp. Biol. Med.* **105,** 177 (1960); J. Patrick and J. Lindstrom, *Science* **180,** 871 (1973).

103. J. S. Flier, C. R. Kahn, J. Roth, and R. S. Bar, *Science* **190,** 63 (1975); C. R. Kahn, K. L. Baird, D. B. Jarrett, and J. S. Flier, *Proc. Natl. Acad. Sci. USA* **75,** 4209 (1978).

104. R. T. McCluskey, *Arthritis Rheum.* **25,** 867 (1982); E. M. Tan, *Adv. Immunol.* **33,** 167 (1982).

105. M. Ziff, in Rose and Mackay, eds., ref. 90, p. 59.

106. N. Miyasaka, W. Seaman, A. Bakshi, B. Sauvezie, V. Strand, R. Pope, and N. Talal, *Arthritis Rheum.* **26,** 954 (1983).

107. J. B. Howie and B. J. Helyer, *Adv. Immunol.* **9,** 215 (1968). See also Rose and Mackay, eds., ref. 90, passim.

108. P. A. Gorer, S. Lyman, and G. D. Snell, *Proc. R. Soc. London* **135,** 499 (1948); R. M. Zinkernagel and P. C. Doherty, *Adv. Immunol.* **27,** 52 (1979); K. Kano, C. J. Abeyounis, and M. B. Zaleski, eds., *Immunobiology of the Major Histocompatibility Complex.* Karger, New York, 1981; J. L. Tiwari and P. I. Teresaki, *HLA and Disease Associations.* Springer, New York, 1985.

109. H. O. McDevitt and B. Benacerraf, *Adv. Immunol.* **11,** 31 (1969); T. A. Gonwa, B. M. Peterlin, and J. D. Stobo, *Adv. Immunol.* **34,** 71 (1983); R. H. Schwartz, *Adv. Immunol.* **38,** 31 (1986).

110. A. Vincent, *Physiol. Rev.* **60,** 756 (1980).

111. See, e.g., A. Bussard, Darwinisme et Immunologie. *Bull. Soc. Fr. Philos.* **77,** 1 (1983).

8

The Donath–Landsteiner Autoantibody: The Incommensurable Languages of Immunological Dispute

Therefore is the name of it called Babel;
because the Lord did there confound the
languages of all the earth. —Genesis 11:9

ONE OF the greatest stimuli to progress in a scientific discipline occurs when opposing theories compete with one another to furnish the intellectual foundation of the science. To the heuristic value of each concept is added the impetus provided by the conflict itself, as the protagonists vie to gather evidence to support their own ideas or to contradict those of their opponents. The secondary literature in the history of medicine contains numerous reports of such conflicts, but little attention has been paid to the linguistic aspects of these disputes. Opposing theories are often associated with different terminologies, whose semantic implications may be unacceptable and even incomprehensible to the other side. The historian of a given dispute may not be able to describe it and its context adequately, unless the languages of debate are fully understood. A particularly apt example of this situation occurred during the early years of immunology and involved a hard-fought conflict between opposing theories of antibody formation and function. It will be seen that failure to appreciate the nature of the different languages employed by the opposing camps may lead to later misinterpretation of their views and of their contributions.

The Donath–Landsteiner Discovery, 1904

In an impressive series of studies commencing in 1899,[1] Paul Ehrlich and Julius Morgenroth sought to identify the constituents and to define

190

the mechanisms involved in the phenomenon of immune hemolysis, which Jules Bordet had only recently described.[2] Such studies involved the immunization of animals with foreign red blood cells, a procedure resulting in an immune serum whose thermostable antibody would collaborate with a thermolabile substance (variously termed complement, alexin, or cytase) to cause the specific destruction *in vitro* of the erythrocyte species employed for immunization. During the course of these studies, Ehrlich and Morgenroth attempted repeatedly to induce the animal to form hemolytic antibodies toxic for *its own* cells, using as the immunizing agent blood from members of the same species or even from the immunized animal itself. These attempts to elicit the formation of *auto*antibodies were uniformly unsuccessful, and at best only *iso*antibodies were detectable, able to agglutinate or to hemolyze the red cells of certain other members of the same species. (Indeed, it was the discovery of isohemagglutinins in the serum of *normal* humans that enabled Karl Landsteiner to describe the ABO blood group system,[3] so important for the later success of human blood transfusion and for forensic medicine. It was this discovery, along with that of the M, N, and P blood groups in humans,[4] that earned Landsteiner the Nobel prize for physiology or medicine in 1931.)

The failure to detect the formation of hemolytic autoantibodies did not disturb Ehrlich unduly. Although he had postulated, in his landmark paper of 1897,[5] that antibody formation was part of the normal physiological process of cellular digestion and so might theoretically be stimulated by autochthonous as well as by foreign substances, he pointed out that "It would be dysteleologic in the highest degree, if under these circumstances self-poisons of the parenchyma—autotoxins—were formed."[6] Thus, "we might be justified in speaking of a *horror autotoxicus* of the organism."[7] When Metalnikoff described the ability of the guinea pig to produce autoantibodies against its own spermatozoa,[8] Ehrlich pointed out that even this did not speak against the concept of *horror autotoxicus,* because even though this autoantibody would attach specifically to the sperm, it appeared incapable of utilizing complement to effect their destruction and was thus not an *autotoxin* "within our meaning."[9]

It was in the context of a widespread acceptance of Ehrlich's dictum that Julius Donath and Karl Landsteiner published their famous study of the mechanism of hemolysis in patients with paroxysmal cold hemoglobinuria (PKH) in 1904.[10] This fascinating but relatively uncommon disease is characterized by acute episodes of intravascular destruction of erythrocytes and an accompanying hemoglobinuria, upon exposure of the patient to the cold. Donath and Landsteiner were able to reproduce this phenomenon *in vitro*, demonstrating that exposure of the patient's (or another human being's) washed red cells to the patient's serum in the cold permitted the fixation of a thermostable substance, whereupon the cells would be hemolyzed on warming by a thermolabile agent available even in normal serum. Here, then, was the first report that appeared to contradict Ehrlich's generalization of *horror autotoxicus*. A naturally occurring disease, paroxysmal hemoglobinuria, seemed to involve the same two agents shown to function in all previous studies of *immune* hemolysis—a thermostable antibody-like substance and a thermolabile complement-like substance. This discovery by Donath and Landsteiner, extended in several subsequent papers over the next 20 years,[11] has been widely acclaimed as the first description of an autoantibody and of an autoimmune human disease.

The importance of the Donath–Landsteiner discovery has been called into question in a recent article by Dietlinde Goltz.[12] In a carefully reasoned reassessment of the Donath–Landsteiner publications, Goltz suggests that in fact the ascription to these authors of the first discovery of autoantibody is erroneous. Donath and Landsteiner, she claims, did not even *themselves* believe that they were dealing with an antibody or even with an immunological phenomenon; nowhere in the early articles do they use the accepted terms "antibody," "*Ambozeptor*," "antigen," or even "immune." Rather, they persist in employing such apparently nonspecific terms as "hemolysin," "lytic substance," "toxin," and "poison." From this, Goltz concludes that Donath and Lendsteiner subscribed to a nonimmunological toxin theory for the pathogenesis of paroxysmal hemoglobinuria and that the "myth of their discovery" is ascribable to the desire of later immunohematologists "to create pioneers and heroes that mark the starting point of their science,"[13]

One of the incidental purposes of this chapter is to demonstrate that Donath and Landsteiner did indeed discover the first autoantibody and that they understood full well what they were about. To this end, it will suffice merely to examine what they *and their contemporaries* thought that they had accomplished in their report and to recall that throughout his career Landsteiner's scientific style was one of extreme conservatism and caution in his writing, rarely speculating beyond the limits of his data. But if this were merely a question of priority in scientific discovery, it would scarcely be of broad interest to either the immunologist or to the historian of medicine. Dr. Goltz's thesis, however, raises a much more fundamental issue for the historian (and sociologist) of science—the need to recognize that at any given time, competing schools in a science may speak completely different scientific languages, which are often incommensurable and which may reflect totally different world views.

At the turn of the century, the dominant language of immunology was that of Paul Ehrlich's side-chain theory. For Ehrlich and his disciples, each of the key words that they employed reflected their understanding of how antibodies are formed *and how they function*. Karl Landsteiner belonged to a different school, that of Jules Bordet and Max von Gruber, and all three violently disagreed with the Ehrlich theories (see Chapter 5). They employed a completely different language, based upon diametrically opposite views of the origin, nature, and workings of the immunological reactants. To seek, therefore, for the Ehrlich terms "antibody" or "amboceptor," or even for the more universal terms "immune" or "antigen," in a Landsteiner paper on paroxysmal hemoglobinuria in 1904 is fruitless, since Landsteiner would not *and could not* have brought himself to use these words at that time. Even though Landsteiner's vocabulary in 1904 may have been different from that of Ehrlich, it was no less broad, and it permitted him no less to express what he intended. An understanding of these different languages of the early immunological dispute is thus crucial for an understanding both of the protagonists and of their technical and philosophical positions. It is equally important for a clear understanding of the nature and value of their contributions.

Linguistic Aspects of the Great Immunological Debate

When Paul Ehrlich advanced his famous side-chain theory of antibody formation and antibody function in 1897,[14] he found it necessary to coin a new vocabulary to describe the various participants in the several immunological reactions under consideration. Each of the terms he employed not only described a discrete physical entity but also carried full semantic implications about how that entity was supposed by Ehrlich to originate and to act. Jules Bordet, on the other hand, disagreed strongly with almost every aspect of Ehrlich's theories and elected to employ a completely different set of terms to describe the same immunological reactants—terms that either reflected his opposing views of the nature of the phenomena or that, at minimum, were semantically noncommittal as to the mode of action of these substances.

The members of each school were loathe to accept and to employ the language of the other school. But while they would not willingly speak one another's language, it is clear that they understood one another's terms and their implications quite well. Thus, in their writings, the Bordet school often refered to the "so-called *Ambozeptor*" or used the phrase "in the terminology of the Ehrlich theory," while the Ehrlich school might write of "the so-called *sensibilisatrice*," or "*Komplement* (= Bordet's *alexine*)." In addition, each school would, in its general reviews of the subject, provide full translation dictionaries for the use of the public at large.[15] It is important to note here that while these two languages might be semantically incommensurable and might lead to certain difficulties of translation at a later time, contemporary participants had perforce to understand the nuances of *all* current languages, in order to remain successfully in the forefront of their discipline.

THE LANGUAGE AND CONCEPTS OF THE EHRLICH SCHOOL

With the discovery by von Behring and Kitasato[16] that antitoxic immunity in tetanus and diphtheria infections could be ascribed to circulating "anti-bodies," perhaps the most significant conceptual problem faced by the young field of immunology was to explain the origin and basis for specificity of these new substances. Paul Ehrlich met this challenge in 1897, by advancing a theory broad enough to encompass all aspects of the formation and mode of action of these newly discovered anti-bodies.[17] On the basis of his extensive earlier work with dyes, he assumed that the neutralizing interaction of antibody and toxin involved a purely chemical union betweeen two chemically defined complementary structures, whose stereochemical "fit" would assure initial binding. Indeed, he named the specific binding site on the antibody molecule the "haptophore group" (Greek *aptein*, to bind to). To explain the provenance of these antibody molecules, Ehrlich advanced a simple explanation. Just as nutrients might be assumed to be ingested by cells by virtue of specific surface receptors (side chains), so toxins should be able to damage only those susceptible cells that carry specific toxin receptors. But the utilization of these receptors should lead to their regeneration by the cells concerned and any overregeneration of receptors would result in their being cast off into the blood, to appear as circulating antitoxin antibody. Here for the first time was a plausible suggestion that not only explained antibody formation and antibody specificity but appeared to integrate the immune response into the more general laws of biology and chemistry.

When Jules Bordet described the phenomenon of immune hemolysis in 1898,[18] Ehrlich was quick to undertake studies of this fascinating new area with his colleague Morgenroth and quick also to integrate his findings into the conceptual framework of the side-chain theory. The thermostable hemolytic antibody was, he suggested, a specialized molecule with not one but two binding sites—one site was a haptophore group specific for the erythrocyte antigen, and a separate site bound the thermolabile substance responsible for lytic action. Although this latter substance had been termed alexin (Greek *aleksein*, to protect) by its discoverer Buchner,[19] Ehrlich chose to call it *Komplement*, since its function appeared to complement that of the anti-erythrocyte antibody. For the antibody itself, Ehrlich chose the terms *Zwischenkörper* (interme-diary body) and *Ambozeptor*, the former term reflecting its role in mediating the interaction of complement and erythrocyte and the latter term describing the presence of two combining sites. Both of these sites were understood by Ehrlich to mediate highly specific and purely chemical interactions.

It will be noted that for Ehrlich, the specific antibody found in the circulation of an animal immunized with the corresponding antigen was a natural *and preexisting* substance, normally present on appropriate cells in the body of the host. Thus, it was easy for the Ehrlich theory to explain another of the current findings that had perplexed immunol-ogists—the presence in hitherto unimmunized animals of small amounts of antitoxins, antibacterial substances, or even substances that would cause the hemagglutinaton or hemolysis of certain erthrocytes. Accord-ing to the Ehrlich theory, these were simply cell receptors that had been prematurely cast off into the circulation of "normal" individuals. For Ehrlich, then, "normal" antibodies and "immune" antibodies (obtained in response to active immunization with antigen) were identical, and the presence of the former in individuals with no known previous exposure to a specific antigenic stimulus posed no particular conceptual problem.

THE LANGUAGE AND CONCEPTS OF THE BORDET SCHOOL

As he continued his exploration of the mechanisms involved in immune hemolysis, Jules Bordet put together a conceptual framework that differed markedly from that of Ehrlich.[20] Bordet was more interested in the functions of antibodies than in their origin, and he rejected Ehrlich's speculations in this latter area as contributing little to one's understand-ing of the basic process.[21] Bordet fought continuously against Ehrlich's theory of a firm chemical interaction between antigen and antibody and suggested rather that the interaction was a physical one, resembling more the adsorption so characteristic of colloids.[22] Bordet viewed the interaction of antibody with erythrocyte as reversible, in opposition to Ehrlich's view of a tight chemical union. Moreover, Bordet suggested that the antibody did not *first* fix complement and then attach to the erythrocyte to effect its hemolysis, as Ehrlich had suggested. Rather, he proposed that the antibody would interact with the erythrocyte to cause a change in the surface pattern—a sensitization—that led to an altered configuration, with a subsequent fixation of complement and hemolysis. For Bordet, anti-erythrocyte antibody was neither *Zwischenkörper* nor *Ambozeptor,* but rather *la substance sensibilisatrice.*[23] Again, he chose to employ Buchner's less committal name *alexine* for the final active factor in hemolysis rather than use Ehrlich's more suggestive term *Komplement.*

The running battle between Bordet and Ehrlich over the nature and activity of hemolytic antibody carried over into an ancillary dispute about complement or alexin. For Ehrlich, the existence of a specific receptor for complement on the antibody molecule implied a specific site on the complement molecule, and thus Ehrlich was logically forced to postulate the presence of many different complements, one for each type of antibody.[24] Bordet, on the other hand, was content with but a single complement in each individual, which would affix to *any* antibody-sensitized erythrocyte in an almost nonspecific manner.[25]

Another aspect of the Bordet–Ehrlich dispute pertinent to our present consideration of their language differences relates to Bordet's concept of the significance of those antibody-like substances found in the serum of normal individuals. For Ehrlich, as I have noted, these were *identical* to those antibodies obtained by active immunization and thus could logically be called "immune" substances or "antibodies." This Bordet would not concede. He (together with Landsteiner) viewed these naturally occurring substances as, at best, primitive precursors from which specific antibody might later be formed following their "adaptation" (*perfectionnement*) by interaction with injected antigen.[26] Thus, *at that time* (at least during the first decade or two of this century), Bordet would no more use the terms immune or antibody in referring to these naturally occurring substances than he would use the term amboceptor in referring to hemolytic antibody.[27]

A final aspect of the Bordet language then current at the Pasteur Institute and among its outside adherents is deserving of attention. It involves the generic terms that Bordet most generally employed in referring to antibodies or antisera capable of destroying cells. While he would occasionally utilize the terms *anticorps* or *hemolysine,* he more frequently in this era called them *cytotoxines.* He makes this abundantly clear in a broad review of the field published in 1900, in which he says:

> We shall employ very frequently the terms "hemolytic sera" or preferably "hemotoxins" to refer to anti-erythrocyte sera. If we adopt this latter word, then the antitoxin against a hemolytic serum will be called an "antihemotoxin." These terms are highly convenient. They were suggested by M. Metchnikoff who, as we know, calls the serum active against spermatozoa a spermotoxin, and that which destroys leukocytes a leukotoxin. The general

term "cytolytic" or "cytotoxic serum" will designate the various immune sera capable of destroying energetically either microbes or other cells (erythrocytes, etc.).[28]

This same terminology was employed again and again in the same volume by other Pasteurians. Thus, Metchnikoff reviewed the general field of anti-cell antibodies in a paper entitled "Sur les Cytotoxines";[29] Besredka wrote on "leukotoxins";[30] Metchnikoff and Besredka collaborated on an article on "hemotoxins";[31] and Metalnikoff described "spermotoxins."[32] In each of these reports, it is abundantly clear that the authors meant specific antibody when using the term toxin and did not imply some sort of nonimmunological toxic action. It is this peculiarly francophone convention and lexicon that Landsteiner chose to employ in his report with Donath on paroxysmal cold hemoglobinuria, language that Goltz interpreted to imply that Landsteiner actually believed in a toxic (in the narrow sense) pathogenesis for the disease. In fact, Landsteiner was only writing in the immunological language of Bordet.

LANDSTEINER'S ALLEGIANCES AND HIS LANGUAGE

Karl Landsteiner's first exposure to immunology came at the hands of Max von Gruber in Vienna, in whose Institute of Hygiene he served as second assistant from January 1896 to October 1897.[33] Gruber was noted for his significant contributions to the new field of serology; but perhaps he was even more noted as one of the foremost and often the most outspoken and vitriolic critics of Paul Ehrlich's theories.[34] Thus, the young Landsteiner's formative period in immunology took place in an environment that was decidedly hostile to Ehrlich's views. It is no wonder, therefore, that the majority of Landsteiner's studies over the next dozen years or so were devoted to experiments often seemingly devised to contradict the basic elements of Ehrlich's theory. He followed the lead of Gruber[35] in claiming that Ehrlich's side-chain theory was too complicated and that the universe of potential antigens and therefore of specific antibodies was too large to be accounted for by *naturally occurring* products.[36] More important, however, Landsteiner developed very early a high regard for the work and the concepts of Jules Bordet, which Bordet reciprocated;[37] and he followed Bordet in arguing variously against Ehrlich that immunological interactions are physical and colloidal rather than chemical,[38] that hemolytic antibody is not a *Zwischenkörper* or *Ambozeptor* with a uniquely determined specificity but a Bordet-type sensitizer,[39] and that the active substances in the serum of normal individuals are not the same as immune antibodies, but at best antibody precursors.[40]

As Mazumder has pointed out,[41] while some of Landsteiner's immunological beliefs (such as that on the colloidal nature of the antigen–antibody interaction) were perhaps more casual and transient, others were deeply rooted in a philosophical worldview that he retained throughout his life. Thus, Landsteiner argued repeatedly against Ehrlich's notion of discrete and uniquely separable specificities for antibody, suggesting instead that a multiplicity of only slightly differing molecules provides a continuous spectrum of cross-reactions more dependent upon quantitative than upon qualitative variations.[42] In this, as Mazumdar shows, Landsteiner's argument with Ehrlich was only the latest engagement in a long-standing philosophical debate between those who joined Leibnitz in arguing for an underlying continuity in a seamless physical world and those who held, with Kant, that Nature is marked by sharp discontinuities in most of its aspects. Ehrlich, in the tradition of the botanist Ferdinand Cohn and the bacteriologist Robert Koch, argued for sharp discontinuities and major qualitative jumps. Landsteiner, in the tradition of the botanist Karl von Nägeli and the bacteriologist Max von Gruber, favored smooth transitions and minor quantitative variation.[43] In the event, it is not surprising that Landsteiner chose to employ, during the early years of this century, the language of Bordet—of continuity, of colloids, and of physical chemistry—rather than Ehrlich's terminology—of discontinuity, of discrete molecules, and of structural organic chemistry.

But no language is static. New terms are continually added, and old terms change their meaning in any developing science. Only an analysis based upon comparative linguistics can reveal what a scientist meant by the words that he employed *at that time*. Thus, close attention must be paid to subtle changes in Landsteiner's vocabulary as the years passed. In his very first publications on hemolysis, Landsteiner referred repeatedly to the work of Gruber and Bordet and denoted the interactants as *sensibilisierende Substanz* and *Alexin,* while studiously avoiding the then-current Ehrlich terms *Ambozeptor, Zwischenkörper,* and *Komplement.*[44] However, just a few years later,[45] he gave up the usage of Bordet's *alexine* in favor of Ehrlich's *Komplement* (apparently feeling that this term, used uniquely by German-language writers, no longer carried with it an unwanted semantic burden). But never thenceforth, in any of his writing, did he utilize the terms *Zwischenkörper* or *Ambozeptor,* unless it was preceded by a modifier such as "*soqenannte*" or followed by the phrase "in the terminology of the Ehrlich school." It was some time before Landsteiner used even the term "*Antikörper,*" preferring instead, in line with French practice, to utilize less committal terms such as "*Antistoffe,*" "agglutinating [or hemolytic] substances," or, in the case of cell-destructive reactions, "cytotoxic sera" or more simply "poisons."

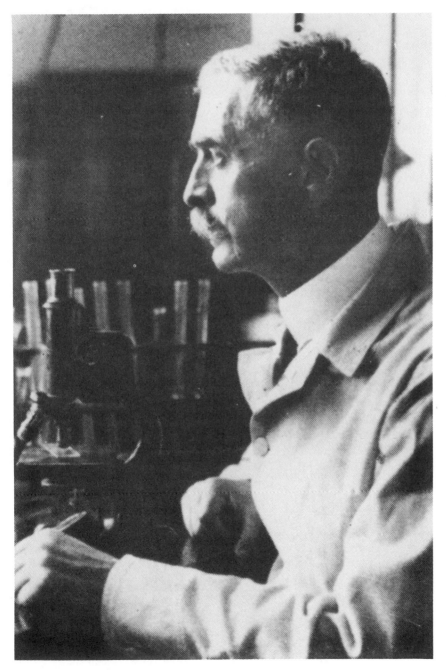

Karl Landsteiner (Courtesy University of Wisconsin Library)

Landsteiner's most notable early contribution to immunology was the demonstration that the serum of normal individuals contains substances (isoagglutinins) capable of clumping the erythrocytes of certain other individuals.[46] He returned again and again to the study of such naturally occurring substances, making it clear from his reports that he felt that their characteristics provided one of the strongest arguments against Ehrlich's ideas. In a series of papers between 1905 and 1907,[47] Landsteiner sought to show that the side-chain concept was improbable, in that these normally occurring substances and "immune antibodies" were not identical, as the theory required. Rather, they differed markedly in their specificity and in their susceptibility to various treatments. Throughout, he was careful to call them "normal agglutinins," "normal hemolysins," or simply "*Normalstoffe*," in contrast to "immune agglutinins" and "*Immunstoffe*." Landsteiner never offered an explanation for the origin of these normal substances; but he suggested that Ehrlich was wrong and that immune antibodies result from the effect of antigen on these normal substances to "adapt" them for greater specificity.[48] Only in his lengthy review of 1909, while still emphasizing the differences between normal and immune agglutinins, does he permit himself to refer to "*die Antistoffe der normalen und Immunsera*"; but he goes on to say that "The specific immune bodies . . . are newly formed during the immunization process, and different from the physiologic antibodies."[49]

This is the very first time in his writings (1909) that Landsteiner, while still protesting their difference, permits himself to refer to these active substances in normal serum as "antibodies." The use of such a term five years earlier, to refer to the presumably naturally occurring agent responsible for hemolysis in paroxysmal cold hemoglobinuria, would have been unlikely and probably even impossible. His extensive publications in this and closely related fields *at that time* show that the word in this special context was not yet in his vocabulary.

Landsteiner's views on the nature of the active agents present in normal sera have other implications for the language that he employed to describe them—*and for the words that he did not employ*. Landsteiner fought Ehrlich, in part, by demonstrating the differences between these normal agents and "immune" antibodies. Landsteiner considered them, in fact, to be the relatively nonspecific stuff of which true specific antibodies are formed. Their presence could therefore not be ascribed to an "immune response," and their activity could not be classified as an "immune reaction." Thus, while admitting the antibody-like function of these normal substances, Landsteiner consistently reserves the term "immune" for the *active* response to defined antigens, introduced to the host either naturally through infection or artificially by immunization.

Similarly, since antigen (i.e., the *gen*erator of *anti*body) was assumed by Landsteiner to act *on* these natural substances, it would be illogical for him to postulate that antigen was also responsible for their presence.

It is evident, then, that the immunological language employed by Karl Landsteiner during the first decade of the century differed markedly from that used by Paul Ehrlich. Each of the key terms used by one school embodied within it a distinctive viewpoint about origin or function and was avoided by adherents of the opposing school. During the ensuing decades, it was the language of Bordet and Landsteiner that substantially disappeared and the language of Ehrlich that survived in large measure and is currently used in modern immunology. Without knowing, therefore, what a given word meant to its user at that time, within the context of his *then-current* conceptual position, the modern reader might easily misconstrue the user's meaning.

Karl Landsteiner's Scientific Style

Throughout his long career, Karl Landsteiner had the reputation among all who knew him for the careful execution of his laboratory studies and for the precision and conservatism with which he wrote up his results for publication. Perhaps he was merely following the lead of his conceptual mentor Jules Bordet, who insisted repeatedly that he himself was not a theorist. Bordet also insisted that any ideas that he had advanced were not even worthy to be called theories but merely represented "a description of the true state of affairs." Landsteiner would rarely argue beyond the strict confines of his data. This restraint was true even in his earliest publications, with one notable series of exceptions! Only when he was attempting to refute Paul Ehrlich would Landsteiner not only employ his data to counter Ehrlich's ideas but also would use them to advance alternative concepts sometimes only weakly supported by the data. Thus, in arguing against Ehrlich's notion of a firm chemical union between antigen and antibody, he speculated about the colloidal nature of the reactants and their physicochemical (adsorptive) combination.[50] Again, in arguing against Ehrlich's side-chain theory of the origin of antibody, he theorized that antibody was formed through the adaptation of "natural antibodies" under the influence of antigen.[51] Only when Ehrlich and Ehrlich's concepts were not at issue was Landsteiner content to let his facts speak for themselves and to curb any impulse toward speculation.

Landsteiner's usual scientific style is perhaps best illustrated in a statement by one of his former students, Dr. John L. Jacobs:

> Dr. Landsteiner had a gift for building patiently, step by step . . . the rigid limitation of his experiments to the exploration of facts (avoiding

theories)—advancing by one limited hypothesis at a time, kept his work close to objective reality . . . In writing papers, Dr. Landsteiner was never ready to put pen to paper until he had definitely established a new fact . . . He limited himself severely to pointing out the highly probable implications and relationships of the facts observed, almost completely omitting opinon and theory. Thus, discussion in Dr. Landsteiner's papers consisted of relating the new fact or facts observed . . . in the manner that held hypothesis in check, to the point that such hypotheses as were advanced, represented only one short step forward with obviously a high probability of accuracy . . . a large element of his genius consisted in the humility with which he would forego the opportunity to draw broad theoretical conclusions in the interest of maintaining a high degree of accuracy and objective reality.[52]

A long-term collaborator of Landsteiner's, Dr. Merrill W. Chase, finds Jacob's assessment of Landsteiner's style highly accurate. Indeed, Chase has suggested that Landsteiner's care in performing and reporting experiments and his general disinclination to theorize were rooted in a basic dread of being proved wrong in anything by his colleagues in the scientific community.[53]

Since the 1904 report by Donath and Landsteiner on paroxysmal cold hemoglobinuria did not directly concern any of Paul Ehrlich's fundamental precepts, it may be reasonable to assume that Landsteiner brought to this paper and to the others on the same subject the conservatism of approach that typified all of his other publications that were not anti-Ehrlich in nature. Thus, one would not expect to find in the report a broad theory on the possible immunological basis for the pathogenesis of this disease, since this had not yet been rigorously proved. Given the nature of his theoretical base and the restraints on language that this imposed, Landsteiner would also not have employed in this paper the immunological key words that an Ehrlich might have used or that a later generation of immunologists might expect.

But did Landsteiner himself actually write the Donath–Landsteiner report of 1904, and does it really reflect well Landsteiner's views on the subject? In answer, one must conclude either that he wrote the paper himself, or (since it is not as tight and crisp as his other writings at the time) that he carefully revised a draft that Donath had written. This conclusion appears warranted, based upon a comparison of the Donath–Landsteiner report with one written earlier in that same year by Donath alone.[54] Donath reported his own study of three cases of paroxysmal cold hemoglobinuria and reviewed at length the various possible mechanisms that may cause the disease. Ruling out various physical mechanisms, Donath then spent seven pages discussing the possibility of the participation of a *hemolysin*, and there is no question that he here meant antibody. He suggested that the attack is elicited by a hemolysin that "like Ehrlich's normal [immune] serum hemolysins, is composed of two components (complement and amboceptor)."[55] Throughout the paper, Donath refers to Ehrlich's theory and uses the Ehrlich terminology *Komplement* and *Ambozeptor*. These are terms that do not appear only a few months later in the paper with Landsteiner. This discrepancy would imply, not that an antibody is ruled out in the latter paper, but more probably that it is Landsteiner who is calling the tune on nomenclature in this joint publication and will neither permit the use of Ehrlich's language nor a theoretical overcommitment not yet fully warranted by the facts.

Contemporary Views of the Donath–Landsteiner Report

In contesting the priority of the Donath–Landsteiner discovery of the first autoantibody, Dietlinde Goltz suggested not only that these authors did not believe that an antibody was involved but also that the attribution was not made until many years later, most notably in the 1940s to 1960s by that most famous of immunohematologists, William Dameshek.[56] But, in fact, Landsteiner repeatedly claimed priority for this discovery, *and his contemporaries readily conceded this claim.*

Despite the limitations imposed upon Landsteiner by his conservative style and by his arcane vocabulary, he could, when the situation demanded, bring himself to employ more explicit language in describing the agent responsible for paroxysmal cold hemoglobinuria. As early as the year following the 1904 report, Landsteiner and Eisler wrote a paper on the isoagglutinins and isohemolysins in normal and diseased patients. They pointed out that, while none of these had been shown to be pathological, "in fact, diseases and even disease symptoms have been shown reliably to be caused directly by auto- and isolysins in a special series of experiments on cases of paroxysmal hemoglobinuria."[57] Again, in a broad review of immunology written in 1910, Landsteiner says that "Donath and Landsteiner found a strongly active hemolysin (autolysin [*sic*]) in the serum of people . . . with paroxysmal cold hemoglobinuria." And then, after outlining the phenomenon itself, he concludes that "The entire event occurs in two separate phases. In the first, the hemolytic '*Immunkörper*' [Landsteiner's quotation marks] is bound to the blood cells . . . in the second phase . . . only the presence of complement is necessary."[58]

The initial report on paroxysmal cold hemoglobinuria by Donath and

Landsteiner attracted much attention. Repeated reference was made thereafter to the phenomenon *and to its interpretation* by numerous authors in both scientific reports and literature reviews. All of these make it quite evident that even if Landsteiner's language might be misinterpreted at a later period, his contemporaries surely understood him. Thus, in 1905, Widal and Rostaine from Paris published on PKH.[59] These authors credited Donath and Landsteiner with the description of an autohemolytic substance in patients' serum; but following the lead of Besredka[60] and the language of Bordet, they claimed that such substances are normally present in *everyone*. Furthermore, they suggested that the proximate cause of the disease is the *absence* of an anti-autohemolytic substance (in modern terms, an anti-antibody). This proposal, according to Landsteiner, was impermissible; and in the Donath–Landsteiner paper of 1908, the Widal–Rostaine thesis was criticized as follows: "it may also be said of the Widal and Rostaine hypothesis that both substances . . . the autohemolytic and the anti-autolytic substance have not until now been experimentally observed . . . such a hypothesis is, however, manifestly superfluous, since one can simply omit the supposed combination (i.e., the anti-autolytic substance) without altering the way of thinking about the phenomenon, and we must accordingly give preference to our interpretation that assumes only the actually observed hemolysin." It is clear from this that Donath and Landsteiner understood that their own explanation of the pathogenesis of paroxysmal cold hemoglobinuria involved a hemolytic autoantibody. Indeed, they even define the putative "antilysin" of Widal and Rostaine in a footnote, as "i.e., *Antiambozeptor, antisensibilisierende Substanz.*"[61]

In the same paper, Donath and Landsteiner also contest the priority for their discovery with the British physician John Eason. Eason had published two papers in 1906,[62] claiming to have discovered the pathogenesis of paroxysmal hemoglobinuria in work purportedly done prior to that of Donath and Landsteiner. Using the Ehrlich language then popular in England, Eason acknowledges that it is his view, *as well as that of Donath and Landsteiner,* that an "intermediary body (Ehrlich's *Zwischenkörper*) anchors to the red blood cell, requires low temperature, and then a rise in temperature sufficient to allow complement to participate in the process."[63] There is, he says, a potential toxin composed of two bodies, one of which possesses the characteristics of amboceptor and the other those of complement. He concludes "that paroxysmal hemoglobinuria is attributable to the activities of an intermediary body (which is, in fact, an immune body to corpuscles of the affected individual)."[64] Here, in unmistakable (i.e., Ehrlich's) language, is a purely immunological explanation of the disease. Do Donath and

Landsteiner take exception to Eason's proposal? On the contrary, they merely state that "Eason joined [himself] to our interpretation of the mechanism of hemolysis,"[65] and contest, not the theory, but Eason's claim to its priority.[66] Indeed, in as explicit a statement as they have permitted themselves thus far, Donath and Landsteiner conclude, "Since the development of the hemolysin is connected to the course of certain infections [most notably syphilis], so does our earlier-mentioned concept become more apt, that the development of autotoxic substances, which are bound to the organism's own cells, can be related to the process of antibody formation, a possibility which, so far as we know, has not previously been discussed."[67]

The recognition that Donath and Landsteiner had described an autoantibody in their 1904 paper was not restricted to Britain and France but was acknowledged even within the "enemy camp" itself. In his review of recent advances written in 1906 expressly for the English edition of his collected works, Ehrlich already referred to Donath and Landsteiner as observing "hemolytic autoamboceptors."[68] Again, Ehrlich's principal disciple Hans Sachs published an extensive review of "Hemolysins and Cytotoxic Sera" in 1906, conceding that "Donath and Landsteiner have produced information of the highest interest, that in the serum of this disease [PKH] an amboceptor is present that acts upon its own red cells."[69] Not only did Sachs concede the concept to Donath and Landsteiner, but he went so far as to dispute their priority! Apparently unwilling to yield too much to an acknowledged opponent, Sachs claims that the fact that "the serum of a hemoglobinuric patient dissolves its own blood cells *in vitro,* i.e., contains an *Autoambozeptor,* has already been reported from other quarters."[70] Sachs repeated this concession to Donath and Landsteiner, and the accompanying counterclaim, two years later in another extensive immunological review.[71]

Other adherents of the Ehrlich school also conceded the autoantibody discovery to Donath and Landsteiner. In an extensive review of cytotoxins, Rössle discussed the general evidence for the existence of autoantibodies and stated that "There are also cases, however, in which direct evidence for the presence of autoamboceptor is splendid. The best known instance concerns paroxysmal hemoglobinuria . . . Already in their first paper, Donath and Landsteiner advanced the conjecture that in paroxysmal hemoglobinuria the production of autotoxic substances (hemolysins) was involved."[72] Rössle concluded the discussion with: "Even in their first report, Donath and Landsteiner called our attention to the possibility that such a substance might be the result of a self-immunization."[73]

In 1909, Meyer and Emmerich published an extensive report on paroxysmal hemoglobinuria,[74] and it is they who are credited by Goltz with advancing the first clear hypothesis of the autoimmune character of paroxysmal cold hemoglobinuria.[75] Meyer and Emerich worked in Munich and spoke the language of Paul Ehrlich. They did indeed expand upon many of the immunological aspects of the mechanism involved, but they claimed no priority for themselves in discussing this concept. Indeed, they referred to the "very pretty and numerous investigations" of Donath and Landsteiner in which "the hemolysin so observed proves to be of a complex nature, composed of a complement destructible at 56°, and a thermostable amboceptor."[76] They conclude their paper with the revealing statement that "In [our] four cases of typical paroxysmal cold hemoglobinuria, the autohemolysin found by Donath and Landsteiner was observed."[77]

It is evident from the foregoing that Donath and Landsteiner did indeed understand from the outset that they were describing an autoantibody and an immunological process, despite the curious terminology they employed. Moreover, *all* of their contemporaries understood precisely what they meant and the full significance of their report. When necessary, they were always quick to translate the crucial terms from the language of Jules Bordet (which Landsteiner employed in 1904 and for some time thereafter) into their own language (most generally that of Paul Ehrlich). In order to compete effectively in the immunological science of the first decade of this century, it was absolutely necessary that a German understand French and that a Francophone understand German. No less important in this science was that a follower of the Bordet school understand "Ehrlichese" and that an adherent of the Ehrlich school understand the language of the Pasteur Institute. The latter language has become substantially extinct and thus may lead to modern difficulties of translation. But fortunately, an appropriate Rosetta stone exists and is available to us throughout the journals of that period.

The Lexicons of Scientific Dispute

The most popular philosophical view of the scientific endeavor during the 1940s and 1950s, advanced most notably by Sir Karl Popper, [78] was that science is unique among intellectual pursuits in building in linear and cumulative fashion an ever-clearer picture of the physical world, and that scientific progress is characterized by a remarkable consensus of view about both fact and theory among its participants. The principal features of this point of view were adopted also by many early sociologists of science, a group led by Robert Merton.[79] The philosophers sought to explain the bases for agreement among scientists by examining their epistemological underpinnings, and they ended up suggesting that all scientists adhere to the same set of logical principles of scientific inference. If these principles are followed rigorously, then scientific consensus is inevitable. The sociologists, for their part, looked to the behavioral rules that govern individual scientists and the scientific community and found that consensus is based upon a set of shared social norms, the observance of which guides all reasonable individuals toward agreement.

This rosy picture of the workings of science has been questioned in recent decades by historian Thomas Kuhn,[80] by philosophers Imre Lakatos[81] and Paul Feyerabend,[82] and by sociologist Michael Mulkay,[83] among others. Pointing to the innumerable instances in science of conceptual debate, they suggest that it may be more important to seek explanations of scientific *disagreement* than of scientific *agreement* and that, indeed, the former may be more productive of scientific progress than the latter. Kuhn points out that when anomalies are encountered in the workings of normal science, a crisis may develop and lead to the proposal of a new "paradigm," with a resulting disagreement and conflict between proponents of the old theory and supporters of the new one.[84] Because the theories are usually incommensurable, the two schools of thought generally have little basis for a reasonable exchange of views. Even if the words employed are the same, they often mean fundamentally different things to the opposing parties, and thus translation is often impossible.

Although Kuhn's approach to the study of scientific dispute has been criticized severely,[85] it is now clear that *dis*sensus constitutes an important aspect of science. It may be instructive to examine Bordet and Landsteiner's dispute with Ehrlich within the context of this larger question. When scientific dissensus arises within a *single* discipline, language problems often arise, in part because old terms may be given new meanings and in part because new concepts may demand new terminology. Such apparently was the case in the neurosciences in arguments between "brain" and "mind," in physics between wave and particle theories of light, in geology between gradualists and saltationists, in chemistry between Priestley and Lavoisier, etc. Sometimes, however, the new concept is so radically different that an entirely new lexicon must be devised, such as that accompanying Einstein's relativity theory and quantum mechanics.

In each instance, theories and lexicons may have been incommensurable, but the historian must be cautious in joining to his conclusion that the theories were mutually incompatible the further conclusion that the respective languages were untranslatable, and thus quite incomprehensible to the opposition. Mutual and total incomprehensibility of language does occasionally occur in scientific dispute, most commonly when the same question is approached by representatives of two distinct scientific disciplines. Perhaps the best instance of this in biology was the decades-long conflict over the driving force for evolution and the basis of speciation, by geneticists on the one hand and field naturalists and paleontologists on the other. As Ernst Mayr has pointed out,[86] the geneticists studied the genotype, argued proximate causes, and evolved a concept of evolutionary speciation based upon saltationism. For their part, the naturalists confined their attention to the phenotype, argued ultimate causes, and arrived at a concept based upon gradualism. Each camp had as its point of departure a scientific training and tradition and a worldview diametrically opposite that of its opponents. Thus both developed not only a set of incommensurable theories but also a set of languages that were incommensurable as well. Communication between the two schools was almost nonexistent for a long period, only in part because they could not understand each other's language. The major factor appears to have been that each thought so little of the other's approach that they felt little need even to attempt the translation.[87]

This was not the case in the immunological dispute discussed in this chapter. Paul Ehrlich and Jules Bordet each had a theory to describe the origin, nature, and mode of action of the major components of the immune response; each theory was based upon quite different philosophical viewpoints; and each man disagreed violently with the other. In turn, each protagonist coined his own lexicon to describe the several substances—terms that carried full semantic implications about the governing theories and were thus incommensurable. The opponents would no sooner accept the other's terms than they would their theoretical origins. And yet, while the languages were incommensurable, they were nevertheless fully understood by all parties to the dispute. How else, in an actively moving discipline, could one be able to plan the next experiment to advance one's own theory or to refute the opponent than by understanding precisely what he had done and what he meant in his report. In this example of immunological dissensus, as perhaps in many other scientific disagreements, incommensurability need not necessarily imply incomprehensibility.[88]

NOTES AND REFERENCES

1. P. Ehrlich and J. Morgenroth, The six landmark communications on hemolysis appeared in *Berl. Klin. Wochenschr.* **36,** 6, 481 (1899); **37,** 453, 681 (1900); **38,** 251, 569 (1901). These also appear in *The Collected Papers of Paul*

Ehrlich, Vol. 2. Pergamon, New York, 1957, in both German and English translation, and in English alone in *Collected Studies on Immunity* (C. Bolduan, trans.). Wiley, New York, 1906.

2. J. Bordet, *Ann. Inst. Pasteur, Paris* **12,** 688 (1898).

3. K. Landsteiner, *Zentralbl. Bakteriol. Orig.* **27,** 357 (1900).

4. K. Landsteiner and P. Levine, *Proc. Soc. Exp. Biol. Med.* **24,** 600 (1926–1927).

5. P. Ehrlich, *Klin. Jahrb.* **60,** 299 (1897). [English translation in Ehrlich, *Collected Papers*, Vol. 2, p. 107.]

6. P. Ehrlich, *Verh. Ges. Dtsch. Naturforsch. Aerzte, 73* (1901). [Reprinted in Ehrlich, *Collected Papers*, Vol. 2, pp. 298–315.]

7. Ehrlich and Morgenroth, ref. 1, 5th communication, p. 255; Ehrlich, *Collected Papers*, Vol. 2, p. 253. See Chapter 7 for a more extensive discussion of *horror autotoxicus* and of autoimmunity.

8. S. Metalnikoff, *Ann. Inst. Pasteur, Paris* **14,** 577 (1900).

9. Ehrlich and Morgenroth, ref. 1, 5th communication, p. 255; Ehrlich, *Collected Papers*, Vol. 2, p. 253n.

10. J. Donath and K. Landsteiner, *Muench. Med. Wochenschr.* **51,** 1590 (1904).

11. J. Donath and K. Landsteiner, *Z. Klin. Med.* **58,** 173 (1906); *Zentralbl. Bakteriol. Parasitenkd.* **45,** 205 (1908a); *Wien. Klin. Wochenschr.* **21,** 1565 (1908b); *Z. Immunitaetsforsch.* **18,** 701 (1913); *Ergeb. Hyg. Bakteriol.* **7,** 184 (1925).

12. D. Goltz, Das Donath–Landsteiner Hämolysin. Die Entstehung eines Mythos in der Medizin des 20 Jahrhunderts. *Clio Med.* **16,** 193 (1982).

13. Reference 12, p. 193, summary.

14. Reference 5. See also Chapter 4.

15. Thus H. Sachs, a disciple of Ehrlich, opened the section on hemolysis in a broad review of cytotoxins [*Handbuch der Technik und Methodik der Immunitätsforschung*, Vol. 2, p. 896. Fischer, Jena, 1909] with definitions as follows: Thermostable substance: *Ambozeptor, Immunkörper, Zwischenkörper* (Ehrlich and Morgenroth); *Substance sensibiliratrice* [*sic*] (Bordet); *Copula* (P. Mueller); *Desmon* (London); *Philocytase, Fixateur* (Metchnikoff); *Präparateur* (Gruber); *Hilfskörper* (Buchner). Thermolabile substance: *Komplement, Addiment* (Ehrlich and Morgenroth); *Alexin* (Buchner, Bordet); *Cytase* (Metchnikoff).

16. E. von Behring and S. Kitasato, *Dtsch. Med. Wochenschr.* **16,** 113 (1890). See also E. von Behring and E. Wernicke, *Z. Hyg. Infektionskr.* **12,** 10, 45 (1892).

17. Reference 5.

18. Reference 2.

19. H. Buchner, *Zentralbl. Bakteriol. Parasitenkd.* **6,** 561 (1889).

20. The best summary of Bordet's general position is provided in his book, *Traité de l'immunité dans les maladies infectieuses.*" Masson, Paris, 1920, passim. The Ehrlich–Bordet dispute is discussed more extensively in Chapter 5.

21. Bordet criticized Ehrlich's theories as being too complex and said of them: "One knows with what luxuriance they have been developed on the fertile ground of immunology, where so much of the unknown still stimulates the imagination and invites audaciously synthetic concepts from the schools desirous of affirming their superiority . . . conceptions that are defended with all of the partisanship that amour-propre mixed with chauvinism so readily inspire"

(Bordet, ref. 20, pp. vi ff.). Bordet's use of the epithet "chauvinism" is carefully chosen. We have commented in Chapter 3 on the contributions of Franco-German enmity to immunological disputes, and Bordet's book was written in Belgium during the First World War.

22. Bordet, ref. 20, p. 546. See also P. M. H. Mazumdar, [*Karl Landsteiner and the Problem of Species 1838–1968* (thesis), Vol. II, pp. 320 ff. Johns Hopkins Press, Baltimore, Maryland, 1976] for a discussion of the broader aspects of the debate about chemical versus physical interactions around the turn of the nineteenth century.

23. J. Bordet, *Ann. Inst. Pasteur, Paris* **14**, 257 (1900).

24. P. Ehrlich and H. Sachs, *Berl. Klin. Wochenschr.* **39**, 297, 335 (1902).

25. J. Bordet, *Ann. Inst. Pasteur, Paris* **15**, 303 (1901).

26. J. Bordet, *Ann. Inst. Pasteur, Paris* **13**, 273, 288 (1899).

27. Much later (1920), Bordet would employ the term *anticorps* to denote these naturally occurring substances (Bordet, ref. 20), but he would continue to protest their differences from "immune" antibodies.

28. Reference 23, p. 257.

29. E. Metchnikoff, *Ann. Inst. Pasteur, Paris* **14**, 369 (1900).

30. A. Besredka, *Ann. Inst. Pasteur, Paris* **14**, 390 (1900).

31. E. Metchnikoff and A. Besredka, *Ann. Inst. Pasteur, Paris* **14**, 402 (1900).

32. Reference 8.

33. P. Speiser and F. G. Smekal, *Karl Landsteiner* (R. Rickett, Engl. trans.). Verlag Brüder Hollinek, Vienna, 1975.

34. The Ehrlich–Gruber debates are discussed in Mazumdar, ref. 22, pp. 222–243. Also in Chapter 5.

35. M. von Gruber, *Muench. Med. Wochenschr.* **48**, 1827, 1924 (1901). Gruber concludes (p. 1927) that "The entire Ehrlich nomenclature must be given up since it is based upon false premises."

36. K. Landsteiner, *Wien. Klin. Wochenschr.* **22**, 1623 (1909). Landsteiner says of Ehrlich's theory: "In reality, this hypothesis does not assist our understanding, it offers no principle that is more simple than the phenomenon itself . . . the physiologic presence of countless substances whose utility to the organism . . . cannot be perceived."

37. Max von Gruber noted, in a letter written in 1908 [*Wien. Med. Wochenschr.* **81**, 309 (1931)] that "His [Landsteiner's] recognition in Austria seems to be hindered by his not belonging to [the school of] Paltauf [a pro-Ehrlich institute in Vienna], and in Germany by his having set himself up against Ehrlich. But in France . . . his reputation is of the highest. Bordet once said to me that in his opinion Landsteiner is the only brilliant mind among Austrian bacteriologists."

38. K. Landsteiner, *Muench. Med. Wochenschr.* **49**, 1905 (1902); L. Landsteiner and N. Jagič, *Muench. Med. Wochenschr.* **50**, 764 (1903); Landsteiner and Jagič, *Wien. Klin. Wochenschr.* **17**, 63 (1904).

39. K. Landsteiner, in *Handbuch der Biochemie* (C. Oppenheimer, ed.), Vol. I. Fischer, Jena, 1910. See also refs. 3 and 36.

40. K. Landsteiner and M. Reich, *Wien. Klin. Rundsch.* **19**, 568 (1905). See also Landsteiner, ref. 39.

41. Mazumdar, ref. 22, pp. 379 ff.; see also P. M. H. Mazumdar, *J. Hist. Biol.* **8,** 115 (1975).

42. Landsteiner, refs. 36 and 39. Landsteiner's continuing search for continuity in antibody interactions is well reflected in his lifelong study of the cross-reactions of related antigens, well summarized in his book, *The Specificity of Serological Reactions* [Harvard University Press, Cambridge, Massachusetts, 1945]. A reprint of the 2nd edition [Dover, New York, 1962] contains Landsteiner's complete bibliography.

43. Mazumdar, ref. 22, pp. 1–12.

44. Reference 3.

45. J. Donath and K. Landsteiner, *Z. Hyg.* **43,** 552 (1903).

46. Reference 3. See also K. Landsteiner, *Wien. Klin. Wochenschr.* **14,** 1132 (1901).

47. Landsteiner and Reich, ref. 40; K. Landsteiner and H. Raubitschek, *Zentralbl. Bakteriol.* **45,** 660 (1907); K. Landsteiner and M. Reich, Ueber den Immunisierungsprozess. *Z. Hyg.* **58,** 213 (1907).

48. Landsteiner and Reich, ref. 47, 1907, pp. 230–231.

49. Landsteiner, ref. 36, p. 1626.

50. Landsteiner, ref. 38. Bordet would later credit Landsteiner with the leading role in this aspect of the dispute with Ehrlich and would claim that "The affinity of adsorption is sufficiently delicate, graduated, and elective, so that the notion of its participation in antigen–antibody reactions is compatible with that of specificity" (Bordet, ref. 20, p. 546).

51. Landsteiner and Reich, ref. 40.

52. Jacobs worked with Landsteiner from 1931 to 1936. The quote is from a letter to Dr. Paul Speiser dated October 31, 1962 published in ref. 33, pp. 119–121.

53. M. W. Chase, personal communication, 1984. Dr. Chase worked closely with Landsteiner at the Rockefeller Institute from 1932 until Landsteiner's death in 1943.

54. J. Donath, *Z. Klin. Med.* **52,** 1 (1904).

55. Reference 54, p. 27.

56. See, e.g., W. Dameshek, R. Schwartz, and H. Oliner, *Blood* **17,** 975 (1961); W. Dameshek, Theories of autoimmunity. In *Conceptual Advances in Immunology and Oncology,* p. 37. Harper, New York, 1963.

57. K. Landsteiner and K. Leiner, *Zentralbl. Bakteriol.* **38,** 548 (1905).

58. Landsteiner, ref. 39, pp. 492–494.

59. G. F. I. Widal and P. Rostaine, *C. R. Seances Soc. Biol. Ses Fil.* **58,** 321, 372 (1905).

60. A. Besredka, *Ann. Inst. Pasteur, Paris* **15,** 785 (1901).

61. Donath and Landsteiner, ref. 11, 1908a, p. 211.

62. J. Eason, *J. Pathol. Bacteriol.* **11,** 167, 203 (1906).

63. Reference 62, p. 176.

64. Reference 62, p. 183.

65. Donath and Landsteiner, ref. 11, 1908a, p. 206.

66. In fact, Leonor Michaelis had published a case of paroxysmal cold

hemoglobinuria in 1901 [*Dtsch. Med. Wochenschr.* **27,** 51 (1901)], in which he speculated on the possible involvement of an autolysin. Michaelis, much involved with immunology at the time, provided no experimental support for this insight and thus received little credit from later workers.

67. Donath and Landsteiner, ref. 11, 1908a, p. 213.

68. Ehrlich, *Collected Studies,* p. 581. Also in *Collected Works,* Vol 2, p. 444.

69. H. Sachs, Lubarsch and Ostertag's *Ergeb. Allg. Pathol.* **11,** 515–644 (1907), p. 565.

70. Reference 69, p. 566. Sachs is referring here to the work of R. Kretz [*Wien. Klin. Wochenschr.* **16,** 528 (1903)] and to G. Mattirolo and E. Tedeschi [G. Acad. Med. Torino **9,** 58 (1903)], which fall far short of providing the evidence for their conjectures that Donath and Landsteiner did.

71. Sachs, ref. 15, pp. 902, 927.

72. R. Rössle, Lubarsch and Ostertag's *Ergeb. Allg. Pathol.* **13,** 124, 228 (1909).

73. Reference 72, p. 250.

74. E. Meyer and E. Emmerich, *Dtsch. Arch. Klin. Med.* **96,** 287 (1909). A brief report had earlier been presented by these authors in *Verh. Ges. Dtsch. Naturforsch. Aerzte, 80 Versammlung* Part II, p. 66. Vogel, Leipzig, 1909.

75. Reference 12, p. 210.

76. Reference 74, p. 289.

77. Reference 74, p. 326.

78. K. Popper, *The Logic of Scientific Discovery.* Basic Books, New York, 1959.

79. R. K. Merton, The normative structure of science. In *The Sociology of Science,* pp. 267 ff. University of Chicago Press, Chicago, Illinois, 1973.

80. T. Kuhn, *The Structure of Scientific Revolutions,* 2nd Ed. University of Chicago Press, Chicago, Illinois, 1970.

81. I. Lakatos, Falsification and the methodology of scientific research programs. In *Criticism and the Growth of Knowledge* (I. Lakatos and A. Musgrave, eds.). Cambridge University Press, London, 1970.

82. P. Feyerabend, *Against Method.* Verso, London, 1978.

83. M. Mulkay, Sociology of the scientific research community. In *Science, Technology, and Society* (H. Spiegel-Rosing and D. J. Price, eds.). Sage, Beverly Hills, California, 1977.

84. Reference 80, pp. 77–91.

85. See, e.g., Lakatos and Musgrave, eds., ref. 81. See also F. Suppe, ed., *The Structure of Scientific Theories.* University of Illinois Press, Urbana, 1971. L. Laudan has summarized the positions in Two puzzles about science: Reflections about some crises in the philosophy and sociology of science. *Minerva* **20,** 253 (1984).

86. E. Mayr, Some thoughts on the history of the evolutionary synthesis. In *The Evolutionary Synthesis* (E. Mayr and W. B. Provine, eds.), p. 1. Harvard University Press, Cambridge, Massachusetts, 1980.

87. It is interesting that they finally did come to an understanding of sorts, in what was called the modern synthesis by Julian Huxley [*Evolution, the Modern Synthesis.* Allen & Unwin, London, 1942]. Some of the history of the famous

meeting that helped to reconcile the parties is described in Mayr and Provine, eds., ref. 86.

88. The dispute between Bordet and Ehrlich was actually never resolved, in the broadest sense. Both made many lasting technical contributions to the field, but their theories were already disbelieved by the 1920s. The fact that Ehrlich's concept would be recast in the now-prevailing paradigm of immunology, the clonal selection theory of antibody formation, was almost accidental; its proponents often did not acknowledge Ehrlich's influence 60 years later (see Chapter 4). No scientific revolution resulted from this debate—immunology *itself* was the revolution that changed the face of nineteenth-century bacteriology and pathology.

9

Allergy and Immunopathology: The Price of Immunity

The conception that antibodies, which should protect against disease, are also responsible for disease, sounds at first absurd.
—Clemens von Pirquet

THE QUOTATION that opens this chapter echoes that of Paul Ehrlich with which the chapter on autoimmunity was introduced. It reflects yet again the contemporary implausibility of the notion that the same mechanisms responsible for defense against infectious disease might also function to embarrass the host. In the dawning years of the twentieth century, those investigators active in the young field of immunology had been brought up, with Metchnikoff and Ehrlich, to view the immune response as a superb Darwinian adaptation. It had evolved, presumably, to defend the organism against an outside world heavily populated by highly pathogenic organisms and virulent toxins. So deeply ingrained was this view of a benevolent immunity that the earliest observations that might have contradicted it were quickly attributed to other causes and mechanisms. Thus, Robert Koch's observations on the hyperreactivity of tuberculous animals to new inoculations of tubercle bacilli (the Koch phenomenon) or to tuberculin were attributed by him to the direct effect of local excesses of bacterial toxins.[1] Again, when Emil von Behring reported in 1893 a "hypersensitivity" to diphtheria toxin in previously immunized guinea pigs, he called it a "paradoxical reaction" and followed Koch's lead in assigning it to the direct cumulative action of the toxin itself,

214

rather than to any component of the acquired immune response.[2] Even
the many workers who studied the formation and activity of a variety of
antitissue iso- and xeno-antibodies (e.g., anti-erythrocyte, anti-
spermatozoa, anti-liver) made little or no connection between these
phenomena and human disease. They appeared to be more interested in
what their results might tell them about antibody formation and
antibody function.

It is not surprising, therefore, that the investigators who first reported
on the phenomena that would open up the field of allergy and
immunopathology and many who first dared to speculate that these
reactions might be an integral part of the "immune" response were not
part of the classical tradition of bacteriological immunology. Paul Portier
and Charles Richet, who described anaphylaxis, were physiologists, as
was Maurice Arthus, who discovered the phenomenon of local anaphylaxis (the Arthus reaction). The discoverers of the third of that famous
triad, serum sickness, were Clemens von Pirquet and Bela Schick, both
pediatricians. As I noted in Chapter 7, it was not long after these initial
discoveries, with such obvious implications for human disease, that (for
other reasons) immunology "shifted gears." It became a predominantly
chemical science, so that it was left primarily to clinicians and later to
experimental pathologists to expand upon these initial findings.

But throughout the course of the slow conceptual development of the
field of allergy, one can detect a continuing and pervasive schizophrenic
approach to the relationship between allergy and immunity, an approach shared by both immunologists and allergists. Just as Ehrlich's
maxim of *horror autotoxicus* inhibited free speculation and progress
toward the understanding of autoimmune diseases, so did the general
Darwinian teleological view of a benign immune apparatus inhibit
acceptance of allergic disease as another facet of the same response. The
continuing desire to keep allergy separate from immunity fostered early
suggestions that substances other than antibodies (such as toxic by-
products of the protein stimulant) were the immediate causes of these
reactions. Even after full acceptance of the role of antibodies, this
contemporary tendency was made evident by the ascription of these
conditions to special classes of antibody (atopic reagins) or to those with
special characteristics (sessile, or cell-bound antibodies). Now, with the
identification of IgE antibodies not only as the agents responsible for so
many allergic diseases but also as full-fledged members of the immunoglobulin family, this same teleological drive may be an important
contributor to the recently accelerated search for some protective role
for this class of immunoglobulins.[3]

Early Observations

Knowledge of the vexing problems of asthma and hay fever is almost as old as recorded history.[4] The clinical signs and symptoms of these conditions were well described by the ancient Greeks and appear also in the Talmud. In the Greek humoralist tradition, these conditions were lumped together with other reactions apparently unique to the individual under the generic term "idiosyncrasies" [Greek *idios*, self; *syncrasis*, a mixture (of the humors)]. From the time of Galen onward, the term was increasingly applied to abnormal reactions to drugs and to such conditions as poison sumac dermatitis and were usually included in discussions of individual *sympathies* and *antipathies*. As the prefix *idio-* implies, these conditions were long felt to arise in the unique constitution of the individual (a conclusion later to be borne out by modern knowledge of the genetic predisoposition to many of these diseases).

It is of interest that Edward Jenner provided a very good description *and illustration* of the wheal and erythema reaction in his 1798 report that introduced anti-smallpox vaccination to the world.[5] In 1839 the French physiologist Magendie described anaphylactic shock and death in dogs repeatedly injected with foreign proteins.[6] Again, in 1894 Simon Flexner provided a clear statement of the basic phenomenon of anaphylaxis in rabbits, reporting that "animals that had withstood one dose of dog serum would succumb to a second dose given after the lapse of some days or weeks."[7]

Two other observations made during this period are of interest. Von Behring, working with diphtheria toxin in 1893, and Richet and Héricourt, working with eel toxin in 1898,[8] reported that animals would suffer enhanced responses and even death following a second dose of toxin too small to injure normal untreated animals. In each case, the phenomenon was interpreted as an increased susceptibility to the direct effects of the toxin; and, indeed, von Behring coined the term hypersensitivity (*Überempfindlichkeit*) to describe these exaggerated reactions.

Little attention was paid to these early reports, or to their implications, until the studies of Portier and Richet[9] caught the attention of the immunological world. In this oft-told study, these physiologists set sail on the yacht of the Prince of Monaco in order to study the mode of action of marine invertebrate poisons in mammals. They furnished careful descriptions of the clinical shock syndrome encountered in dogs given otherwise innocuous doses of the toxin, after previous experience with the same substance. Employing a somewhat questionable etymology, they named this new phenomenon *anaphylaxis* (to express its antithesis to the more familiar term for protection, *prophylaxis*). It is not widely appreciated that credit for this discovery ought to be shared also by Theobald Smith, who independently in 1902 studied analogous anaphylactic shock reactions in the guinea pig. Smith, however, failed to publish his results and only communicated them to Paul Ehrlich several years later.[10] Ehrlich assigned the task of following up these studies to his colleague, Richard Otto, who published studies on *"das Theobald Smith'sche Phänomen"* in the years that followed.[11]

Now that investigators had been alerted to the hyperreactivity that might accompany the injection of foreign proteins, a series of new phenomenological observations on analogous responses rapidly followed, with concomitant reevaluations and reinterpretations of earlier observations. Thus, in 1903, Maurice Arthus described the heightened local hemorrhagic and necrotic response to repeated intradermal injections of protein antigens,[12] soon named the Arthus reaction. In 1906, von Pirquet and Schick reanalyzed the now well-established observation that certain patients receiving diphtheria or tetanus antitoxic serum might suffer strange systemic and local symptoms, and they named it serum sickness.[13] For the first time, they identified this disease as the product of immunological mechanisms. In order to describe these and related phenomena, they coined the term "allergy" (Greek *allos ergos,* altered reactivity) to set these responses apart from the customary minimal reactions expected of such otherwise innocuous substances.

Given the impetus provided by these widely publicized observations, many other investigators undertook the study of these interesting reactions and made important contributions to their phenomenological description and to the discussion of their causes. Foremost among these, in addition to Otto, were Rosenau and Anderson, who published an extensive series of paper on the quantitative and qualitative analysis of anaphylactic reactions.[14] In addition, significant contributions were made by other investigators such as Gay and Southard,[15] Auer and Lewis,[16] Biedl and Kraus,[17] Friedberger,[18] and Vaughan.[19]

Finally, the human conditions of hay fever and asthma were brought into this newly expanding immunological fold and joined conceptually to the new knowledge of anaphylaxis and allergy. In 1906, Alfred Wolff-Eisner made the connection between hay fever and a hypersensitivity state or reaction in the immunological sense,[20] and in 1910 Samuel J. Meltzer did the same for asthma.[21]

The Debate on Mechanisms of Allergy

DIRECT TOXICITY

One of the earliest concepts of anaphylaxis held that it was the result of the action of a potent toxin, either present intact in the injected material or split from its components by enzymatic action. Since many of his original observations were obtained using marine invertebrate toxins, Richet initially postulated that the material actually contained two active substances: *thalassin,* which was of only modest toxicity and would induce immunity; and *congestin,* which far surpasses the original poison in toxicity and leads to "hypersensitiveness" by cumulative action.[22] Once it became known that even normal serum might serve to sensitize for and induce anaphylactic shock, Gay and Southard suggested that all sera capable of eliciting anaphylaxis contain such a toxic substance, which they called *anaphylactin.*[23] Vaughan, however, maintained that the active toxin could not be present in a free state but rather was a toxic cleavage product of the injected protein.[24] He suggested that the cleavage process is so slow initially that a first injection would generally not lead to a systemic response; but "the cells learn from this lesson." A second injection results in the rapid liberation of large amounts of toxin, thereby causing the typical shock syndrome.

As further knowledge of the specificity of anaphylactic reactions was gained and especially after the demonstration that anaphylactic sensitivity, like protective immunity, might be passively transferred using the serum of sensitized animals,[25] the involvement of antigen–antibody interactions became more likely and a direct toxin theory less likely. But as late as 1921, Maurice Arthus could claim a clear separation between anaphylaxis and immunity and conclude, "Thus, we may absolutely separate these two states and deny that they may be two different manifestations of a single and same state."[26]

SPECIAL ANTIBODIES: "MISDIRECTED" IMMUNITY

I noted earlier in Chapter 8 that the French school of immunologists—the followers of Jules Bordet—were given to a freer and more exuberent speculation than were their German counterparts, who adhered to the doctrines of Paul Ehrlich. Workers at the Pasteur Institute in Paris felt unfettered by the tight doctrinaire strictures imposed by Ehrlich's side-chain theory, and it was predominantly they who led the way in proposing that antibodies might play the significant role in mediating anaphylaxis, a view that no firm adherent of Ehrlich's theory would share until years later. Their position is well illustrated in an extensive review on anaphylaxis by Ehrlich's student, Richard Otto, in 1909. After summarizing the increasingly strong evidence implicating circulating antibody in the pathogenesis of anaphylaxis, Otto finally credits the theory with "a certain likelihood," especially in view of the passive transfer experiments, but finally ends up on the fence, saying that "one must on this basis be cautious in using the term antibody."[27]

The most elaborate theory implicating an antibody in the development of anaphylaxis was that of Alexandre Besredka. In the French vernacular, the antibody was called a *sensibilisine*. The offending serum was held to contain a *sensibilisinogène* (antigen), which would stimulate the production of its corresponding antibody. Then, in a curious reprise of his anti-antibody immunoregulation theory of a few years earlier (see Chapter 10), Besredka postulated that the offending serum also contained an "anti-sensibilisin" (apparently not an antibody in this case) whose interaction with the sensibilisin antibody (purportedly attached to cells of the central nervous system) would result in the shock syndrome. This theory, supported initially by Richet and by Robert Doerr,[28] represents an interesting transition between the dualistic theories of Gay and Southard and of Vaughan (in which antigen and toxin coexist in the injected material but specific antibody plays no role in anaphylaxis) and the unitarian theories to be described later, in which the antigen–antibody interaction is held to account for all aspects of the response.

In all of the considerations of the mediation of allergic reactions by "special" types of antibodies, perhaps none set the tone for the next 50 years quite so well as that of J. R. Currie in 1907. He employed the term "supersensitization" to denote the state of preparedness for anaphylactic shock and assumed, with others, that specific antibodies (precipitins) are the active factors. But, suggested Currie, two different antibodies may be formed against the same antigen, one protective and one destructive, "because these [sensitizing substances] are not normal noxious agents introduced through normal channels." He goes on to say:

> But, if the active principle is introduced into the system neither through the customary channels nor under the form of a micro-organism, whose power for mischief depends upon its liberty to grow and multiply, the procedure is out of accord with the course of nature, and the defensive powers of the animal, adapted to cope with natural infections, are somewhat at fault in their method of dealing with the artificial invasion . . . Extraneous sera appear to belong to an order of substances which effect immunization, not by inducing insusceptibility of tissue cells, but by means of an accelerated reaction [allergy], which may thus be regarded as the expression of a misdirected defense, a formal but useless immunity.[29]

Here, in the expression "a formal but useless immunity" was a view that several generations of immunologists and allergists would fall back upon in trying to defend the notion that protective immunity and destructive allergy might both depend upon the same central mechanisms. The concept of a specific, although somewhat special type of antibody was extended also to the Arthus reaction by Charles Nicolle in his study of this phenomenon in 1907.[30] This attempt to set apart the antibody responsible for these deleterious responses was repeated often, by the assignment of special names to the "allergic antibody" such as cytotropic or cytophilic antibody or atopic antibody. The antibodies responsible for allergy in man were given the special name *reagins* (not to be confused with the so-called reaginic antibody in the Wassermann test for syphilis), presumably in yet another attempt to set them apart from the more usual antibodies associated with defensive immune responses. Even IgE, when first discovered, was implied to be a special type of antibody unrelated to protective immune responses.

THE UNITARIAN APPROACH

As might be expected from any young field in conceptual ferment, adherents could be found for each plausible theory, and even for many implausible ones. One of the earliest and strongest voices to be raised on behalf of the role of "ordinary" antibodies in allergic reactions was that of Clemens von Pirquet. In his book with Schick on serum sickness, von Pirquet assumed automatically that "precipitins" are the causative agents. It is the clinician and not the classically trained bacteriologist–immunologist that is able to say:

> The conception that antibodies, which should protect against disease, are also responsible for the disease, sounds at first absurd. This has as its basis the fact that we are accustomed to see in disease only the harm done to the [host] and to see in the antibodies solely antitoxic [protective] substances. One forgets too easily that the disease represents only a stage in the development of immunity, and that the organism often attains the advantage of immunity only by means of disease. Thus, a mild disease leads to immunity in the normal way, and since the entry of non-multiplying agents (serum) into the body seldom takes place in nature, serum sickness represents, so to speak, an unnatural (artificial) form of disease.[31]

In his 1911 book, *Allergy*, von Pirquet expanded upon this thesis. He suggested that the *immune precipitate* of antigen and antibody is the pathogenic factor. "This explanation involves also a new conception of the antibody . . . A disease might be due indirectly to an antibody, an

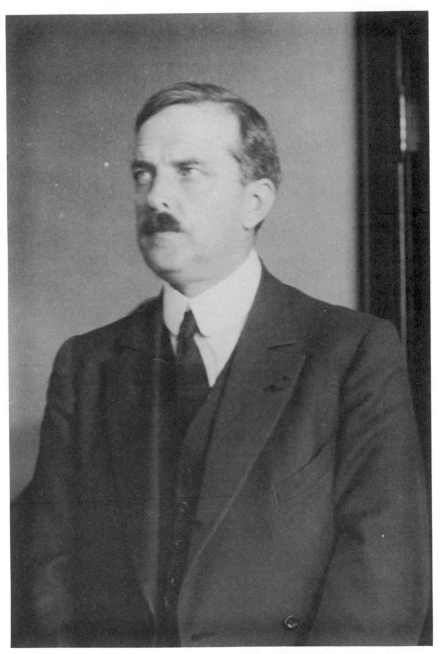

Clemens von Pirquet (Courtesy National Library of Medicine)

idea to which at that time [1906] adherents of the school of Ehrlich, like Kraus, took strong exception."[32] Pirquet, in Vienna, was not bothered by the possibility that antibodies may be toxic as well as protective. Indeed, he pointed out that the symptoms of infectious diseases in general are not entirely due to the action of the microorganisms *per se,* because the host takes an active part in the production of most of the symptoms through the interaction of *its* products with those derived from the infecting agent. This statement is a broad view of disease pathogenesis that echoes the theories of Metchnikoff and assigns to the phenomenon of allergy a respectable position in the immunological schema; taking the bad with the good, it is at once a harmful by-product of the immune response and a potential contributor to the development of protective immunity.

This latter view of allergy as a step on the road to immunity was taken up during those early years by several other investigators. In one of their papers, Rosenau and Anderson suggest that "resistance to disease may be largely gained through a process of hypersusceptibility."[33] They expand further upon this view in their monograph on anaphylaxis written in 1906. They freely grant a role to antibody in the pathogenesis of anaphylaxis and declare that "whether this increased susceptibility is an essential element or only one stage in the process of resistance to disease, must now engage our attention." They eventually conclude that "we cannot escape the conviction that this phenomenon of hypersusceptibility has an important bearing on the prevention and cure of certain infectious processes."[34] Finally, even Charles Richet reached the same conclusion, despite his apparent support of Besredka's ideas. As he pointed out, anaphylaxis can be stimulated by far smaller doses and much more rapidly than can protective immunity and thus may enhance the production of protective antitoxins. He concludes that "anaphylaxis appears to us then, in the final analysis, to be a process of rapid *defense* and above all of *defense against small doses* . . . Put in another way, *immunity can be established because anaphylaxis has taken place* [his italics]."[35]

The name of Clemens von Pirquet is associated by most historians and immunologists only with the naming of the disease serum sickness and with the coinage of the term allergy. What is not generally appreciated is the remarkable quality of his early clinical and experimental observations and the full significance of his interpretations of the data collected. His contribution is nowhere better illustrated than in his interpretation of the pathogenesis of serum sickness in man, illustrated in Fig. 9.1. This diagram is taken from his book, *Allergy,* published during his brief tenure as professor of pediatrics at the Johns Hopkins Medical School.

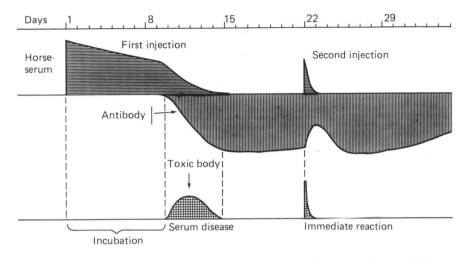

Fig. 9.1. von Pirquet's concept of the steps in the development of serum sickness in man. (From *Allergy,* ref. 32, p. 53.)

From the very outset, von Pirquet had no difficulty in assigning to precipitating antibody the key role in the development of serum sickness, and, indeed, he correctly identified immune complexes (which he called toxic bodies) as the active agent. Almost in anticipation of a later generation's interest in immune complex disease, he also described many of the clinical accompaniments of such conditions, including glomerulonephritis, arthropathy, and such systemic changes as a drop in serum complement levels. But his diagram is even more revealing. In this description of the time course of the response to intravenous horse serum, he correctly attributed the initial incubation period to the time necessary to activate the immune system for the production of antibody. He recorded the initial slow (metabolic) disappearance of antigen during this period, followed by a much more rapid immune elimination phase with the onset of antibody formation. It is precisely at this time that immune complexes are formed, said Pirquet, accompanied by an active disease process. There is then a remission, after antigen has been completely eliminated and immune complexes are no longer being formed. A second injection of antigen leads to an abrupt lowering of serum antibody levels, with rapid disappearance of free antigen, the formation of significant amounts of immune complex, and an immediate exacerbation of the disease process.

Here in a nutshell is summarized the type of phenomenological observation that would occupy so many investigators in the decades immediately following the Second World War—a prescient analysis of causes and effects for which von Pirquet has received little credit. Von Pirquet's interest in the pathological effects of antigen–antibody complexes was pursued by many investigators—most notably by Fred Germuth[36] and Frank Dixon[37]—and the role of these complexes in the pathogenesis of many different disease processes has been amply demonstrated.

THE CELLULAR THEORY: CYTOTROPIC ANTIBODY

Once it became generally accepted that specific antibody was somehow involved in the pathogenesis of various allergic reactions, the debate on mechanism became interestingly reminiscent of the earlier humoralist–cellularist debate on the basis of acquired immunity (see Chapter 3). For their part, those who favored the cellularist view pointed to the fact that anaphylactic shock could often be induced in animals in the absence of detectable circulating antibody, and they proposed that the small amounts of antibody required were in fact affixed to the surface of appropriate target cells. There, any subsequent interaction with specific antigen would result in cell damage or death and a consequent shocklike syndrome. Additional support for this view was adduced by the observation that in passive anaphylaxis, a certain minimal time was required before which shock could not be induced by antigen administration. During this time, the passively administered antibody disappeared almost completely from the circulation, and it was assumed that the refractory period was that required by antibody to take up residence on target cells.

Perhaps the strongest support for this view was found in the experiments of Schultz,[38] who in 1910 excised portions of intestine from sensitized guinea pigs, suspended them in a bath of Ringer's solution, and observed vigorous contraction of the isolated muscle upon exposure to specific antigen. These observations were confirmed and extended by Dale,[39] who substituted strips of uterus from sensitized guinea pigs for the intestinal preparation (whence the name Schultz–Dale phenomenon).

With the demonstration that an anaphylactic shock-like syndrome can be induced by intravenous administration of histamine,[40] the humoral approach to anaphylaxis appeared to find strong support. However, the subsequent demonstration that histamine is a normal constituent of many tissues[41] tended to neutralize somewhat the implications of this observation, since the cellular release of histamine might be one of the consequences of the interaction of antigen with cell-bound antibody.[42]

THE HUMORALIST VIEW: ANAPHYLATOXIN

The observation that initially stimulated an interest in a humoral effector mechanism in anaphylaxis was that of Friedemann in 1909.[43] He showed that the characteristic symptoms of acute anaphylactic shock could be obtained by injecting into the guinea pig the mixture of an antigen and its homologous antibody, following a brief period of incubation *in vitro*. This view was championed in a series of subsequent publications by Friedberger.[44] The interpretation given to this phenomenon was very much in accord with Ehrlich's then-popular theories. It was supposed that the reduction in circulating complement that accompanies anaphylactic shock was due to its fixation onto antigen–antibody complexes. The complement thus activated would exercise its putative enzymatic activity and engage in proteolysis, the breakdown products of which would constitute the toxic substances (*anaphylatoxins*). These would account for the various local and systemic symptoms that accompany the shock syndrome. This view was tempered somewhat by later observations that sera could be rendered toxic in the same sense by a variety of other procedures in which antigen and antibody played no part. Thus, anaphylatoxins may be produced by incubating normal sera with kaolin, barium sulfate, talc, starch, or agar, among others. In addition, similar shocklike syndromes could be induced with a variety of other substances, including the heterophile Forssman antibody, peptone, and even the simple chemical histamine, as indicated earlier.[45] Because of the heterogeneity of these experimental models and their likely lack of relationship to the "true" anaphylaxis mediated by antibody, these reactions were grouped together under the rubric of *anaphylactoid* reactions.

Progress in Allergy: The Clinical Discipline[46]

I have noted earlier, in several contexts, that the period after World War I saw a shift from biological to more chemical approaches to the study of immunity. The disease–related aspects of antigen–antibody interactions were more and more left to clinicians, while most laboratory-oriented immunologists chose to follow the lead of Landsteiner, Heidelberger, Marrack, and Wells in studying antibody formation and the chemistry of antigen–antibody interactions. This development was not without its advantages, for it helped to foster the independent development of a new clinical specialty, allergy, with its own agenda and its own distinctive avenues of research. When a Division of Immunology was established in 1919 at Cornell Medical College (the first such unit in the United States), its leadership was entrusted to Robert A. Cooke, the prototypical clinical allergist, who organized a combination of laboratory and clinical studies that would provide the academic model for the new field of allergy. One of Cooke's first actions at Cornell was the appointment of Arthur F. Coca (the founding editor of the American *Journal of Immunology*) to his staff. Cooke and Coca contributed significantly to the development of allergy as a scientific discipline. It was Cooke who introduced to the allergy clinic the intradermal (actually intracutaneous) skin test for the etiological diagnosis of allergic conditions, and Coca who pioneered in the purification of allergenic extracts for use in such tests. Together, Coca and Cooke attempted to classify the various hypersensitivity states and to distinguish among such conditions as hay fever, contact dermatitis, serum sickness, and experimental anaphylaxis in animals.[47] In recognition of the fact that hay fever and asthma in man might be genetically controlled, they coined the term *atopy* to set these conditions apart from other types of allergic conditions.

Coca and Cooke were also instrumental in the founding in 1924 of the Society for the Study of Asthma and Allied Conditions (called the "Eastern" Society, to distinguish it from the "Western" Society for the Study of Hay Fever, Asthma, and Allergic Diseases).[48] It is interesting that when Arthur Coca founded the Allergy Roundtable Discussion Group in New York,[49] all of its members were clinicians. Not until 1949 was a Ph.D. "basic scientist" invited into the group. This was Merrill W. Chase, in apparent recognition of his pioneering work with Karl Landsteiner on the passive transfer of tuberculin hypersensitivity and of poison ivy-type contact dermatitis.

One of the more important contributions to the practical study and theoretical understanding of human allergies came in 1921 from Carl Prausnitz and Heinz Küstner.[50] Küstner was exquisitely sensitive to the cooked flesh of certain fish, but fish extracts failed to demonstrate the presence of precipitating antibodies in his serum. However, when a little of this serum was injected into Prausnitz's skin, a typical wheal and erythema hypersensitivity reaction could be elicited 24 hours later by local administration of the appropriate allergen. Here, finally, was the demonstration of the ability to transfer passively this human allergic condition, which strongly implicated antibody by analogy with other passive transfer reactions. Moreover, the persistence of this local hypersensitivity for more than four weeks after transfer implied a tight binding of the antibody involved to neighboring cells, thus reinforcing earlier speculations on so-called cytophilic antibodies.

With the discovery of a new class of immunoglobulins, IgA, in the late 1950s,[51] it was thought for a time that these might be the elusive reaginic antibodies responsible for human atopic allergies.[52] However, the report by Loveless in 1964 of allergy in an IgA-deficient patient[53] and subsequent failure to transfer wheal and flare activity with purified IgA preparations led to the demise of this theory. Then in the mid-1960s the husband-and-wife team of Kimishige and Teruko Ishizaka prepared an antiserum to a reagin-rich fraction from the serum of a person showing extreme hypersensitivity to ragweed and demonstrated that this antibody would neutralize the Prausnitz–Küstner transferability of allergy with the patient's serum. Upon purification of the antibody, it was found that it would not react with any other known immunoglobulin class and was given the name γ-E (for erythema) globulin,[54] since renamed IgE. Independently of the Ishizakas, Johanssen and Bennich isolated from a myeloma patient an atypical immunoglobulin, which they called IgND (after the patient's initials).[55] They went on to demonstrate that the serum of patients suffering from asthma or hay fever exhibited elevated levels of IgND, and it was soon concluded that this new class of human serum immunoglobulins was identical to IgE and was the true mediator of the biological and immunological features formerly ascribed to reaginic antibodies.

With the discovery of IgE antibodies and with improved methods for the isolation and purification of various allergens,[56] it has more recently been possible to work out many of the mechanisms and pharmacological pathways involved in human allergic conditions.[57] Thus, IgE antibodies have the specialized ability to bind tightly to basophils and mast cells, and their interaction with specific allergen on those cell surfaces has been shown to result in degranulation and the release of histamine and other agents that cause directly the symptoms of disease.

DESENSITIZATION

Not long after the discovery of anaphylactic shock, it was observed that those sensitized animals that escaped death following the administration of large doses of specific antigen were unable for some time thereafter to respond to newly administered antigen with the development of a shock syndrome. Moreover, sensitized animals given repeated doses of antigen too low to provoke clinical symptoms would also develop this refractory state.[58] This was termed "immunity to anaphylaxis" by some investigators,

and "anti-anaphylaxis" by Besredka and Steinhardt.[59] The interpretation of the phenomenon was similar in all cases, however. Besredka, whose theory of the mechanism of anaphylaxis involved the
interaction of antigen with antibody (sensibilisin) bound to the surface
cells of the nervous system, postulated that the antibody became
"saturated" with antigen and thus could not react further.[60] Those who
claimed that the primary stimulus for anaphylaxis resulted from an
antigen–antibody interaction within the circulation suggested similarly
that these precipitins were saturated with antigen and unable to participate further in the elaboration of shock-inducing substances. The
relatively short duration of the refractory state was generally attributed
to renewal of the supply of free antibody over the next days or weeks, so
conditions for the induction of anaphylaxis would be reestablished.

While some such explanation seemed to be at least partially valid in
the case of anaphylactic shock in the guinea pig, for example, it did not
appear to offer an acceptable explanation for the occasional success
obtained by clinicians in their efforts to desensitize patients suffering
from hay fever or susceptible to allergic reactions to insect stings. This
approach involves a regimen of subcutaneous injections of purified
pollen allergens or insect venom, beginning with doses too feeble to
support a clinical response. The dose is then slowly increased until
"desensitization" is achieved. The recent understanding of the existence
of different classes of immunoglobulin, with different biological functions, has provided a more compelling explanation for the process of
desensitization. It is no longer believed that the antibodies responsible
for atopic allergy in man (IgE) are neutralized and thus prevented from
acting; rather it is postulated that the production of specific antibodies of
other immunoglobulin classes (blocking antibodies) is stimulated during
the "desensitization" series of injections.[61] Such antibodies compete with
IgE for the allergen, thus inhibiting the type of interaction that would
result in the release of those pharmacological mediators responsible for
the allergic disease being treated. Desensitization is, therefore, something of a misnomer; the end result is the neutralization of allergen
before it can embarrass the host, rather than neutralization of the culprit
antibody.

The Concept of "Allergy of Infection"

Tuberculosis, the "white plague," was one of the leading scourges of the
nineteenth-century industrialized western world. Thus, when Robert
Koch identified the tubercle bacillus as the responsible etiological agent
in 1882,[62] at a time when he and Louis Pasteur were demonstrating that

many important infectious diseases might be controlled by preventive vaccination, the world looked forward to the conquest of this deadly disease. Koch's announcement[63] at an international congress in 1890 of a cure for tuberculosis was received, understandably, with a thrill of anticipation. The material that he proposed to employ was an extract of the broth used to culture tubercle bacilli, which he called tuberculin, and it was hoped that this bacterial product might serve both as a therapeutic agent to cure those already infected and as a vaccine to induce immunity. Unfortunately, neither of these aspirations was realized; the material was incapable of inducing acquired immunity to later infection by the organism, and its use in tuberculous patients proved to be extremely harmful. Intravenous injection of tuberculin in such patients often led to reactivation of old tubercles (the focal reaction) and to severe systemic reactions and occasionally death. But accompanying all of these disappointing results was an observation that would prove extremely valuable in the future—the discovery that small amounts of tuberculin administered into the skin of tuberculous patients resulted in a local inflammatory dermal reaction that would allow the positive diagnosis of this infectious process. This finding was quickly seized upon by other workers, and a variety of other diagnostic applications of tuberculin were advanced, including the cutaneous reaction of von Pirquet,[64] the percutaneous reaction of Moro,[65] the intradermal reaction of Mantoux,[66] and the conjunctival ophthalmoreaction of Calmette.[67]

In the absence of any knowledge in the early 1890s of a relationship between such hypersensitivity reactions and the mechanisms of immunity, it is understandable that Koch should attribute such responses to tuberculin (as he attributed the heightened response of tuberculous animals to the subcutaneous administration of tubercle bacilli—the Koch phenomenon) to the incremental toxic effect of these inocula on tissues already saturated with the toxins thought to accompany tubercular infection. However, with the description in the opening years of the twentieth century of anaphylaxis, the Arthus reaction, and serum sickness, the mechanism of the tuberculin skin test was reinterpreted as an antibody-mediated "anaphylaxis," most notably by von Pirquet.[68] Given the ubiquity and importance of tuberculosis in contemporary society and the clear-cut nature of the results obtained with the tuberculin test, it is not surprising that this disease should become the prototype for studies of the relationship between allergy and immunity in infectious processes or that the tuberculin test should provide the focus for the future distinction to be made among different allergic mechanisms. Indeed, the tuberculin reaction was viewed as so archetypal that the term "tuberculin-type hypersensitivity" was long used to characterize all reactions of this type, only later giving way to such terms as "delayed-type hypersensitivity" and finally "cellular immunity."

EARLY SPECULATIONS

I have already noted that as early as 1906, von Pirquet and Schick attempted a grand conceptual unification of all of the phenomena of allergy, including anaphylaxis, serum sickness, the tuberculin and other cutaneous reactions, and even the exanthems that accompany certain infectious diseases. These authors held that all of these responses were antibody-mediated and that allergy in general was but a step on the road to immunity. This view was questioned only a few years later by Edward Baldwin, in the specific context of the tuberculin test and of hypersensitivity in tuberculosis.[69] Baldwin pointed to the fact that reactions to tuberculin were accompanied by fever, while *hypo*thermia generally accompanies anaphylactic shock. More telling, however, was Baldwin's argument about the oft-noticed inability to transfer typical tuberculin reactivity by passive transfer of serum, whereas the passive transfer of anaphylactic sensitivity is usually accomplished with ease. Baldwin also called attention, apparently for the first time, to differences in the passive transfer of hypersensitivity from mother to fetus *in utero*. As he says:

> When we consider our results upon the progeny of tuberculous and [anaphylactically] sensitized females [animals] respectively there is an argument for a difference, because of the absence of any appreciable sensitiveness in the young of the former and the very great susceptibility of the latter. Clinical experience on the newly born from tuberculous mothers also indicates a lack of cutaneous and fever sensitiveness transmitted to the child, which is hard to understand if acute anaphylaxis and tuberculin hypersusceptibility have a common origin and mode of development.[70]

While admitting that true anaphylactic sensitivity may be induced with bacterial products, Baldwin concluded that "enough is shown in these experiments to indicate a difference between the infected animals and those simply anaphylactic, in relation to Koch's old tuberculin applied in this way."[71]

The implications of Baldwin's work and the significance of his conclusions appear to have made little impression at the time. This disregard is perhaps best illustrated by the absence of any mention of Baldwin's work in Hans Zinsser's comprehensive book, *Infection and Resistance*,[72] published in 1914. Zinsser was actively interested in this field, and he was usually dependably encyclopedic in his reviews. But, even though he did write a chapter in this book on "bacterial anaphylaxis," his emphasis was on the relationship of hypersensitivity to pathogenesis and to immunity in infectious diseases. He did not suggest that the tuberculin and analogous reactions might be set apart from other forms of anaphylaxis.

Zinsser was not long in coming around to the view that basic differences do exist between the skin tests exhibited by tuberculous animals and those sensitized with protein for anaphylaxis; indeed, he soon became one of the foremost champions of the view that the hypersensitivity that accompanies infection is unique. After Calmette had insisted on the separation of tuberculin reactivity from anaphylaxis—in a widely read 1920 book, *Bacillary Infection and Tuberculosis*[73]—Zinsser published a series of papers[74] pointedly addressing these differences. In these papers he argued forcefully that different mechanisms must be at work.

The basis for the conceptual separation of tuberculin sensitivity and anaphylactic sensitivity advanced by Zinsser may be summarized in the following points.

1. Conditions of induction. Anaphylactic sensitivity may be induced by administration of almost any protein substance by almost any route, whereas active infection with live organisms is required to induce typical skin reactivity to tuberculin in tuberculosis, to typhoidin in typhoid fever, to mallein in glanders, and to abortin in brucellosis; dead organisms or their extracts generally fail to induce this reactivity.

2. The timing of the skin reaction. Perhaps for the first time, Zinsser in 1921 applied the (still currently used) terms "immediate" skin reaction to anaphylaxis and "delayed" to the tuberculin-type of skin reaction. The former starts in a few minutes and fades after a few hours, whereas the latter does not commence until 4 to 5 or more hours after testing and may not reach its highest development until about 48 hours.

3. Clinical signs. Anaphylactic reactions in the skin are characterized by a wheal of edema and a flare of hyperemia without residual local tissue damage, whereas tuberculin-type reactions are more often indurated and, where intense, may be accompanied by hemorrhage and central necrosis.

4. Temperature changes. As a rule, systemic reactions to tuberculin and similar substances are accompanied by a rise in the temperature of the host, while systemic anaphylactic reactions lead to a depression in body temperature.

5. Passive transfer of hypersensitivity. I have already cited earlier, in a discussion of the studies of Baldwin, the most important components of this argument. Indeed, it is only in 1921 that the now-converted Zinsser can say that "Baldwin's work is fundamental."[75]

From this point onward, the notion that some special mechanism of hypersensitivity was associated with infectious processes in general, and with tuberculin-type reactions in particular, was central to the formulation of experiments and to the interpretation of results in this area. There developed, for a time, almost a mystique about the nature of the infectious process that could engender so unique a form of allergic response, reflected in part in the oft-used term "allergy of infection."

THE RELATIONSHIP OF ALLERGY TO IMMUNITY

With the development of the notion that infectious diseases might be accompanied by a peculiar form of allergic response that not only appeared to exacerbate the disease but also had other deleterious consequences, an old and vexing dilemma was raised anew. How could these hypersensitivities, now so clearly a component of the general immunological response, be conceptually integrated into a biological function so obviously evolved for the benefit and protection of the individual? As noted earlier, when simple anaphylaxis was considered, the easiest and most teleologically pleasing answer was to conclude with von Pirquet that hypersensitivity is merely a step (and even an important one) in the development of immunity.

The old debate was renewed in the context of tuberculin-type hypersensitivity and of the pathogenesis of infectious diseases. On one side, the foremost advocates of the position that hypersensitivity may be a protective component of the immune response were Dienes[76] and Topley and Wilson.[77] These authors pointed to the fact that the local allergic reaction and especially the granulomatous responses that often accompany it (most notably the tubercle in tuberculosis) may serve an important function in walling off the infection and restricting the spread of the pathogenic organism. Furthermore, in view of the lack of relationship between tuberculin sensitivity and circulating antibody, they assumed that the "antibodies" responsible for tuberculin hypersensitivity are cell-bound. In line with Ehrlich's theory, these antibodies (receptors) merely await the appearance of antigen to stimulate their exuberant release to provide for added humoral immunity. If this happens to be accompanied by a local hypersensitivity reaction, then, they implied, that is a small price to pay for the protection it affords. As Topley and Wilson put it:

> There seems to be no valid reason for excluding resistance to tuberculosis from this general picture. Our present knowledge is compatible with the

view that allergy represents a stage in the development of immunity when the antibodies are concentrated mainly on the surface of the cells, whereas so-called immunity is a stage further on, when there is a considerable amount of free antibody in the circulation, and the local disturbances caused by the meeting of antigen and antibody in the tissues are therefore less severe."[78]

This view of an essentially benign role for tuberculin-type hypersensitivity was challenged by one of the world's foremost authorities on tuberculosis, Arnold Rich. In a long series of studies from his laboratory, summarized in his impressive book *The Pathogenesis of Tuberculosis,*[79] Rich argued against the view that hypersensitivity and immunity are closely related. He cited the lack of obvious relationship between the level of tuberculin skin reactivity and the resistance to infection or the spread of disease in both man and experimental animals. He also made the following points: simple hypersensitive inflammation is incapable of preventing the early spread of bacteria in the absence of specific acquired resistance; immunity can be established without concomitant hypersensitivity; immunity can be passively transferred without transfer of hypersensitivity; and acquired resistance remains intact both in man and in lower animals after the abolition of hypersensitivity by desensitization.[80] He felt able to conclude with the dogmatic statement that "up to the present, *hypersensitive inflammation has never been satisfactorily shown to be necessary for the successful operation of acquired immunity at any stage of any infection under any condition whatsoever*" [his italics].[81]

The continuing desire to integrate allergy and immunity into a teleological pleasing single mechanism rose yet a third time, during the rebirth of interest in the 1950s and 1960s in delayed-type hypersensitivity. With the demonstration that "pure" delayed hypersensitivity to protein antigens[82] is followed by active antibody formation[83] and that delayed hypersensitive guinea pigs, though not yet forming antibody, are primed to yield an anamnestic antibody response,[84] it was once again speculated by Pappenheimer et al.[85] that delayed hypersensitivity might constitute an "early" or "immature" stage in the cellular mechanism of antibody formation. Final resolution of this relationship, however, had necessarily to await newer findings on cell–cell interactions and on the differentiation pathways of these cells—findings that were not long in coming.

Progress on Delayed (Tuberculin)-Type Hypersensitivity

The interest in tuberculin-type hypersensitivity reactions and in the mechanisms responsible for its peculiar features were couched initially in the terms and in the context of infectious disease processes, as I noted earlier. Soon, however, new information would appear that would significantly broaden the interest in and implications of this phenomenon.

HYPERSENSITIVITY TO BLAND PROTEINS

It was in 1929 that Louis Dienes first showed that tuberculin-type hypersensitivity was not restricted to substances of bacterial origin.[86] He injected egg albumin directly into the tubercles of tubercular animals and demonstrated that they would then develop typical "delayed" hypersensitivity skin reactions to the bland protein itself. This finding was quickly followed up by similar studies at the hands of Jones and Mote[87] and of Simon and Rackeman.[88] With the introduction of Freund's adjuvant,[89] a mixture containing emulsions of antigen with dead mycobacteria, Uhr, Salvin, and Pappenheimer were able to show that delayed hypersensitivity could also be obtained by immunizing with minute amounts of simple proteins or with antigen–antibody complexes.[90] Skin reactions in such sensitized animals, elicited with specific antigen, were characterized by a similar time course of development, by similar histopathological changes (save for the necrotic component), and by the same temperature rise in the systemic reaction so characteristic of the reaction to tuberculin. During the same period, Benacerraf and Gell showed that similar delayed hypersensitivity responses could be elicited by hapten–protein conjugates.[91] These studies were accompanied by two important new findings. First, it was discovered that the delayed hypersensitivity state induced by such bland proteins could easily be desensitized without untoward systemic reactions by simple intravenous administration of specific antigen. So different was this from previous experience with the difficulty of desensitizing tuberculous individuals with tuberculin that Raffel and Newell argued that this was not typical *tuberculin*-type hypersensitivity and should be placed in a separate category called "Jones–Mote hypersensitivity."[92]

The second curious finding that emerged from these studies was the demonstration by Benacerraf and Gell[93] of the "carrier effect." Even though the delayed skin reaction appeared to be specific for the simple chemical hapten employed, the skin reaction was elicited only when that hapten was attached to the same carrier protein employed for sensitization. In contrast to anti-hapten antibodies, which interact with the hapten regardless of the protein to which it is attached, the delayed hypersensitivity mechanism seemed to "see" the hapten and its neighboring carrier protein as a single entity. This finding led to the speculation that the combining site responsible for delayed hypersensitivity reactions might be larger than that on the surface of the normal antibody molecule. The demonstration of a carrier effect in delayed-type hypersensitivity would constitute one of the more important stimuli to the discovery of the role of cell–cell cooperation in the production of antibodies.

HISTOPATHOLOGICAL STUDIES

In addition to the more obvious differences in the clinical symptoms that accompany immediate and delayed hypersensitivity reactions, significant differences were also found on the cytological level. It was Dienes and Mallory[94] who first pointed out that the most prominent cytological feature of the tuberculin reaction was the intense infiltration with mononuclear cells and that polymorphonuclear infiltration was probably only secondary and in proportion to the degree of epithelial necrosis. In contrast, the picture of passive anaphylactic skin reactions in animals was a rapidly developing edema and hyperemia, quickly followed by intense polymorphonuclear infiltration. These studies were taken up and extended by Rich and co-workers,[95] who emphasized the presence of large numbers of lymphocytes in these delayed inflammatory infiltrates. (It was undoubtedly the significant presence of these cells of unknown function that prompted Rich's plaint in 1950, "The lack of more adequate information regarding the function of the lymphocyte is one of the most lamentable gaps in medical knowledge."[96])

The next significant step was taken by Gell and Hinde,[97] who not only confirmed the predominantly mononuclear nature of the delayed skin test but also pointed out two additional features: first, that the temporal progression of Arthus skin reactivity shows a transition from an initial immediate-type skin response to a later cytological picture more typical of the delayed-type response; and second, that significant local plasmacytosis and antibody formation would follow on the heels of the delayed hypersensitivity skin test. The significance of such cytological studies both to distinguish among different forms of hypersensitivity as well as to provide leads for the study of mechanism were then emphasized in a series of detailed histopathological studies by Waksman,[98] whose work so importantly pointed up the new directions of study of what would soon be called *cellular* immunity. The distinctive cytology of this delayed-type hypersensitivity reaction was amply confirmed by the extensive studies of Turk et al.[99] and the similar cytological characteristics of contact dermatitis reactions were made clear by the studies of Flax and Caulfield[100] and of Turk et al.[101]

PASSIVE TRANSFER OF DELAYED HYPERSENSIVITY

I have already mentioned that one of the characteristics that differentiated immediate- from delayed-type hypersensitivities was the ease with which the former could be passively transferred by serum, a characteristic not shared by the latter phenomenon. It was not until 1942 that Landsteiner and Chase were able to demonstrate the passive transfer into a naive recipient of reactivity, with material from a guinea pig that was contact-hypersensitive to picryl chloride.[102] This transfer was accomplished with live peritoneal exudate cells from the donor. These cells were injected intraperitoneally into the recipient. Twenty-four hours later, a positive skin test could be elicited by application of picryl chloride to the skin of the recipient. No such transfer could be obtained using the fluid phase from the exudate or with peritoneal exudate cells that had been killed prior to transfer. These results were confirmed by Stavitsky[103] and by Haxthausen,[104] who showed that transfer could also be effected using peripheral blood leukocytes. The generality of this system of passive transfer of delayed-type hypersensitivity using cells was made clear a few years later when Chase, using a similar method, showed that tuberculin sensitivity could be transferred passively.[105] Mitchison[106] demonstrated analogous passive transfer of transplantation immunity with cells, and similar demonstrations were made subsequently in other model systems.[107] (A number of very early studies had suggested that passive transfer of tuberculin hypersensitivity could be attained using defibrinated blood or ground-up lymph nodes and spleen of tuberculous guinea pigs,[108] but in most of these instances it is not clear that the sensitization observed was truly passively acquired; active primary sensitization may have been produced by means of tubercle bacilli in the mixture transferred.)

One of the important consequences of these passive transfer studies came with the use of donor cells marked with radioactive labels. It was shown from a number of different laboratories[109] that the proportion of specifically sensitized cells at the site of a passively induced delayed skin test or allograft rejection reaction is minimal. These studies implied that only a small specific immunological trigger might be required to initiate a predominantly nonspecific train of inflammatory events.

Stimulated by the rise of interest in the passive transfer of delayed-type hypersensitivity, H. S. Lawrence in 1954 claimed that tuberculin hypersensitivity could be passively transferred to tuberculin-negative recipients using an *extract* of sensitized donor peripheral blood leukocytes.[110] Subsequent reports showed a similar passive transfer of delayed hypersensitivity to diphtheria toxoid, to coccidioidin, and to other stimulants of delayed-type reactions,[111] with a specificity that implied that these "transfer factors" were indeed informational molecules. They have since been shown to be of relatively low molecular weight and resistant to DNase and RNase; but little progress has been made in elucidating the mechanism of information carriage or of information transfer to the recipient in this unique passive transfer system.

RELATIONSHIP TO OTHER PHENOMENA

I have already noted that, predominantly on the basis of histopathological criteria, Waksman in 1959 stressed the importance of delayed hypersensitivity in the pathogenesis of a variety of autoimmune diseases, a view that has since been amply confirmed (see Chapter 7). Even before this, the role of such cellular mechanisms had been extended to include a variety of other important biological systems. Thus, contact dermatitis had been brought within the fold of typical delayed-type hypersensitivities; in this disorder sensitization is accomplished by the coupling of the active chemical or its metabolic intermediaries to proteins of the skin.[112] Indeed, it was the successful passive transfer of contact sensitivity with cells that helped to establish this approach as one of the principal criteria for the identification of the delayed-type hypersensitivity state.

Delayed-type hypersensitivity has also been implicated as the distinctive characteristic of a number of viral diseases and even as an important contributor to their pathogenesis. Typical delayed hypersensitivity skin reactions can be demonstrated to vaccinia, herpes simplex, mumps, and measles viruses.[113] Indeed, it is now apparent that the measles rash is not so much the primary disease itself as the delayed hypersensitive response to dermal virus and in fact accompanies clearance of virus from the body. The primary disease, as seen in immunodeficient individuals, is a serious giant-cell pneumonia, so the symptoms seen in normal individuals may be considered more a part of the cure than of the disease itself. Perhaps the best-studied example of the role of delayed hypersensitivity mechanisms in the pathogenesis of a viral disease may be seen in the case of lymphocytic choriomeningitis infection in mice.[114] This infection is characterized in normal animals by a severe inflammatory infiltrate of the meninges and choroid plexus, whereas the immunosuppressed or immunologically tolerant animal shows no such pathological changes. The brains of such animals, while harboring large amounts of virus, show no disease, but passive transfer of specifically sensitized T cells to such animals leads to typical choriomeningitis.

Early in his studies of allograft rejection, Peter Medawar was impressed by the predominance of mononuclear cells rather than polymorphonuclear leukocytes in skin allografts in the process of rejection.[115] While Medawar initially believed in an Arthus-type mechanism of rejection (see Chapter 11), this cytological evidence was later taken as an indication that the process is related to delayed-type hypersensitivity, a suggestion confirmed by the demonstration that transplanation immunity could be transferred with cells rather than with serum. Further evidence for the relationship was produced when Brent, Brown, and Medawar showed[116] that guinea pigs that had rejected a skin graft would show a delayed hypersensitivity reaction to subsequent intradermal injection of an extract of lymph node or spleen cells from the same donor, with all of the temporal and histological features of a typical tuberculin reaction. Subsequent studies on the *in vivo* graft versus host reaction[117] and the *in vitro* mixed lymphocyte reaction[118] showed that these were indeed caused, like allograft rejection itself, by the response of lymphoid cells to the histocompatibility antigens of the other partner to the reaction.

SORTING OUT THE MECHANISMS

Lymphocyte Subset Functions. It was the ability experimentally to induce defects in the immune response that first pointed the way to the assignment of different immunological functions to different subsets of lymphocytes. The demonstration that the bursa of Fabricius exercises (at least in birds) an important supervisory role over antibody formation[119] and that the thymus in mammals appears to control delayed hypersensitivity responses[120] led to the first functional division of lymphoid cells into T (thymus-dependent) cells and B (bursa-dependent or bone marrow) cells.[121] The former group includes those effector cells responsible for tuberculin-type skin reactions and allograft rejection; the latter comprises that developmental line of lymphoid cells responsible for antibody formation, the ultimate differentiated form of which is the plasma cell. Since then, as additional functions have been delineated, new subsets of T lymphocytes have been defined, usually characterized not only by function but by distinctive cell surface markers as well.[122] In their expanding role as regulators of immune responses, helper and suppressor T cells have been identified. (It is the requirement that helper T cells interact with the protein carriers of haptenic determinants that resolved the paradox of the "carrier effect" mentioned earlier.) To perform the several effector functions of T lymphocytes, other distinctive subsets have been identified, such as cytotoxic T cells.

Cell–Cell Intercommunications. During the course of studies on the mechanisms responsible for tuberculin-type hypersensitivity, Rich and

Lewis in 1933 first demonstrated a curious response to antigen *in vitro* on the part of mononuclear cells from tuberculin-sensitive animals.[123] Whereas cells normally migrate out of explanted bits of spleen in culture, such migration can be inhibited by the addition of specific antigen—in this case, tuberculin. These studies were extended by George and Vaughan,[124] who studied the inhibition of migration by tuberculin of sensitized cells in capillary tubes. Further studies by David[125] and by Bloom and Bennett[126] helped to clarify the nature of this response and to open up a new dimension in the study of cellular-immune reactions. These investigators showed (1) that the phenomenon was immunologically specific; (2) that it was the migration of macrophages that was inhibited; (3) but that it was an antigen—lymphocyte interaction that initiated the inhibition; (4) that only very small numbers of sensitized lymphocytes were required to affect the activity of large numbers of macrophages; and (5) that the response was mediated by a small, nonspecific molecule released by the activated lymphocyte (called migration inhibition factor or MIF). Here was a mechanism of intercellular communication and of amplification that helped to explain why so few specific cells are required in a tuberculin skin test site or in the rejection of a tissue allograft. Here also was the cue to begin the search for other such intercellular signals, which resulted in the finding of a number of different monocyte-derived signal substances (monokines) and lymphocyte-derived substances (lymphokines and interleukins).[127] Each of these physiologically active substances has a more or less well defined role in the evolution of immunogenic inflammatory reactions and in the protective and deleterious consequences of such reactions.

Other Immunopathological Processes

I have noted, in the foregoing pages, many examples of the way in which immunology was reoriented along more biological and medical lines in the years following the Second World War. This shift was especially marked during the late 1950s by the surge of interest in diseases *caused* by the immune response, as is well attested to by the many reviews, symposia, and books devoted for the first time to this subject.[128] One of the landmarks of the period was Gell and Coombs's *Clinical Aspects of Immunology*, in which the authors proposed a new breakdown of immunopathological processes into four distinct categories, which has since proved extremely popular.[129] Their type I reactions include all of the phenomena of anaphylaxis as well as human atopic allergies; type II reactions include antibody- (and complement-) mediated, membrane-destructive reactions such as immune hemolysis and bacteriolysis; type III reactions include those attributable to the effects of immune complexes; and type IV those reactions variously termed tuberculin-type, delayed-type, or cellular-immune reactions. Since I have already addressed many of the disease processes and models covered by this classification, it may only be necessary here to fill in briefly some of the blank spaces in the picture, with special emphasis on those immunopathological processes that do not fit into the simple categories proposed.

LYMPHOPROLIFERATIVE DISEASES

Just as the organized lymphoid tissues of the body (the spleen and regional lymph nodes) respond to antigenic stimulus with an intense lymphoid cell proliferation and germinal center formation, so may the same response occur in other tissues following chronic stimulation by antigen. This picture is a prominent component of diseases like Hashimoto's thyroiditis, in which a significant portion of the normal thyroid may be replaced by widespread lymphoid proliferation, plasmacytosis, and massive germinal center formation. Perhaps the best example of this process is seen in the blinding disease trachoma,[130] wherein the essentially noncytopathogenic organism *Chlamydia trachomatis* grows almost benignly in the conjunctival epithelium but induces in the subepithelial tissues a chronic immunogenic inflammatory response with typical germinal center formation and surrounding mantles of T and B cells. Although reactions of this type must necessarily be placed in the category of immunopathological disease, they appear to be little more than the usual immune response that is expected of an organized lymphoid tissue subjected to chronic antigenic stimulus but that, in an ectopic and sensitive location, may present as serious disease.

LOCAL ORGAN HYPERSENSITIVITY

It was Alexandre Besredka[131] who first called attention to the possibility that active immune responses might be localized to specific organs or special regions of the body, with possible important implications not only for host immunity to infection but also for immunopathological disease as well. This view was taken up in the 1930s by Beatrice Seegal and co-workers,[132] who showed that the injection of antigen into an isolated organ like the eye could lead to the development of a local hypersensitivity such that each subsequent systemic administration of antigen induces an exacerbation of a potentially blinding ocular inflammatory disease. A similar mechanism occurring in the joints is thought to contribute to certain forms of arthritis. It has been suggested[133] that such processes may be nothing more than the establishment in the affected tissues of specific immunological memory of the antigen involved. Just as lymphadenitis accompanies the booster antibody response in the lymph node, so might local inflammation (and clinical disease) accompany a booster antibody response in these ectopic locations.

Immunological Deficiency Diseases

I have thus far limited my discussion of immunopathological processes to those induced *by* the immune system. The discussion would not be complete, however, without mention of pathological processes *of* the immune system. Having already mentioned the important role of plasmacytomas in helping to define the nature of the antibody molecule, I will pass over other tumors of lymphoid cell lines and restrict this discussion to those immunological *deficiency* diseases that have helped to sort out the complex mechanisms of the immune response. For the purposes of the historical record, only a brief account of origins will be given for each area discussed; more recent developments may be obtained from the numerous reviews that address these issues.[134]

SELECTIVE IMMUNOGLOBULIN DEFICIENCIES

The first defect of production of a single immunoglobulin class was that of IgA, reported in 1964 by Rockey *et al.*[135] Despite its importance as a component of the secretory immune system, IgA-deficient patients are often clinically normal. The condition may be inherited through either a dominant or an autosomal recessive trait, may be due to a defect in chromosome 18, or may be acquired secondary to certain drug therapies, to viral infection, or to lymphoid malignancies.

Isolated IgM deficiencies are rare, perhaps as a result of the inability of further Ig class maturation and therefore the complete lack of all protective antibodies in such individuals. The first cases of this condition were reported by Hobbs *et al.*,[136] in two brothers whose father also showed low serum IgM.

Selective IgG deficiencies have also been reported.[137] The several subclasses of IgG are variously affected: one patient lacked IgG1 and 2; another IgG1, 2, and 4; another IgG1, 2, and 3; and a fourth lacked IgG2 and 4. The bases for these defects are unkown.

B CELL DEFECTS

Sex-linked hypogammaglobulinemia was first described by Bruton in 1952.[138] In this condition, there is a dearth of B lymphocytes, but most T cell functions appear to be normal. Patients with this condition have repeated, severe bacterial infections but handle most viral infections normally. The generally accepted cause of this disease is an arrest in the normal maturation of pre-B cells,[139] although others suggest that the pre-B cell may produce an abnormal and functionally useless μ chain in those afflicted.[140]

Hypogammaglobulinemia may be acquired later in life;[141] and even though patients present with many of the same symptoms as the X-linked form, they often show additional complications such as polyarthritis, autoimmune disease, and gastrointestinal disorders. The causes of this condition are probably multiple, some apparently genetic in nature and others arising secondary to lymphoproliferative tumors.

T CELL DEFECTS

The prototypical example of a defect in T cell function was reported by DiGeorge in 1965,[142] although Good and Varco had previously described a similar situation associated with thymoma in 1955.[143] B cell function and immunoglobulin levels are usually normal in such cases, but all typical T cell reactions are reduced or absent. A related condition was described by Nezelof[144] and apparently was due to an autosomal recessive defect. Other T cell defects have been described, due variously to deficiencies in enzymes such as nucleoside phosphorylase and adenosine deaminase, to the absence of HLA-A and -B antigens (the bare lymphocyte syndrome), or to other causes.

SEVERE COMBINED IMMUNODEFICIENCY

The first cases involving a defect in both B and T cell function were reported by Glanzmann and Riniker in 1950.[145] They termed it essential lymphocytophthisis, but it is now known as Swiss-type agammaglobulinemia, or severe combined immunodeficiency disease. Views of the pathogenesis of this disease complex are 3-fold: it may be due to a primary defect in thymic function, to a biochemical defect that prevents normal maturation of both T and B cells, or to an inability of stem cells to differentiate appropriately into T and B cell precursors. Recent experience with acquired immune deficiency syndrome (AIDS) has shown that a virus may, by infecting and destroying specific subsets of lymphoid cells at an early stage in their differentiation, cause an analogous disease state.[146]

COMPLEMENT

Since complement has played such an important role in the advancement of our understanding of the functions of the immunological apparatus (namely, immune hemolysis, opsonization, anaphylaxis, and immune complex pathology), it may be well to pause here to review briefly the history of this complicated set of physiological processes.

The Complement System.[147] It was Nuttall who in 1888 first pointed out the existence in normal serum of a protective substance,[148] soon called alexin by Buchner and complement by Ehrlich, who presciently assigned to it an enzymatic function. Its true significance was only shown a decade later by Bordet,[149] who demonstrated its crucial role in immune hemolysis (and, by implication, in bacteriolysis).

Ferrata in 1907[150] showed that hypotonic solution would separate complement into two inactive fractions, called midpiece and endpiece (later the basis for complement components one and two). The third component of complement (C3) was discovered in conjunction with the finding that complement might be inactivated by cobra venom[151] or yeast.[152] A fourth component was found during studies examining the ability of ammonia to inactivate the hemolytic activity of fresh serum.[153] Then, beginning in the 1960s, "classical" C 3 was shown to comprise a congeries of individual components and conversion products,[154] whose end effect is the result of a cascade of combinations and enzymatic alterations of the different components.[155] The existence of an alternative pathway for the activation of complement was heralded by the studies of Pillemer and Ecker on the effect of yeast on complement.[156] Pillemer described a new substance, *properdin,* which was held to be a significant contributor to natural (nonantibody) immunity.[157] It has since been shown that various bacterial polysaccharides can activate C3 directly and thus initiate the alternative pathway to the complement cascade.[158]

A new facet of the complement story (and a justification of the old view that complement plays an important role in anaphylaxis) came with the reports that by-products of the activation of C3 and C5 are significant pharmacological contributors to inflammation.[159] Here at last was the long-elusive anaphylatoxin that had so fascinated an earlier generation of workers.

Complement Deficiencies. A strain of complement-deficient guinea pigs was described first in the 1920s by Hyde,[160] but unfortunately the colony was lost and the precise nature of the defect remains unknown. The first case of complement deficiency in a human was reported in 1960 by Silverstein.[161] This person was an adult (in fact, an immunologist) who, despite a severe deficiency in the second component of complement, was clinically normal. Numerous other cases have since been reported, usually showing autosomal codominant inheritance.[162]

Deficiencies in most of the components of the complicated pathway of complement activation have been reported.[163] As might be expected, defects in the components up to C5 are often (*but not invariably*) accompanied by systemic disease and increased susceptibility to infection, whereas deficiencies in the components that function later in the pathway are generally without significant consequence. A possible defect in the alternative pathway has also been described.[164]

Conclusions

New scientific concepts have often won acceptance with difficulty, especially when they appeared to conflict with teleologically pleasing arguments in favor of the old view. Thus, Ptolemaists (and churchmen) found Copernicus's theory of the solar system unacceptable, and atomists found it difficult to believe that their "ultimate indestructible particle" was composed of subunits and could be fissioned. Similarly, early immunologists brought up to believe in an immune response evolved for the protection of the host found it hard to acknowledge that disease might result from its workings. Instead, they sought other explanations for allergic and immunopathological processes, other mechanisms, or other "abnormal" antibodies or modes of antibody participation. Even now, when modern developments have shown how all of these factors are intimately tied together in close interrelationship, one can still detect in modern writings on the subject a certain unease about the pathological aspects of the "immune" response that harks back to the views of an earlier time. The immunopathologist, given his training, sees no problem here, but many of the rest retain at least a trace of that old schizophrenic feeling when contemplating the problems of that almost oxymoronic expression "immunological disease."

NOTES AND REFERENCES

1. R. Koch, *Dtsch. Med. Wochenschr.* **17**, 101 (1891). See also R. Koch, *Dtsch. Med. Wochenschr.* **16**, 756, 1029 (1890); **17**, 1189 (1891).
2. E. von Behring, *Dtsch. Med. Wochenschr.* **19**, 389, 415, 543 (1893).
3. Byron Waksman recounts (personal communication, 1987) that Louis Dienes pointed out to him many years ago that the sequence of events leading to the elucidation of the role of special antibodies (reagins and later IgE) in allergic and parasitic diseases depended very much on the development of immunology in industrial societies. In the tropics and among primitive cultures, parasitic diseases were so prominent that immunological progress *there* would likely have taken a far different course—the discovery of IgE and its relationship to

protective immunity against parasites would probably have occurred much sooner.

4. A highly detailed compendium of developments in all aspects of allergy will be found in H. Schadewaldt, *Geschichte der Allergie,* 4 vols. Dustri-Verlag, Düsseldorf, 1979.

5. E. Jenner, *An Inquiry into the Causes and Effects of the Variolae Vaccinae . . .* Sampson Low, London, 1798.

6. Magendie, *Vorlesungen über das Blut.* Krüpp, Leipzig, 1839; cited by J. Morgenroth, in Ehrlich's *Collected Studies in Immunity,* p. 332. Wiley, New York, 1906.

7. S. Flexner, *Med. News* **65,** 116 (1894).

8. J. Héricourt and C. Richet, *C. R. Seances Soc. Biol. Ses Fil.* **50,** 137 (1898).

9. P. Portier and C. Richet, *C. R. Seances Soc. Biol. Ses Fil.* **54,** 170 (1902).

10. The story of these events is told by R. Otto in his initial paper on the subject in *Von Leuthold-Gedenkenschrift,* p. 153. Berlin, 1906. See also R. Otto, Über Anaphylaxie und Serumkrankheit, in Kolle and Wassermann's *Handbuch der pathogenen Mikroorganismen,* p. 231. Fischer, Jena, 1909.

11. See ref. 10 and especially Otto's summary in his chapter in Kolle and Wassermann, p. 239.

12. M. Arthus, *C. R. Seances Soc. Biol. Ses Fil.* **55,** 817 (1903).

13. C. von Pirquet and B. Schick, *Die Serumkrankheit.* Deuticke, Vienna, 1906. [English translation: *Serum Sickness.* Williams & Wilkins, Baltimore, Maryland, 1951.]

14. M. J. Rosenau and J. F. Anderson, Bull. No. 36, Hyg. Lab., Washington, D.C., 1906; *J. Am. Med. Assoc.* **42,** 1007 (1906).

15. F. P. Gay and E. E. Southard, *J. Med. Res.* **16,** 143 (1907); **18,** 407 (1908); **19,** 1 (1908).

16. J. Auer and P. A. Lewis, *J. Am. Med. Assoc.* **53,** 458 (1909); *J. Exp. Med.* **12,** 151 (1910).

17. A. Biedl and R. Kraus, *Z. Immunitaetsforsch.* **7,** 205, 408 (1910).

18. E. Friedberger, *Muench. Med. Wochenschr.* **57,** 2628 (1910); E. Friedberger and S. Mita, *Z. Immunitaetsforsch.* **9,** 362, 453 (1911).

19. V. C. Vaughan, *J. Am. Med. Assoc.* **47,** 1009 (1906); V. C. Vaughan and S. M. Wheeler, *J. Infect. Dis.* **4,** 476 (1907).

20. A. Wolff-Eisner, *Das Heufieber.* Munich, 1906.

21. S. J. Meltzer, *Trans. Assoc. Am. Physicians* **25,** 66 (1910); *J. Am. Med. Assoc.* **55,** 1021 (1910).

22. C. Richet, *Bull. Soc. Biol.* **55,** 246, 1073 (1903); **56,** 302 (1904); *Ann. Inst. Pasteur, Paris* **21,** 497 (1907).

23. Reference 15, 1907.

24. Vaughan, ref. 19.

25. C. Nicolle, *Ann. Inst. Pasteur, Paris* **21,** 128 (1907); R. Otto, *Muench. Med. Wochenschr.* **54,** 1665 (1907); U. Friedemann, *Muench. Med. Wochenschr.* **54,** 2414 (1907); R. Doerr and V. K. Russ, *Z. Immunitaetsforsch.* **3,** 181, 706 (1909). The passive transfer of anaphylactic sensitivity from mother to newborn was also

demonstrated at this time by M. J. Rosenau and J. F. Anderson, Bull. No. 36, Hyg. Lab., Washington, D.C., 1907.

26. M. Arthus, *De l'Anaphylaxie à l'Immunité*, p. 285. Masson, Paris, 1921.

27. Reference 10, 1909.

28. R. Doerr, Die Anaphylaxie. In Kraus and Levaditi's *Handbuch der Technik und Methodik der Immunitätsforschung*, pp. 856–894. Fischer, Jena, 1909.

29. J. R. Currie, *J. Hyg.* **7**, 35, 58 (1907).

30. Nicolle, ref. 25.

31. Reference 13, p. 119.

32. C. von Pirquet, *Allergie*. Springer-Verlag, Berlin, 1910. [English translation: *Allergy*. Am. Med. Assoc., Chicago, Illinois, 1911.]

33. Reference 14, *J. Am. Med. Assoc.*

34. Reference 14, Bull. Hygienic Lab., p. 7.

35. C. Richet, *Ann. Inst. Pasteur, Paris*, **21**,497, 524 (1907).

36. F. G. Germuth, J. Exp. Med. **97**, 257 (1953); F. G. Germuth and G. E. McKinnon, *Bull. Johns Hopkins Hosp.* **101**, 13 (1957).

37. W. O. Weigle and F. J. Dixon, *Proc. Soc. Exp. Biol. Med.* **99**, 226 (1958); F. J. Dixon, *Harvey Lect.* **58**, 21 (1963).

38. W. H. Schultz, *J. Pharmacol. Exp. Ther.* **2**, 221 (1910).

39. H. H. Dale, *J. Pharmacol. Exp. Ther.* **4**, 167 (1913).

40. H. H. Dale, *Bull. Johns Hopkins Hosp.* **31**, 257, 310 (1920); H. H. Dale and P. P. Laidlaw, *J. Physiol. (London)* **52**, 355 (1919).

41. H. H. Dale, *Lancet* **i**, 1179, 1233, 1285 (1929).

42. The role of histamine in mediating many of the typical local symptoms of allergic reactions was especially well pointed out by T. Lewis, *The Blood Vessels of the Human Skin and Their Responses*. Shaw, London, 1927. Lewis called the active factor "H-substance."

43. U. Friedemann, *Z. Immunitaetsforsch.* **2**, 591 (1909).

44. E. Friedberger, *Berl. Klin. Wochenschr.* **47**, 1490, 1922, 2303 (1910); *Z. Immunitaetsforsch.* **3**, 787 (1910).

45. A review of the many substances that might mimic anaphylactic shock is presented in a series of papers by P. J. Hanzlik and H. T. Karsner, *J. Pharmacol. Exp. Ther.* **14**, 379, 425, 449, 479 (1920); **23**, 173 (1924).

46. The development in America of the clinical discipline of allergy is well summarized in the fiftieth anniversary issue of the *Journal of Allergy and Applied Immunology* [**64**, 306–474 (1979)], with an article by Merrill Chase on Cooke and Coca, one by Max Samter on future prospects for the field, and a lengthy history of the institutionalization of the discipline by Sheldon Cohen.

47. A. F. Coca and R. A. Cooke, *J. Immunol.* **8**, 163 (1923). See also A. F. Coca, M. Walzer, and A. A. Thommen, *Asthma and Hay Fever in Theory and Practice*. Thomas, Springfield, Illinois, 1931.

48. The story of the founding of and developments within and between the Eastern and Western Societies is recounted by S. G. Cohen, *NER Allergy Proc.* **5**, 247, 342 (1984).

49. See L. Tuft, *NER Allergy Proc.* **6**, 279 (1985).

50. C. Prausnitz and H. Küstner, *Zentralbl. Bakteriol.* **86**, 160 (1921).

51. J. F. Heremans, M. T. Heremans, and H. W. Schultze, *Clin. Chim, Acta* **4,** 96 (1959).

52. J. F. Heremans and J. P. Vaerman, *Nature (London)* **193,** 1091 (1962).

53. M. H. Loveless *Fed. Proc.* **23**(2), 403 (1964). See also J. H. Rockey, L. A. Hanson, J. F. Heremans, and H. G. Kunkel, *J. Lab. Clin. Med.* **63,**205 (1964).

54. K. Ishizaka and T. Ishizaka, *J. Allergy* **37,** 169 (1966); **38,** 108 (1966).

55. S. G. O. Johanssen and H. Bennich, *Immunology* **13,** 381 (1967).

56. L. Berrens, *The Chemistry of Atopic Allergens.* Karger, Basel, 1971.

57. A. B. Kay, K. F. Austen, and L. M. Lichtenstein, eds., *Asthma: Physiology, Immunopharmacology, and Treatment.* Academic Press, Orlando, Florida, 1984.

58. See, e.g., refs. 10 and 14; A. Besredka and E. Steinhardt, *Ann. Inst. Pasteur, Paris* **21,** 117, 384 (1907).

59. Besredka and Steinhardt, ref. 58.

60. A. Besredka, *Ann. Inst. Pasteur, Paris,* **21,** 384 (1907); **22,** 496 (1908).

61. R. A. Cooke, J. H. Barnard, S. Hebald, and A. Stull, *J. Exp. Med.* **62,** 733 (1935).

62. R. Koch, *Berl. Klin. Wochenschr.* **19,** 221 (1882).

63. Reference 1.

64. C. von Pirquet, *Berl. Klin. Wochenschr.* **48,** 644, 699 (1907).

65. E. Moro and A. Doganoff, *Wien. Klin. Wochenschr.* **20,** 933 (1907); E. Moro, *Muench. Med. Wochenschr.* **55,** 216 (1908).

66. C. Mantoux, *Presse Med.* **18,** 10 (1910).

67. L. C. A. Calmette, *C. R. Hebd. Seances Acad. Sci.* **144,** 1324 (1907).

68. Reference 13; von Pirquet's ideas were further expanded and given additional substance in his book *Klinische Studien über Vakzination und Vakzinale Allergie.* Deuticke, Leipzig, 1907.

69. E. R. Baldwin, *J. Med. Res.* **22,** 189 (1910).

70. Reference 69, p. 252.

71. Reference 69, p. 238.

72. H. Zinsser, *Infection and Resistance.* Macmillan, New York, 1914.

73. A. Calmette, *L'Infection Bacillaire et la Tuberculose.* Masson, Paris, 1920.

74. H. Zinsser, *J. Exp. Med.* **34,** 495 (1921); H. Zinsser and J. H. Mueller, *J. Exp. Med.* **41,** 159 (1925).

75. Zinsser, ref. 74, p. 499.

76. L. Dienes, *Arch. Pathol.* **21,** 357 (1936).

77. W. W. C. Topley and G. S. Wilson, *The Principles of Bacteriology and Immunity,* 2nd Ed., pp. 911 ff., 1044 ff. William Wood, Baltimore, Maryland, 1938.

78. Reference 77, p. 1047.

79. A. R. Rich, *The Pathogenesis of Tuberculosis,* 2nd Ed. Thomas, Springfield, Illinois, 1951.

80. Reference 79, p. 565.

81. Reference 79, p. 568.

82. J. W. Uhr, S. B. Salvin, and A. M. Pappenheimer, Jr., *J. Exp. Med.* **105,** 11 (1957); S. B. Salvin, *J. Exp. Med.* **107,** 109 (1958).

83. Salvin, ref. 82; S. B. Salvin and R. F. Smith, *J. Exp. Med.* **109,** 325 (1959); B. Benacerraf and P. G. H. Gell, *Immunology* **2,** 53 (1959).

84. Salvin and Smith, ref. 83; S. Sell and W. O. Weigle, *J. Immunol.* **83,** 257 (1959).

85. A. M. Pappenheimer, Jr., M. Scharff, and J. W. Uhr, In *Mechanisms of Hypersensitivity* (J. H. Shaffer, G. A. LoGrippo, and M. W. Chase, eds.), p. 417. Churchill, London, 1959. See also P. G. H. Gell and B. Benacerraf, *Adv. Immunol.* **1,** 319 (1961).

86. L. Dienes, *J. Immunol.* **17,** 531 (1929); L. Dienes and E. W. Schoenheit, *Am. Rev. Tuberc.* **20,** 92 (1929).

87. T. D. Jones and J. R. Mote, *N. Engl. J. Med.* **210,** 120 (1934).

88. F. A. Simon and F. M. Rackeman, *J. Allergy* **5,** 439 (1934).

89. J. Freund and K. McDermott, *Proc. Soc. Exp. Biol. Med.* **49,** 548 (1942); J. Freund, *Am. J. Clin. Pathol.* **21,** 645 (1951).

90. Uhr *et al.,* ref. 82.

91. B. Benacerraf and P. G. H. Gell, *Immunology* **2,** 53 (1959).

92. S. Raffel and J. M. Newell, *J. Exp. Med.* **108,** 823 (1958).

93. Reference 91. See also S. B. Salvin and R. F. Smith, *Proc. Soc. Exp. Biol. Med.* **104,** 584 (1960); B. Benacerraf and B. B. Levine, *J. Exp. Med.* **115,** 1023 (1962); P. G. H. Gell and A. M. Silverstein, *J. Exp. Med.* **115,** 1037 (1964).

94. L. Dienes and T. B. Mallory, *Am. J. Pathol.* **8,** 689 (1932).

95. These studies are well summarized by Rich ref. 79.

96. Reference 79, p. 600.

97. P. G. H. Gell and J. T. Hinde, *Int. Arch. Allergy Appl. Immunol.* **5,** 23 (1954). These local reactions were called "progressive immunization reactions" to reflect their maturation toward abundant local antibody production.

98. B. H. Waksman, Experimental allergic encephalomyelitis and the "auto-allergic" diseases. *Int. Arch. Allergy Appl. Immunol.* **14,** Suppl., 1959; B. H. Waksman, *Medicine (Baltimore)* **41,** 93 (1962).

99. J. L. Turk and C. J. Heather, *Int. Arch. Allergy Appl. Immunol.* **27,** 199 (1965); J. L. Turk, C. J. Heather, and J. V. Diengdoh, *Int. Arch. Allergy Appl. Immunol.* **29,** 278 (1966). A fine summary of this and other aspects of delayed hypersensitivity will be found in J. L. Turk, *Delayed Hypersensitivity.* North-Holland Publ., Amsterdam, 1967.

100. M. H. Flax and J. B. Caulfield, *Am. J. Pathol.* **43,** 1031 (1963).

101. J. L. Turk, E. J. Rudner, and C. J. Heather, *Int. Arch. Allergy Appl. Immunol.* **30,** 248 (1966).

102. K. Landsteiner and M. W. Chase, *Proc. Soc. Exp. Biol. Med.* **49,** 688 (1942).

103. A. B. Stavitsky, *Proc. Soc. Exp. Biol. Med.* **67,** 225 (1948).

104. H. Haxthausen, *Acta Derm.-Venereol.* **31,** 659 (1951).

105. M. W. Chase, *Proc. Soc. Exp. Biol. Med.* **59,** 134 (1945).

106. N. A. Mitchison, *Nature (London)* **171,** 267 (1953).

107. For example, transfer of sensitivity to streptokinase in the rabbit by W. J. Warwick, O. Archer, and R. A. Good, *Proc. Soc. Exp. Biol. Med.* **105,** 459 (1960); to tuberculin in man by H. S. Lawrence, *Proc. Soc. Exp. Biol. Med.* **71,** 516 (1949);

to a variety of contact sensitizers in man by W. L. Epstein and A. M. Kligman, *J. Invest. Dermatol.* **28,** 291 (1957).

108. See, e.g., H. F. Helmholtz, *Z. Immunitaetsforsch.* **3,** 370 (1909); O. Bail, *Z. Immunitaetsforsch.* **4,** 470 (1910).

109. J. S. Najarian and J. F. Feldman, *J. Exp. Med.* **118,** 341 (1963); J. L. Turk and J. Oort, *Immunology* **6,** 140 (1963); R. T. McCluskey, B. Benacerraf, and J. W. McCluskey, *J. Immunol.* **90,** 466 (1964); R. A. Prendergast, *J. Exp. Med.* **119,** 377 (1964).

110. H. S. Lawrence, *J. Clin. Invest.* **33,** 951 (1954). See also H. S. Lawrence, *Adv. Immunol.* **11,** 196 (1969).

111. H. S. Lawrence and A. M. Pappenheimer, Jr., *J. Exp. Med.* **104,** 321 (1956); F. T. Rapaport *et al.*, *J. Immunol.* **84,** 358 (1960).

112. The early work is summarized by K. Landsteiner, *The Specificity of Serological Reactions,* pp. 197 ff. Dover, New York, 1962. See also M. Sulzberger and R. L. Baer, *J. Invest. Dermatol.* **1,** 45 (1938).

113. J. F. Enders, S. Cohen, and L. W. Kane, *J. Exp. Med.* **81,** 119 (1945); H. M. Rose and E. Molloy, *Fed. Proc.* **6,** 432 (1947); O. Urteaga, H. Wagner, and A. Chavez, *Arch. Peru. Patol. Clin.* **16,** 113 (1962). See also refs. 13 and 68.

114. E. Traub, *Science* **81,** 298 (1935); J. Hotchin, *Cold Spring Harbor Symp. Quant. Biol.* **27,** 479 (1962); G. A. Cole, N. Nathanson, and R. A. Prendergast, *Nature (London)* **238,** 335 (1972); M. J. Buchmaier, R. M. Welsh, F. J. Dutko, and M. B. A. Oldstone, *Adv. Immunol.* **30,** 275 (1980).

115. P. B. Medawar, *J. Anat.* **78,** 176 (1944); R. E. Billingham, L. Brent, and P. B. Medawar, *Proc. R. Soc. London, Ser. B* **143,** 58 (1954).

116. L. Brent, J. B. Brown, and P. B. Medawar, *Lancet* **ii,** 561 (1958); *Proc. R. Soc. London, Ser. B* **156,** 187 (1962).

117. M. Simonsen, *Acta Pathol. Microbiol. Scand.* **40,** 480 (1957); S. C. Grebe and J. W. Streilein, *Adv. Immunol.* **22,** 120 (1976); *Immunol. Rev.* **88** (1985).

118. The mixed lymphocyte reaction was first described by B. Bain, M. Vas, and L. Lowenstein, *Blood* **23,** 108 (1964). The topic is reviewed by B. Dupont, J. A. Hansen, and E. J. Yunis, *Adv. Immunol.* **23,** 107 (1976).

119. B. Glick, T. S. Chang, and R. G. Jaap, *Poultry Sci.* **35,** 224 (1956); N. L. Warner, A. Szenberg, and F. M. Burnet, *Aust. J. Exp. Biol. Med.* **40,** 373 (1956); N. R. Warner and A. Szenberg, in *The Thymus in Immunobiology* (R. A. Good and A. E. Gabrielson, eds.), p. 395. Harper (Hoeber), New York, 1964.

120. J. F. A. P. Miller, *Lancet* **ii,** 748 (1961); B. D. Janković, B. H. Waksman, and B. G. Arnason, *J. Exp. Med.* **116,** 159 (1962); R. A. Good *et al.*, *J. Exp. Med.* **116,** 773 (1962).

121. H. N. Claman, E. A. Chaperon, and R. F. Triplett, *Proc. Soc. Exp. Biol. Med.* **122,** 1167 (1966); A. J. S. Davies *et al.*, *Transplantation* **5,** 222 (1967); J. F. A. P. Miller and G. F. Mitchell, *J. Exp. Med.* **128,** 801, 821 (1968).

122. It was N. A. Mitchison [in *Immunological Tolerance* (M. Landy and W. Braun, eds.), p. 149. Academic Press, New York, 1969] who first showed T and B cell cooperation in antibody formation. The first T lymphocyte differentiation marker was described by A. E. Reif and J. M. V. Allen, *J. Exp. Med.* **120,**

413 (1964); M. C. Raff and H. H. Wortis, *Immunology* **18,** 931 (1970). Subsequently, many others have been described, as reviewed by I. F. C. McKenzie and T. Potter, *Adv. Immunol.* **27,** 179 (1979); *Immunol. Rev.* **82** (1984).

123. A. R. Rich and M. R. Lewis, *Bull. Johns Hopkins Hosp.* **50,** 115 (1933). Rich and Lewis believed that the antigen was directly cytotoxic for sensitized cells, but B. H. Waksman and M. Matoltsy [*J. Immunol.* **81,** 220 (1958)] later showed that the effect was one of cell (macrophage) stimulation.

124. M. George and J. H. Vaughan, *Proc. Soc. Exp. Biol. Med.* **111,** 514 (1962).

125. J. R. David, *Proc Natl. Acad. Sci. USA* **56,** 72 (1966).

126. B. R. Bloom and B. Bennett, *Science* **153,** 80 (1966).

127. S. Cohen, E. Pick, and J. J. Oppenheim, eds., *Biology of the Lymphokines.* Academic Press, New York, 1979; R. E. Rocklin, K. Bendtzen, and D. Greineder, *Adv. Immunol.* **29,** 56 (1980).

128. See, e.g., the reviews by Waksman (ref. 98) and Turk's book on delayed hypersensitivty (ref. 99). Perhaps the most influential markers of this new interest were P. Grabar and P. Miescher, eds., *Immunopathology.* Benno Schwabe, Basel, 1959; H. S. Lawrence, ed., *Cellular and Humoral Aspects of the Hypersensitivity States.* Harper (Hoeber), New York, 1959; J. H. Shaffer, G. A. LoGrippo, and M. W. Chase, eds., *Mechanisms of Hypersensitivity.* Little, Brown, Boston, Massachusetts, 1959; G. E. W. Wolstenholme and M. O'Connor, eds., *Cellular Aspects of Immunity,* Ciba Foundation Symposium. Little, Brown, Boston, Massachusetts, 1959.

129. P. G. H. Gell and R. R. A. Coombs, *Clinical Aspects of Immunology,* 2nd Ed., p. 575. Blackwell, Oxford, 1968.

130. P. Dhermy, G. Coscas, R. Nataf, and J. Levaditi, *Rev. Int. Trachome* **44,** 295 (1967); A. M. Silverstein and R. A. Prendergast, in *Morphological and Aspects of Immunity* (K. Lindahl-Kiessling *et al.,* eds.), p. 583. Plenum, New York, 1971.

131. A. Besredka, *Ann. Inst. Pasteur, Paris* **33,** 301, 557, 882 (1919); **34,** 361 (1920); **35,** 421 (1921). See also A. Besredka, *Immunisation Locale; Pansements Spécifiques.* Masson, Paris, 1925; *Les Immunités Locales.* Masson, Paris, 1937.

132. B. C. Seegal, D. Seegal, and D. Kohorazo, *J. Immunol.* **25,** 207 (1933).

133. A. M. Silverstein, in *Immunopathology of Uveitis* (A. E. Maumenee and A. M. Silverstein, eds.). Williams & Wilkins, Baltimore, Maryland, 1964.

134. See, e.g., G. L. Asherson and A. D. P. Webster, *Diagnosis and Treatment of Immunodeficiency Diseases.* Blackwell, Oxford, 1980; F. Aiuti, F. Rosen, and M. D. Cooper, eds., *Recent Advances in Primary and Acquired Immunodeficiencies.* Raven, New York, 1986.

135. J. H. Rockey L. A. Hanson, J. F. Heremans, and H. G. Kunkel, *J. Lab. Clin. Med.* **63,** 205 (1964).

136. J. R. Hobbs, R. D. G. Milner, and P. J. Watt, *Br. Med. J.* **iv,** 583 (1967).

137. P. H. Schur, *et al., N. Engl. J. Med.* **283,** 631 (1970).

138. O. C. Bruton, *Pediatrics* **9,** 722 (1952).

139. E. R. Pearl *et al., J. Immunol.* **120,** 1169 (1978)

140. J. Schwaber *et al., Nature (London)* **304,** 355 (1983).

141. C. A. Janeway, L. Apt, and D. Gitlin, *Trans. Assoc. Am. Physicians* **66**, 200 (1953).

142. A. M. DiGeorge, *J. Pediatr. (St. Louis)* **67**, 907 (1965); A. M. DiGeorge, in *Immunologic Deficiency Diseases in Man* (D. Bergsma, ed.). Natl. Found., New York, 1968.

143. R. A. Good and R. L. Varco, *J. Lancet.* **75**, 245 (1955).

144. C. Nezelof, *Arch. Fr. Pediatr.* **21**, 897 (1964).

145. E. Glanzmann and P. Riniker, *Ann. Pediatr. (Basel)* **175**, 1 (1950).

146. See, e.g., *Prog. Allergy* **37** (1986); G. Geraldo *et al.*, eds., *Recent Advances in AIDS and Kaposi's Sarcoma.* Karger, Basel, 1987.

147. A useful historical review of the complement system has been written by M. M. Mayer, *Complement* **1**, 2 (1984).

148. G. Nuttall, *Z. Hyg.* **4**, 353 (1888).

149. J. Bordet, *Ann. Inst. Pasteur, Paris* **12**, 688 (1899).

150. A. Ferrata, *Berl. klin. Wochenschr.* **44**, 368 (1907).

151. H. Ritz, *Z. Immunitaetsforsch.* **13**, 62 (1912).

152. A. F. Coca, *Z. Immunitaetsforsch.* **21**, 604 (1914).

153. J. Gordon, H. R. Whitehead, and A. Wormall, *Biochem. J.* **20**, 1028, 1036 (1926).

154. H. J. Rapp, *Science* **127**, 234 (1958); W. D. Linscott and K. Nishioka, *J. Exp. Med.* **118**, 795 (1963); K. Inoue and R. A. Nelson, Jr., *J. Immunol.* **96**, 386 (1966).

155. See ref. 148. See also M. M. Mayer, *Proc. Natl. Acad. Sci. USA* **69**, 2954 (1972).

156. L. Pillemer and E. E. Ecker, *J. Biol. Chem.* **137**, 139 (1941).

157. L. Pillemer, *Trans. N.Y. Acad. Sci.* **17**, 526 (1955). See also W. D. Ratnoff's interesting description of the history of the properdin controversy [*Perspect. Biol. Med.* **23**, 638 (1979–1980)].

158. O. Götze and H. J. Müller-Eberhard, *Adv. Immunol.* **24**, 1 (1976); D. T. Fearon, *Crit. Rev. Immunol.* **1**, 1 (1979); D. T. Fearon and K. F. Austin, *N. Engl. J. Med.* **303**, 259 (1980).

159. H. S. Shin *et al.*, *Science* **162**, 361 (1968); L. M. Lichtenstein *et al.*, *Immunology* **16**, 327 (1969). See also T. E. Hugli and H. J. Müller-Eberhard, *Adv. Immunol.* **26**, 1 (1978).

160. R. R. Hyde, *J. Immunol.* **8**, 267 (1923); *Am. J. Hyg.* **15**, 824 (1932).

161. A. M. Silverstein, *Blood* **16**, 1338 (1960).

162. P. J. Lachmann, *Boll. Ist. Sieroter, Milan.* **53**, Suppl., 195 (1974).

163. P. J. Lachmann and F. S. Rosen, *Springer Semin. Immunopathol.* **1**, 339 (1978); V. Agnello, *Medicine (Baltimore)* **57**, 1 (1978).

164. J. F. Soothill and B. A. M. Harvey, *Arch. Dis. Child.* **51**, 91 (1976); *Clin. Exp. Immunol.* **27**, 30 (1977).

10

Anti-antibodies and Anti-idiotype Immunoregulation, 1899–1904

Everything of importance has been said before by someone who did not discover it.
—Alfred North Whitehead

I T HAPPENS occasionally in science that a discovery is made or a concept is advanced long before its full implications can be assessed or its utility exploited. It may then sink into oblivion, only to be "rediscovered" and put to use decades or even centuries later. It matters little that the original concept may have been based upon erroneous premises or upon misinterpretations of fact, so long as its heuristic value impelled its adherents to develop it further along some logically consistent and useful lines. The result of such an enterprise might even be classed, at a later date, as a milestone in the history of the science. Thus, in geography, the ancient Greeks considered the earth to be a sphere on the basis of purely aesthetic reasons, since the sphere was the most perfect of all solids. But the (to us) inadequate basis for this speculation did not prevent Eratosthenes from concluding, in the third century B.C., that the logical consequence of a spherical earth should be that the sun's elevation at any moment would differ to two different observers standing in line with it. From this he was able to measure the circumference of the earth with an accuracy not improved upon for almost two millennia.[1] This concept of a round earth, and Eratosthenes' logical extension of its implications, faded from view, to be rediscovered by the demands of sixteenth century transoceanic voyages.

Perhaps the best-known instance of a "premature" theory in the field of immunology was Paul Ehrlich's side-chain theory of 1897.[2] This model was, for all practical purposes, the first natural selection theory of antibody formation. It dominated the field for perhaps a decade or so, only to fall into disrepute and nearly be forgotten for half a century until Niels Jerne[3] and Macfarlane Burnet[4] gave the selective theory of antibody formation its modern form and appeal. Indeed, it was the success of the clonal selection theory that refocused attention on Ehrlich's imaginative concept and stood witness to his creativity and prescience. But Ehrlich's side-chain theory was more than a concept of antibody formation; it speculated broadly also (within the obvious limitations of contemporary scientific knowledge) about the structure and function of antibody.[5] Implicit in the side-chain theory was an even more startling conceptual anticipation of the future—that the binding site of an antibody is a unique structure and might be immunogenic; that an anti-antibody might be formed against the specific site; that the shape of the anti-antibody combining site would be that of the corresponding antigen for which the original antibody was specific; and that this complex of antibodies and anti-antibodies might serve a very important immunoregulatory role in protecting against such undesirable events as autoimmunization.

All of these consequences of the side-chain theory, and more, were recognized and explicitly developed between 1899 and 1902 by the imaginative and implacably logical Paul Ehrlich, with occasional contributions also by Jules Bordet, Alexandre Besredka, and others. Here, save for the nomenclature, was a theory of idiotypes and anti-idiotypes, of mirror images, and of network immunoregulation that anticipated the modern development of this subject by almost 70 years and that has hardly been improved upon on the theoretical level. Never mind that the earlier version was based upon experiments later shown to be flawed technically, that it was based upon fatal misinterpretations of the data, and that it died ignominiously within a very few years. It testifies nevertheless to the vitality of the early years of immunology and to the imaginative approaches of its founders.

The full flavor and significance of the early work on anti-antibodies can best be appreciated by comparing it with modern developments in the theory and practice of the science of idiotypes. I shall, therefore, preface this look at the past with a brief review of the present status of this field.

Idiotypes and Anti-idiotypes, 1963–1985

The first significant stirrings of modern interest in anti-antibodies date from the 1950s and owe their origins to three different lines of attack.

The first was purely theoretical and stemmed from the fertile imagination of Victor Najjar.[6] Najjar assumed that the interaction of antibody with antigen leads to a change in molecular conformation that is immunogenic, leading to the development of a "cascade" of further anti-antibody reactants to the first and then to subsequent immune complexes, the entire process finally achieving a steady state. This speculation appears to have been the first modern hint at the existence of an immunoregulatory network that might function by self-stimulation and *internal* controls.

The second approach to the study of anti-antibodies was sparked by the growing interest in autoimmune diseases and especially by the growing realization that rheumatoid factor might in fact be an anti-antibody. This proposal was made initially by Milgrom and Dubiski,[7] who suggested also that the agglutinins for erythrocytes sensitized with incomplete antibody might be "anti-antibodies." They further postulated that the immune globulins of the individual's own body may become antigenic, presumably because the antibody becomes denatured upon interaction with antigen, and that this process might be the basis for the development of the putatively pathogenic rheumatoid factor. These studies were followed up by numerous other investigators,[8] all of whom were able to demonstrate that animals could mount an immune response to denatured autologous gamma globulin.

The third approach to anti-antibodies, and ultimately the most productive of all, originated in the earlier discovery that the immunoglobulins of humans and experimental animals possess genetically determined antigenic markers, or *allotypes*.[9] These are based upon unique sequences of amino acids in the polypeptide chains of immunoglobulins, whose composition and structure were even then being elucidated.[10] In the continuing search for new allotypes, three laboratories almost simultaneously discovered the phenomenon of idiotypy. From one direction, Jacques Oudin and Mauricette Michel in France[11] and Philip Gell and Andrew Kelus in England[12] noted the development of antibodies with peculiar characteristics in animals isoimmunized with bacteria coated with specific antibody. These had none of the characteristics of anti-allotypes, which usually react with most immunoglobulins of certain other individual animals; rather, these new antibodies reacted only with those antibodies specific for the bacterial carrier employed. Thus, not only were they anti-antibodies, but indeed they appeared to react with the immunogenic combining site of the antibody employed for immunization. In the terminology of the increasingly popular clonal selection theory of Burnet, Gell and Kelus were the first to suggest that this was, in fact, an "anti-clone antibody," reactive with a unique antibody combining site. They called the immunogen a "private" antigenic determinant, to distinguish it from the more public antigenic determinants constituted by allotypic markers. Oudin soon coined the term idiotype[13] to characterize this distinction more precisely.

A somewhat different point of departure was employed by Henry Kunkel and his colleagues[14] in arriving at the same conclusions as those of Oudin and Michel and of Gell and Kelus. Myeloma proteins and those of certain macroglobulinemias had been shown to possess the characteristics of individual (monoclonal) antibodies and to show unique antigenic specificities.[15] These workers therefore immunized rabbits with purified and fairly homogeneous preparations of human antidextran and anti-levan antibodies. Several of the rabbits produced anti-antibodies specific only for the individual antibody employed for immunization. Clearly, each of these three groups had discovered anti-idiotypic antibodies, although the identity of the "new" antigenic determinant with the antibody combining site had yet to be firmly established.

In 1966, Gell and Kelus reviewed the then-still-limited literature on autoantibodies and idiotypes and speculated with impressive foresight on two aspects that would later loom large in this field. In a discussion of the possible biological significance of autoanti-idiotypes, they pointed out their relevance to our understanding of the mechanisms of autoimmunity and of immunological tolerance. As they said, "It is hard to believe that it [the body] can regularly react to 'private' determinants on its own antibodies, not so much because the process would be self-destructive as that it would lead to an infinite regress of anti-antibody production."[16] Here is yet another hint that each anti-idiotype is itself an idiotype, able to stimulate a further progression of immune responses at each stage. They suggested, however, that the immunogenicity of the idiotype may be quite low, thus cutting short the infinite regress at an early stage. Gell and Kelus further proposed in this review that self-tolerance to idiotypic determinants, in the sense of a Burnetian clonal deletion, does not provide an adequate explanation, since "it would entail the elimination of a number of clones equal to the number of possible antibodies."[17] This is the first intimation that the universe of potential anti-idiotypes may equal in size the universe of possible antibodies.

Despite the many fascinating problems posed by idiotypes and anti-idiotypes, this area did not yet grip the collective imagination of immunologists, and only modest progress was forthcoming for almost a decade.[18] It remained for Niels Jerne to rephrase the questions and the possibilities in another of his landmark speculative ventures, first hinted at in 1971[19] and then developed more fully in 1974. This was his network concept of the immune system. Here was a theory in which idiotypes and anti-idiotypes play the central role not only in determining the ultimate size of the immune-response repertoire but also in furnishing a mechanism for the internal regulation of these responses.

JERNE'S NETWORK THEORY, 1974

In reviewing the pertinent data up to that point, Jerne[20] called special attention to three aspects that he felt were especially significant: (1) A given antibody combining site structurally determines a set of immunogenic regions (idiotopes) in the variable region of the immunoglobulin molecule. (2) The idiotope collective (the idiotype) forms an "internal image" of and interacts with the antigenic site (epitope) against which it is formed; but it reacts also with a corresponding set of anti-antibodies (the anti-idiotopes) whose formation it may stimulate, thus forming a network of ever increasing size. (3) The immune response is a measure of the balance that may exist at any time between active stimulus and active suppression, i.e., the result of an immunoregulatory network in which idiotypes and anti-idiotypes act upon both T and B lymphocytes. (The reader will wish to compare Jerne's formulation with one by Jean Lindenmann,[21] apparently stimulated by informal communications from Jerne himself. Lindenmann noted that the antibody combining site contains a "negative image" of its respective antigen and that the anti-idiotype, which he called a *homobody*, contains a "positive image" of the antigen. These form a network of interconnecting molecules which, Lindenmann suggested, "may have broad biological significance.")

It is difficult to overstate the extent of the interest and research activity generated by Jerne's concept. For almost the first time, it was suggested that the production of autoantibodies against self-antigens might be the normal state of affairs rather than the exception. Again, the idiotype–anti-idiotype network offered an appealing alternative molecular model to explain immunoregulation and the suppression of autoimmune phenomena, in place of the increasingly popular cell-dynamic model based upon the positive and negative contributions of T lymphocytes.[22] (Acceptance of the idiotype network theory of immunoregulation has not been universal. Melvin Cohn[23] has summarized the position of those who maintain that cellular interactions and intercellular signals contribute more to the regulation of the immune response than do the molecular interactions of idiotypes and anti-idioptyes.)

By analogy with earlier demonstrations that anti-allotypes can suppress the development of individual allotypes, it was quickly confirmed

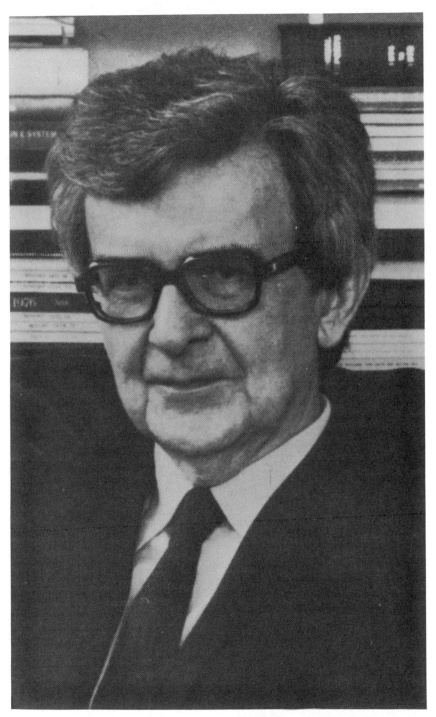

Niels Jerne (Courtesy National Library of Medicine)

that anti-idiotypic antibodies may also suppress the production of specific idiotypes.[24] From this, it followed that passive administration of anti-idiotypic antibody might suppress specifically those immune responses to antigen that are characterized by a preponderance of certain idiotopes, although such responses may also be enhanced by anti-idiotypes under special conditions.[25] Further, idiotypes were found on both helper and suppressor T cells as well as on B cell membrane receptors,[26] a finding suggesting that autoanti-idiotype antibody might contribute also to the regulatory function of these lymphocyte subsets.

Autoanti-idiotypes were also found to be routinely present in association with autoimmune disease states such as systemic lupus erythematosus,[27] thyroid disease,[28] hemolytic anemias,[29] and autoimmune interstitial nephritis.[30] This association implied, as Jerne had predicted, that autoanti-idiotypes might play a central role in the mechanism of self-tolerance and in the suppression of autoimmunity, a prediction that has been confirmed experimentally.[31] The speculation that the anti-idiotype should look like a positive image of the antigen and mimic it was also confirmed[32] and as such could contribute to either positive or negative immunoregulation of the immune response, with possible applications also for use as vaccines. Thus, the full implications of Jerne's network theory were realized, in that internal self-regulation of the immune response, *independent of the presence of antigen*, was a possibility now almost fully realized.

Many other investigators contributed to the development of the idiotype–anti-idiotype story on the theoretical as well as on the technical level. The numerous reviews and symposium proceedings of the last several years not only record their names and contributions but also illustrate the degree to which this relatively new field has captured the attention of an entire generation of immunologists.[33]

In order to appreciate fully the conceptual achievements of those engaged in anti-antibody research at the turn of the last century (to be recounted later) it may be well to keep in mind the salient aspects of the modern approach to this problem: (1) The antibody combining site (the idiotype) is unique and may itself constitute a new immunogenic site. (2) The new antibody combining site may stimulate the formation of autoantibody against it (the autoanti-idiotype). (3) The idiotype presents an internal image of the antigenic site, and the anti-idiotype is structurally similar to and may act in place of antigen. (4) The interaction of idiotypes and anti-idiotypes may constitute an effective molecular regulatory system, one of whose principal activities may be to inhibit the development of pathological autoimmune processes.

The Background to Anti-antibodies, 1890–1899

At the time that Emil von Behring and Shibusaburo Kitasato discovered antibodies in 1890,[34] infectious diseases were generally thought to be mediated by bacterial toxins, and protective antibodies were viewed solely as antitoxins. This view was strengthened by Ehrlich's demonstration that circulating antibodies could be induced even against plant toxins such as ricin and abrin.[35] The discovery of immune hemolysis by Bordet in 1899[36] appeared to confirm further the generalization that most destructive processes of interest to the bacteriologist–immunologist were toxic in nature, except that in this instance the antibody itself was the toxin. Indeed, Bordet and others repeatedly referred to hemolytic antibody as a "hemotoxin"; and when other anti-cell or anti-organ antibodies were discovered, they were variously termed spermotoxins, neurotoxins, leucotoxins, and so on.[37]

The finding that "immunity" responses could be engendered by the cellular elements of the mammalian body as well as by bacteria caused little surprise in the late 1890s, for by this time it had generally become accepted that the immune response was part of a larger, normal physiological process for the digestion and disposal of unwanted substances. As early as 1884, Metchnikoff had postulated that the immune response had evolved from primitive digestive functions, serving now to break down and to mitigate the effects of invading bacteria.[38] Of course, Metchnikoff assigned to the phagocyte the principal role in this process and extended it also to the disposal of effete cells of the animal's own body. With the rise of interest in antibodies, Metchnikoff's disciple Alexandre Besredka extended the concept to include the contribution of hemolytic antibody toward the disposal of worn-out erythrocytes.[39] In a similar manner, Ehrlich utilized the same approach in his side-chain theory of antibody formation, postulating that all antibodies are physiological products that play an important part in the *normal* economy of the cell and of the body.[40]

EHRLICH'S SIDE-CHAIN THEORY, 1897

The major aspects of Paul Ehrlich's side-chain theory of antibody formation have been described extensively elsewhere[41] and need not be treated here in great detail. For the present purposes, it will suffice to recall the principal premises upon which Ehrlich based his concept: (1) antibodies are naturally occurring substances that serve as receptors on the cell surface; (2) the specificity of antibody for antigen is determined by a unique stereochemical configuration of atoms that permits the antibody to bind tightly and chemically to its appropriate antigen; (3) the number of different combining site structures available is so great that each one differs from the others, with little or no cross-reactions among them; and (4) in order to induce active antibody formation, it is only necessary that appropriate receptors be present on the cells for antigen to interact with them and so stimulate their overproduction and liberation into the blood. Thus, the antibody, as first conceived by Ehrlich, appeared to be a rather nondescript blob of cytoplasm *with only one distinguishing feature*—a highly organized combining site (the haptophore group) that defined its specificity and thus its ability to bind to antigen.

With the subsequent discovery of immune hemolysis and of the participation of complement, Ehrlich expanded his theory to define hemolytic antibody as an "amboceptor," this time with two chemically defined combining sites, one for antigen and one for complement.[42] But if the combining site for antigen is a unique structure with a unique specificity, then so also should be the combining site for complement. This proposal implied that just as there exists a multiplicity of different antigens, each defining and being defined by a distinctive combining site on antibody, so there should also be a multiplicity of different complements, one for the complementophile group on each different antibody.[43] Furthermore, in order for antibody to interact with antigen or with complement, its combining site must recognize and attach to a complementary, structurally defined combining site on its partner. These conclusions were among the first of the many logical extensions that Ehrlich and his followers formulated to expand upon the rather simple premises initially embodied in his side-chain theory.

It was the further application of the side-chain theory and of Ehrlich's inexorable logic to the question of anti-antibodies that invites comparison with modern theories of idiotypic interactions and immunoregulation.

THE CONCEPTUAL POSITION OF JULES BORDET

In contrast to Ehrlich, who was concerned primarily with the origin of antibodies and the chemical basis for their specificity, Bordet was more interested in their mode of action and biological implications. He took exception to almost every aspect of Ehrlich's theories and to the conclusions that Ehrlich drew from them.[44] Where Ehrlich argued for a stereochemical basis for specificity and a firm union between antigen and antibody, Bordet concluded that the antigen–antibody union was reversible and a physical one that was based upon colloid-adsorptive processes.[45] It was especially in their ideas about the mechanism of immune hemolysis that the two investigators differed most sharply. Ehrlich's theory demanded, in addition to a specific haptophore group for antigen, an equally specific complementophile group to mediate the firm interaction of antibody with complement. Bordet denied this and suggested that the role of antibody was rather to "sensitize" the erythrocyte, whereupon complement would be fixed nonspecifically and in consequence permitted to effect the destruction of the erythrocyte.[46] Thus, while Ehrlich's logic seemed to require a multiplicity of different complements within a given serum, Bordet was content with but a single complement acting wherever required.[47]

Perhaps the most interesting difference between Ehrlich and Bordet lay in their scientific styles. One gets the impression from reading Ehrlich that he was by far the more doctrinaire of the two. Having advanced his side-chain theory, he (and his students) applied it relentlessly to each new observation and at each step advanced a new modification or *ad hoc* hypothesis to help to fit the new information into the old theoretical mold. This tendency is best illustrated by Ehrlich's attempt to explain the shape of the diphteria toxin–antitoxin neutralization curve, which required him to predict the existence, not only of a toxoid, but of a low affinity "toxon" and of alpha and beta modifications of proto-, deutero-, and tritotoxins of differing affinities.[48] Bordet, on the other hand, appears to have been more the pragmatist and always claimed that he was less a theoretician than a describer of "the true state of affairs." Although he was firmly committed to his sensitization theory of immune hemolysis, contradictory data generally found him prepared to give up a previous conclusion quite readily and to seek a new explanation for the phenomenon.

This difference in scientific styles between Ehrlich and Bordet is important to our story of anti-antibodies. Each investigator undertook to produce and to study anti-antibodies in 1899, to help bolster his own position and undermine that of his opponent. In their very first mention of anti-antibodies,[49] Ehrlich and Morgenroth suggested that these entities would provide further evidence for the multiplicity of amboceptors; and they later utilized the same approach to help prove the existence of a multiplicity of complements. Bordet, for his part, felt that anti-antibodies would prove the unity of complement, a position that he also stated explicitly in his paper on this subject.[50] But it is this very difference in scientific styles that helps to explain the different roles played by Ehrlich and Bordet in the development of the anti-antibody story over the next five years. Ehrlich, the more rigid theorist, would be responsible for an impressive theoretical construct involving (to employ the terminology of a later era) idiotypes, anti-idiotypes, and internal and external images of antigen. Bordet would make little contribution to these theories; rather, it would be he who would pursue the problem experimentally and finally provide the data to show that the entire theory was erroneous and based upon a misinterpretation of the facts.

Anti-antibodies, 1899—1904

Our story of the first discovery of anti-antibodies starts in 1898, with the almost simultaneous demonstration by Kossel in Germany[51] and Camus and Gley in France[52] that a protective antibody could be formed against the hemolytic toxin present in eel serum. Here was an antitoxin analogous to those formed against diphtheria or tetanus toxins, but one whose protective action could be demonstrated in the test tube in a system where the specific target of the toxic antibody (the erythrocyte) was established beyond question. This observation was immediately seized upon by Bordet and by Ehrlich and Morgenroth, who independently concluded that if an antibody could be prepared against hemolytic eel toxin, then it should surely be possible to prepare a similar neutralizing antibody against the hemotoxic antibody found in the serum of animals immunized with erythrocytes. Suiting action to speculation, both laboratories immunized animals of an unrelated species with whole anti-erythrocyte serum and quickly reported the finding of an "anti-antibody" that would inhibit the destructive action of the hemolytic antibody employed for immunization.

THE ANTIBODY-COMBINING SITE AS IMMUNOGEN

In their "Second Communication on Hemolysis" in 1899, Ehrlich and Morgenroth record the theoretical basis for these experiments: "This antibody, formed by an immunity reaction, thrusts itself into the hemotropic group [combining site] of the *Zwischenkörper* and thus deflects it from the erythrocyte. Our attempts, based on these premises, to produce an isolated [specific] antibody for some of the lysins have thus far been unsuccessful."[53] It was not that they were unable to demonstrate inhibition of hemolysis with their putative anti-antibody, but that the inhibition was not restricted to the species of erythrocyte employed to obtain the hemolytic antiserum. Since the hemolysis of many different species of erythrocytes was inhibited by the anti-antibody, the demands of the side-chain theory forced Ehrlich and Morgenroth to conclude that the hemolytic serum must contain a multiplicity of antibodies against various erythrocytes and therefore must stimulate a correspondingly large number of anti-antibodies.

The theoretical basis for the action of anti-antibodies was expanded upon during the following year in Ehrlich's Croonian Lecture before the Royal Society, in which he pointed out that "the lysin, be it bacterial lysin or hemolysin (i.e., immune body plus complement), possesses altogether three haptophore groups, of which two belong to the immune body and one to the complement. Each one of these can be bound by an appropriate anti-group. Three anti-groups are thus conceivable any one of which, by uniting with one of the haptophore groups of the lysin, can frustrate the action of the lysin."[54]

Jules Bordet interpreted his results on anti-antibodies somewhat differently. While concluding that the immune serum that he obtained by immunizing with a hemolytic antiserum might contain anti-antibodies specific for the *sensibilisateur* as well as anti-*alexine* antibodies (to use Bordet's terminology for hemolysin and complement), he argued that his results proved the unity of complement rather than its multiplicity. How else could one explain the ability of a rabbit anti-guinea pig hemolytic serum to neutralize all complement activity of guinea pigs, but not that of other species?[55]

[The modern reader will already have detected the basic flaw in these experiments. In 1899, hemolytic antisera were prepared by immunizing animals with defibrinated *whole blood,* so that antibodies would have been formed against many of the serum components as well as against the erythrocytes present in the inoculum. Similarly, "anti-antibodies" were prepared by immunizing with *whole immune serum;* thus, a variety of complement-fixing antiproteins would be formed. But in 1899, the only antibodies recognized were against bacterial toxins and cellular elements such as erythrocytes, which were known (according to Ehrlich's side-chain theory) to contain specific receptors. Almost nothing was known about the composition of normal serum, so Ehrlich or Bordet were justified *at that time* in expecting antibody formation only against those immunogenic receptors they assumed to be present. In normal defibrinated blood, only the erythrocyte receptors were assumed to be immunogenic, whereas in an immune serum, immunogenicity could only be assumed for the combining sites on specific antibody or on complement.]

AUTOANTI-ANTIBODY IMMUNOREGULATION

Bordet's observations on anti-antibodies were quickly extended by his colleague at the Institut Pasteur, Alexandre Besredka.[56] Arguing from

Elie Metchnikoff's idea that immunity is due to the normal processes of digestion and that antibodies assist in the destruction of injected foreign cells, Besredka asked why antibodies are not formed against the cells of one's own body during their destruction. Why, for example, are auto-hemolytic antibodies not formed during the erythrophagocytosis of effete red blood cells in the spleen? Besredka's answer to this was that they are! Why, then, does this not cause continual hemolysis of all erythrocytes? Because, claimed Besredka, the body normally makes an anti-antibody against *every* potentially threatening autoantibody, thus interfering with its destructive activity.

Besredka justified his thesis by citing a series of experiments on hemolytic antibodies formed in species A against the erythrocytes of species B, utilizing complement from any other species. He showed that A anti-B serum lyses the washed erythrocytes of B, but that the addition of normal B serum inhibits this hemolytic action. However, sera from other species (C, D, etc.) exhibit no similar inhibitory effect. Furthermore, B's serum will inhibit the hemolysis of an anti-B-erythrocyte serum formed in any other species as well. From these data, Besredka concluded (1) that all normal sera contain anti-antibodies that protect their own erythrocytes from immune hemolysis; (2) that he had demonstrated the specificty of these anti-antibodies; (3) that the anti-antibody is not an anti-complement; and (4) that Ehrlich was wrong about the multiplicity of amboceptors—all anti-B hemolysins are identical, since they are all inhibited by the anti-antibody normally present in every B serum.

When Besredka suggested in 1901 that autoantibody formation was the norm, with its pathogenicity controlled by the countervailing production of autoanti-antibodies, the existence of *any* type of autoantibody production had not yet been formally demonstrated. Indeed, Ehrlich had expressed the common view that while theoretically possible, the formation of destructive autoantibodies was "dysteleologic" and unlikely. This point of view was epitomized in Ehrlich's famous dictim of *horror autotoxicus*.[57] However, in 1904, Julius Donath and Karl Landsteiner published the first clear-cut description of a destructive auto-antibody causing serious disease in man[58]—the autohemolysin responsible for paroxysmal cold hemoglobinuria (PKH). Ehrlich and his followers conceded at once that this phenomenon was a probable exception to the rule.[59] Besredka's adherents, however, offered up an alternative explanation based upon autoanti-antibody immunoregulation. They suggested[60] that Donath and Landsteiner were wrong in ascribing the disease to the *presence* of autohemolysins, since according to Besredka's theory everyone produced them. The defect in PKH, they claimed, was due to the *absence* in these patients of the regulatory autoanti-antibodies that normally inhibit spontaneous hemolysis.

Besredka's concept of the existence of autoanti-antibodies and of their immunoregulatory role appears to have been a purely speculative leap of the imagination; Paul Ehrlich, on the other hand, arrived at the same conclusions simply by pursuing the inner logic of his side-chain theory. In 1899, Morgenroth had shown that animals inoculated with the enzyme rennin would invariably produce anti-rennin antibodies.[61] But rennin is presumably one of the normal constituents of the animal's digestive tract, so the formation of an "autoantibody" against a self-constituent could conceivably compromise the well-being of the host. Ehrlich and Morgenroth returned to this question the following year and proposed a thought-experiment to explain the apparent paradox.[62] Here is the logical extension of the side-chain theory in its most elegant form.

Suppose that a hypothetical antigen α is injected into an animal, then two consequences are possible according to Ehrlich and Morgenroth. If the animal lacks group α, then the specific site α on the injected antigen will seek out its corresponding receptor on the surface of the host's cells, react with the combining sites on these receptors, and thus stimulate the formation of anti-α antibodies. This is the usual course of the immune response. Suppose, however, that the immunized animal possesses antigenic group α within its body, as is the case with rennin. Anti-α antibodies will still be formed, but these will now appear as "autoanti-bodies." But these circulating antibodies with combining sites specific for antigenic group α will themselves find cells with α receptors on their surface (i.e., presumably those cells responsible for the original production of that antigen). Such cells will be stimulated to produce additional α molecules for release into the circulation. But not only is α the original antigen, it is also functionally the autoanti-antibody able to combine specifically with the anti-α combining site to prevent its toxic action. Thus, an interactive network is established involving antigen, specific antibody, anti-antibody (= antigen), and so forth, all of which presumably reach a steady-state, self-regulated equilibrium to suppress autoimmune disease.

In this example of Ehrlich and Morgenroth's, one sees epitomized both Ehrlich's inexorable logic and the full sweep of this turn-of-the-century theoretical construct. The antibody combining site is a unique structure and may stimulate the formation of a specific autoanti-antibody; the antibody contains the negative image of antigen, and the anti-antibody contains the positive image of antigen; and finally, a self-regulating network may be established to prevent self-intoxication.

THE IMAGES OF ANTIGEN

The foregoing discussion has already made it abundantly clear that Ehrlich viewed the interaction of antigen with antibody as the combination of two complementary stereochemical structures—the specific combining site on antibody and the immunogenic site on antigen. This required, in effect, that the structure of the antibody combining site present as a "negative image" of the antigen. Indeed, the diagrams published by Ehrlich and Morgenroth to represent these interactions make this conclusion explicit. Figure 10.1A shows a cartoon representation of different antibody combining sites, each with a unique shape into which the corresponding antigen will fit to mediate combination. Ehrlich

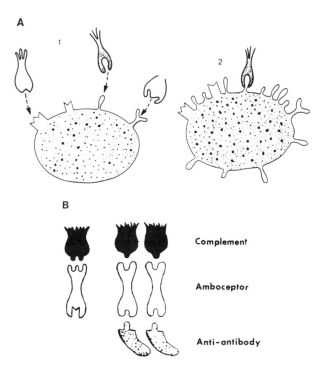

Fig. 10.1. The Ehrlich conceptualization of antibody–antigen and antibody–complement binding sites in cartoon form. (A) Each antigen has a unique stereochemical structure that is matched by the specific combining site on antibody, in the form of a "negative image." (From ref. 5.) (B) Similar unique structures define antibody–complement "image" of the antigen. (Adapted from Ehrlich, ref. 2, p. 289.)

extended this concept to include the individuality of the different combining sites for complements (Fig. 10.1B), upon which he based his prediction of the existence of a multiplicity of different complements. According to these diagrams, the "anti-antibody" contains a "positive image" of the antigen in question.

In their "Third Communication on Hemolysis," Ehrlich and Morgenroth defined clearly the conditions necessary for antibody formation. Cell-surface receptors for the antigen must be present, for "if . . . an organism lack receptors . . . the first essential for the production of an antibody will be wanting. In the development or non-development of antibodies, we shall have an indication of the presence or absence of receptors."[63] It is clear also, as these authors point out, that in order for a hemolytic antibody to function, antigenic receptors must be present on the target erythrocytes. But if an antibody is injected into an animal and finds appropriate receptors, then logic demands that anti-antibody be formed, and this is precisely what Ehrlich and Morgenroth report. It will be recalled here that for Ehrlich, the only identifiable structure on either antigen or antibody is the specific combining site. Thus, the anti-antibody is an anti-haptophore group and therefore, by definition, the positive image of the antigen combining site. The anti-antibody is in fact nothing less than the freed antigenic receptor itself! (While Ehrlich never says so explicitly, it is evident from this discussion that the two partners in the interaction of antigen and antibody cannot readily be distinguished. Either of them may be called the antibody, implying the active combining factor, and the other the antigen, implying the passive partner.)

The notion that the anti-combining site of antibody should be antigen itself was taken up by Pfeiffer and Friedberger[64] with extremely surprising results. These authors immunized a rabbit with goat anti-cholera serum, and obtained an antiserum that appeared to neutralize the anti-cholera antibodies employed for immunization. By studying the quantitative relationships between the anti-antibody and the original antiserum, they were able to show that the former was not an anti-complement but an antibody against the original anti-cholera antibody. But such an anti-antibody would be, according to Ehrlich's theory, the antigenic determinant present originally on the cholera vibrio—a substance that surely should not be present on the cells of higher animals. While somewhat perplexed by these findings, Pfeiffer and Friedberger were forced to conclude that "from the present state of our knowledge, there is left no other remaining possibility than to conclude, in defiance of theory, the existence of anti-antibody in our serum."

August von Wassermann drew a similar conclusion from the logical imperatives of the Ehrlich theory and attempted to apply this to clinical practice in a most interesting manner.[65] In his case, Wassermann had developed an anti-complement, i.e., an antibody of presumed specificity for the unique binding site on the complement "molecule." On the assumption that immunization with this anti-complement would result in its binding to complement receptors on the surface of appropriate cells, he sought to immunize animals with this anti-complement "in the expectation of producing thereby, according to the applicable laws of immunity, an increase in the production of the respective complement, and thus a heightened resistance, or in such animals better therapeutic results." In the event, Wassermann's attempt did not succeed, and no increase in complement titer resulted, although the experiment appeared nevertheless to be firmly based upon the inner logic of Ehrlich's side-chain theory. Indeed, in discussing Wassermann's experiment, Ehrlich's student Hans Sachs pointed out that the anti-complement combining site should in fact have the character and structure of the complementophile group on amboceptor.[66] It should theoretically be possible, therefore, to employ anti-complement antibody for the production of specific anti-amboceptor. The theory is here carried one step further and demonstrates clearly the understanding by these investigators of the reciprocal nature of specifically interacting combining sites, where positive and negative images of a given structure would alternate at each succeeding stage of the immunization process.

The Demise of Anti-antibody Theories, 1901–1905

The discovery of anti-antibodies and speculations about their significance stimulated a flurry of investigations,[67] of which we have mentioned here only the most prominent. But as new data appeared, it quickly became evident that the original interpretations required major modification. Somehow, the specificities of these "anti-antibodies" did not always obey the logical predictions of Ehrlich's theory. Thus, as early as 1900, Bordet showed that an antiserum against guinea pig complement would neutralize all guinea pig complement activity, but not that of other species.[68] He argued from his observation that Ehrlich was wrong in suggesting a multiplicity of different complement specificities and that, in fact, there exists but a single type of complement within the given species. Similarly, Pfeiffer and Friedberger showed in 1902 that the inhibitory action of an "anti-amboceptor" extends to all of the amboceptors of the species, and they suggested on the basis of that result that the anti-amboceptor (which they assumed to be directed against the complementophile receptor) had to be nonspecific.[69] Faced with this objection, Ehrlich was forced to retreat from his original stand and to allow that "we must assume that all the amboceptors of the same animal species are at least partly similar in structure so far as the complementophile apparatus is concerned. In a way, therefore, the amboceptor bears the stamp of the animal species from which it derives."[70] Here is the first concession by Ehrlich not only that a haptophore group (combining site) might not be a unique structure but indeed that these active molecules might possess immunogenic species markers in addition to their specific combining sites.

In the end, it was Bordet who sounded the death knell of the anti-antibody theory, and this by means of two major experimental contributions. The first of these was the discovery in 1901 of the complement fixation test by Bordet and Gengou.[71] Hitherto, complement had been considered to function only in conjunction with anti-erythrocyte and antibacterial antibodies, to effect the lysis or death of these target cells. Now, numerous workers were able to show that *any* protein or bacterial antigen might fix complement in the presence of its specific antibody.[72] This finding led Neisser and Sachs to show that complement fixation might be employed for the determination of proteins for forensic purposes,[73] and Detré[74] and Wasserman *et al.*[75] to show that this approach might also be employed for the diagnosis of syphilis and other infectious diseases.

Complement fixation was therefore entirely nonspecific, as Bordet had originally claimed. The activity of many of the so-called anti-antibodies represented not specific anti-complements but a nonspecific complement fixation due to the presence of unrelated antigen–antibody interactions in the test mixtures employed. These data forced Ehrlich almost to give up completely his belief in antibodies specific for complement or its combining site on amboceptor, and to confess that "in this case, therefore, the anticomplement action is brought about by the interaction of two components, one present in the serum of the immunized animal and the other in the serum of that animal species whose serum was used for immunization. It is clear, of course, that here the dissolved albuminous substances, not the complements, were the antigens. This being the case, the demonstration of anticomplements produced by immunization becomes extremely difficult."[76] Thus was the possibility of an anti-antibody specific for the combining site on complement, or for the complementophile site on amboceptor, laid to rest.

It now remained for Bordet to disprove the existence of an anti-antibody specific for the *antigen* combining site, and this he did in a major publication in 1904.[77] In this paper, Bordet refuted the thesis of Ehrlich and Morgenroth that the anti-antibody might be directed against the specific combining site by showing (1) that the putative anti-antibody appears to neutralize *all* of the antibodies (hemolysins, bacteriolysins, etc.) produced in the species employed to stimulate the anti-antibody; (2) that one can obtain an inhibitory "anti-hemolysin" by injecting into an animal of another species even normal serum, preabsorbed with erythrocytes to remove natural antibodies; and (3) that the so-called anti-hemolysin will not neutralize hemolysins active against the same erythrocytes but formed in a third animal species. Bordet concluded from these results that the action of "anti-antibodies" is not directed against the specific site on the immunizing antibody; that the "anti-antibody" is not the positive image of the original antigen; and that it is in fact directed against something (not further specified) in the immunizing serum that is characteristic of the species.

This was the final nail in the coffin of anti-antibody theories. By 1905, such concepts were no longer seriously considered or experimentally pursued by most workers in the field. Those who held out the longest were the members of Ehrlich's school of immunology, but even Hans Sachs (who had assumed the role of spokesman for this group when Ehrlich's interests shifted to chemotherapy) was forced slowly to concede the earlier conceptual errors, in a series of major reviews on hemolysis and hemolysins.[78]

Conclusions

It must remain a tribute to the breadth of Ehrlich's side-chain theory of 1897 that within it lay the seeds of a concept of idiotypes, anti-idiotypes, and anti-idiotype immunoregulation that would foreshadow modern developments in this area by almost 80 years. It is, further, a reflection of the greatness of Ehrlich's intellect that he was able to extract from this theory all of its logical implications and to construct a conceptual edifice that anticipated in almost every major respect those features of idiotype–anti-idiotype phenomenology that have been elucidated during the past dozen years. What is most surprising about the earlier theoretical construct is not that it was subsequently disproved, but rather that is was so completely effaced from the collective memory of immunologists that no mention of it is to be found in modern writings in this field.[79]

NOTES AND REFERENCES

1. D. J. Boorstin, *The Discoverers*, pp. 94 ff. Random House, New York, 1983.
2. P. Ehrlich, *Klin. Jahrb.* **60,** 299 (1897). [English translation in *The Collected Papers of Paul Ehrlich*, Vol. 2, pp. 107–125. Pergamon, New York, 1957.

3. N. K. Jerne, *Proc. Natl. Acad. Sci. USA* **41,** 849 (1955).

4. F. M. Burnet, *Aust. J. Sci.* **20,** 67 (1957); *The Clonal Selection Theory of Antibody Formation.* Cambridge University Press, London, 1959.

5. See Ehrlich's Croonian Lecture before the Royal Society, *Proc. R. Soc. London* **66,** 424 (1900). See also Chapter 4.

6. V. A. Najjar and J. Fisher, *Science* **122,** 1272 (1955); V. A. Najjar, *Physiol. Rev.* **43,** 243 (1963).

7. F. Milgrom and S. Dubiski, *Nature (London)* **179,** 1351 (1957); S. Dubiski, *Folia Biol.* (Krakow) **6,** 47 (1958). See also F. Milgrom, S. Dubiski, and G. Wozniczko, *Nature (London)* **178,** 539 (1956).

8. J. L. Abruzzo and C. L. Christian, *J. Exp. Med.* **114,** 791 (1961); R. T. McCluskey, F. Miller, and B. Benacerraf, *J. Exp. Med.* **115,** 253 (1962); R. C. Williams, Jr. and H. G. Kunkel, *Ann. N.Y. Acad. Sci.* **124,** 860 (1965).

9. J. Oudin, *C. R. Hebd. Seances Acad. Sci.* **242,** 2606 (1966); R. Grubb, *Acta Pathol. Microbiol. Scand.* **39,** 195 (1956).

10. S. Cohen and R. R. Porter, *Adv. Immunol.* **4,** 287 (1964); T. J. Kindt, *Adv. Immunol.* **21,** 35 (1975).

11. J. Oudin and M. Michel, *C. R. Hebd. Seances Acad. Sci.* **257,** 805 (1963).

12. P. G. H. Gell and A. Kelus, *Nature (London)* **201,** 687 (1964).

13. J. Oudin, *Proc. R. Soc. London, Ser. B* **166,** 207 (1966).

14. H. G. Kunkel, M. Mannik, and R. C. Williams, *Science* **140,** 1218 (1963). See also H. G. Kunkel, *Harvey Lect.* **59,** 219 (1965).

15. R. J. Slater, S. M. Ward, and H. G. Kunkel, *J. Exp. Med.* **101,** 85 (1955).

16. P. G. H. Gell and A. Kelus, *Adv. Immunol.* **6,** 461, 476 (1967).

17. Reference 16, p. 476.

18. Apart from the original laboratories of discovery, only those of Lindermann (see below, ref. 26), of Cosenza and Köhler (see below, ref. 24), and of Alfred Nisonoff made a significant early commitment to idiotypology, from which emerged important contributions to the field and an extensive review as early as 1971 [J. E. Hopper and A. Nisonoff, *Adv. Immunol.* **13,** 57 (1971)].

19. N. K. Jerne, in *Ontogeny of Acquired Immunity.* Elsevier, New York, 1972.

20. N. K. Jerne, *Ann. Immunol. (Paris)* **125C,** 373 (1974); *Harvey Lect.* **70,** 93 (1974).

21. J. Lindenmann, *Ann. Immunol. (Paris)* **124C,** 171 (1973).

22. N. A. Mitchison, in *Immunological Tolerance* (M. Landy and W. Braun, eds.), p. 149. Academic Press, New York, 1969. See also D. H. Katz and B. Benacerraf, *Adv. Immunol.* **15,** 1 (1972).

23. M. Cohn, *Cell. Immunol.* **61,** 425 (1981).

24. While Jerne's network concept provided a rational theoretical basis for immunoregulation, it was in fact preceded by isolated reports of anti-idiotype suppression of the immune response: see, e.g., M. G. Lewis, T. M. Phillips, K. B. Cook, and J. Blake, *Nature (London)* **232,** 52 (1971); H. Cosenza and H. Köhler, *Proc. Natl. Acad. Sci. USA* **69,** 2701 (1972); D. A. Hart, A. L. Wang, L. L. Pawlak, and A. Nisonoff, *J. Exp. Med.* **135,** 1293 (1972); L. L. Pawlak, D. A. Hart, and A. Nisonoff, *J. Exp. Med.* **137,** 1442 (1973). See also M. I. Greene, M. J. Nelles, M. S. Sy, and A. Nisonoff, *Adv. Immunol.* **32,** 253 (1982).

25. K. Eichman and K. Rajewsky, *Eur. J. Immunol.* **5,** 661 (1975).

26. The pioneering work on the idiotypes of lymphocyte receptors was done by H. Ramseier and J. Lindenmann [*Pathol. Microbiol.* **34,** 379 (1969); *Transplant. Rev.* **10,** 57 (1972); *Immunol. Rev.* **34,** 50 (1977)]. See also R. Woodland and H. Cantor, *Eur. J. Immunol.* **8,** 600 (1977); A. Nisonoff, T. J. Shyr, and F. L. Owen, *Immunol. Rev.* **34,** 89 (1977).

27. N. I. Abdou, H. Wall, H. B. Lindsley, J. F. Halsey, and T. Suzuki, *J. Clin. Invest.* **67,** 1297 (1981).

28. M. Zanetti and P. Bigazzi, *Eur. J. Immunol.* **11,** 187 (1981).

29. P. L. Cohen and R. A. Eisenberg *J. Exp. Med.* **156,** 173 (1982).

30. E. G. Neilson and S. N. Phillips, *J. Exp. Med.* **155,** 179 (1982).

31. H. Wigzell, H. Binz, H. Frischknecht, P. Peterson, and K. Sege, in *Genetic Control of Autoimmune Disease* (N. R. Rose, P. Bigazzi, and N. L. Warner, eds.), p. 327. Elsevier, New York, 1978; K. Rajewsky and T. Takemori, *Annu. Rev. Immunol.* **1,** 569 (1983); K. Rajewsky, T. Takemori, and C. E. Müller, *Prog. Immunol.* **5,** 533 (1983); G. J. Thorbecke, B. S. Bhogal, and G. W. Siskind, *Immunol. Today* **5,** 92 (1984).

32. K. Eichman, *Adv. Immunol.* **26,** 195 (1978); K. Rajewsky and K. Eichman, *Contemp. Topics Immunobiol.* **7,** 67 (1977).

33. In addition to those listed above, see also J. Urbain, C. Wuilmart, and P. A. Cazenave, *Contemp. Top. Mol. Immunol.* **8,** 113 (1980); C. A. Janeway, in *Strategies of Immune Recognition* (E. Sercarz and A. J. Cunningham, eds.), pp. 157–177. Academic Press, New York, 1980; C. Bona, ed., *Lymphocyte Regulation by Antibodies.* Wiley, New York, 1981; G. Möller, ed., Idiotypic Networks. *Immunol. Rev.* **79** (1984); C. A. Janeway, E. Sercarz, and H. Wigzell, eds., *Immunoglobulin Idiotypes.* Academic Press, New York, 1981; C. A. Bona and H. Kohler, eds., Immune Networks. *Ann. N.Y. Acad. Sci.* **418,** (1983); M. I. Greene and A. Nisonoff, eds., *The Biology of Idiotypes.* Plenum, New York, 1984; H. Kohler, J. Urbain, and P. Cazenave, eds., *Idiotypy in Biology and Medicine.* Academic Press, New York, 1984.

34. E. von Behring and S. Kitasato, *Dtsch. Med. Wochenschr.* **16,** 1113 (1890); E. von Behring and E. Wernicke, *Z. Hyg. Infektionskr.* **12,** 10, 45 (1892).

35. P. Ehrlich, *Dtsch. Med. Wochenschr.* **17,** 976, 1218 (1891).

36. J. Bordet, *Ann. Inst. Pasteur, Paris* **12,** 688 (1899).

37. A significant portion of Vol. 14 of *Ann. Inst. Pasteur, Paris* was devoted to immune "cytotoxins." The Francophone use of these terms and, indeed, of a completely different immunological vocabulary from that of most of their German colleagues has led to later misinterpretations, especially of the work of Karl Landsteiner; see discussion in Chapter 8.

38. E. Metchnikoff, *Virchows Arch.* **96,** 177 (1884). Metchnikoff elaborated his theory more fully in *Lectures on the Comparative Pathology of Inflammation.* Keegan, Paul, Trench, Trübner, London, 1893. [Reprinted by Dover, New York, 1968.]

39. A. Besredka, *Ann. Inst. Pasteur, Paris* **15,** 785 (1901).

40. Reference 2.

41. See, e.g., J. Parascandola and R. Jasensky, *Bull. Hist. Med.* **48,** 199 (1974); L. P. Rubin, *J. Hist. Med.* **35,** 397 (1980). A detailed summary of Ehrlich's side-chain theory has been presented in Chapter 4.

42. Ehrlich, ref. 5; P. Ehrlich and J. Morgenroth, *Berl. Klin. Wochenschr.* **36,** 6 (1899). [English translation in P. Ehrlich, *Collected Papers,* Vol. 2, p. 150.]

43. P. Ehrlich and J. Morgenroth, *Berl. Klin. Wochenschr.* **36,** 481 (1899) [English translation in P. Ehrlich, *Collected Papers,* Vol. 2, p. 165]; P. Ehrlich and H. Sachs, Berl. Klin. Wochenschr. **39,** 297, 335 (1902).

44. The Ehrlich–Bordet debates are discussed more fully in Chapter 5.

45. Bordet's position is best summarized in his famous book, *Traité de l'immunité dans les maladies infectieuses.* Masson, Paris, 1920.

46. J. Bordet, *Ann. Inst. Pasteur, Paris* **14,** 257 (1900).

47. J. Bordet, *Ann. Inst. Pasteur, Paris* **15,** 303 (1901).

48. P. Ehrlich, *Berl. Klin. Wochenschr.* **40,** 793, 825, 848 (1903).

49. Ehrlich and Morgenroth, ref. 43.

50. J. Bordet, *Ann. Inst. Pasteur, Paris* **13,** 273 (1899); **14,** 257 (1900).

51. H. Kossel, *Berl. Klin. Wochenschr.* **35,** 152 (1898).

52. L. Camus and E. Gley, *Ann. Inst. Pasteur, Paris* **13,** 779 (1899).

53. Ehrlich and Morgenroth, ref. 43, p. 170.

54. Ehrlich, ref. 5. See also Ehrlich, *Collected Papers,* Vol. 2, p. 94.

55. Reference 50.

56. Reference 39.

57. P. Ehrlich and J. Morgenroth, *Berl. Klin. Wochenschr.* **38,** 251 (1901). [English translation in P. Ehrlich, *Collected Papers,* Vol. 2, p. 253.]

58. J. Donath and K. Landsteiner, *Muench. Med. Wochenschr.* **51,** 1590 (1904).

59. P. Ehrlich, *Collected Papers,* Vol. 2, p. 444; H. Sachs, Lubarsch and Ostertag's *Ergeb. Allg. Pathol.* **11,** 515-644 (1907) p. 565.

60. G. F. I. Widal, and P. Rostaine, *C. R. Seances Soc. Biol. Ses Fil.* **58,** 321, 372 (1905).

61. J. Mogenroth, *Zentralbl. Bakteriol.* **26,** 349 (1899).

62. P. Ehrlich and J. Morgenroth, *Berl. Klin. Wochenschr.* **37,** 453 (1900). [English translation in P. Ehrlich, *Collected Papers,* Vol. 2, p. 205.]

63. Reference 62, p. 208.

64. R. Pfeiffer and E. Friedberger, *Berl. Klin. Wochenschr.* **39,** 4 (1902).

65. A. von Wassermann, *Z. Hyg. Infektionskr.* **37,** 173 (1901).

66. H. Sachs, *Ergeb. Allg. Pathol. Anat.* **7,** 714, 768 (1901).

67. See, e.g., P. T. Müller, *Zentralbl. Bakteriol.* **29,** 175, 860 (1901); F. Wechsberg, *Z. Hyg. Infektionskr.* **39,** 171 (1902).

68. Reference 46.

69. Reference 64.

70. P. Ehrlich, *Collected Papers,* Vol. 2, p. 445.

71. J. Bordet and O. Gengou, *Ann. Inst. Pasteur, Paris* **15,** 289 (1901).

72. O. Gengou, *Ann. Inst. Pasteur, Paris* **16,** 734 (1902); C. Moreschi, *Berl. Klin. Wochenschr.* **42,** 1181 (1905); **43,** 100 (1906); F. Gay, *Zentralbl. Bakteriol.* **39,** 603 (1905); R. Muir and W. B. M. Martin, *J. Hyg.* **6,** 265 (1906).

73. M. Neisser and H. Sachs, *Berl. Klin. Wochenschr.* **42,** 1388 (1905).

74. L. Detré, *Wien. Klin. Wochenschr.* **19,** 619 (1906).

75. A. von Wassermann and C. Bruck, *Dtsch. Med. Wochenschr.* **32,** 449 (1906);

A. von Wassermann, A. Neisser, C. Bruck, and A. Schucht, *Z. Hyg.* **55,** 451 (1906).

76. P. Ehrlich, *Collected Papers,* Vol. 2, p. 446.

77. J. Bordet, *Ann. Inst. Pastuer, Paris* **18,** 593 (1904).

78. Sachs, ref. 59; Kraus and Levaditi's *Handbuch der Technik und Methodik der Immunitätsforschung,* Vol. II, pp. 895–1075. Fischer, Jena, 1909; Kolle and Wassermann's *Handbuch der Pathogenen Mikroorganismen,* Vol. II(2), pp. 793–946. Fischer, Jena, 1913.

79. To the best of our knowledge, R. S. Schwartz [*Prog. Allergy* **35,** 1 (1984)] is alone in having hinted that Ehrlich's work with "anti-immune body" resembled modern anti-idiotype interests.

11

Transplantation and Immunogenetics

*One of the distinguishing marks of modern
science is the disappearance of sectarian
loyalties . . . Isolationism is over; we all
depend upon and sustain each other.*
—P. B. Medawar

IN HIS essay "Two Conceptions of Science,"[1] Medawar suggests that biology before Darwin was almost all
facts and that the difficulty of dealing with an ever-increasing factual
load caused the scientist to become ever narrower and more specialized
(read isolationist). One of the characteristics of modern science is the
willingness—indeed, the necessity—of the practitioner to cross disciplinary boundaries. This trend has surely accelerated in the biomedical
sciences since the 1960s, and immunology has been one of the more
important catalysts of this change. The molecular biologist studies the
immunoglobulin gene superfamily; the oncologist studies T and B cell
subsets; the internist and neurologist study autoimmune diseases and
HLA predispositions; and everyone uses monoclonal antibodies and
immunoassays. Indeed, it is becoming increasingly more difficult to
know how to identify oneself in the now perhaps outmoded disciplinary
terms.

Just as one of the advantages of recent ecumenism is the rapid
exchange of information among disciplines, so one of the disadvantages
of early isolationism was the lack of recognition of significant conceptual
advances in other disciplines. Perhaps the best example of this radical
shift in the way that science operates is to be found in the history of the
transplantation of tissues and organs. Five separate specialities are
involved in this story, each with its own agenda. The surgeons had for
centuries been attempting various types of transplantation, and by the

275

First World War had more than hinted at the immunological explanation for their failures; it was they who would help to stimulate the renaissance in transplantation following the Second World War. The tumor specialists wanted to understand and to cure cancer, and to this end they studied transplantable tumors. By 1916, these workers had described substantially all of the phenomenology and "rules" of graft acceptance and rejection as we understand them today, but no one paid attention. The Mendelian geneticists entered the picture in the 1920s and 1930s and began to characterize histocompatibility in scientific terms; it was their next generation that would define the full significance of the HLA complex. After the Second World War, a group of biologists (led by zoologist Peter Medawar) became interested in transplantation; it was they who provided the scientific base upon which modern transplantation biology is built. Finally, those who might have called themselves immunologists paid little attention to this early work; they only entered the fray in the late 1950s and early 1960s, in yet another reflection of the major shift that occurred in immunology, from chemical to more biological interests.

I shall, in this chapter, outline the early history of tissue transplantation. I shall also attempt to explain, in terms of the shifting aspirations and disappointments within the several disciplines, why the "laws of transplantation" had to be discovered twice within the space of some 40 years.

Transplantation Biology

THE SURGEONS BEGIN

In 1597, the famous surgeon Gaspare Tagliacozzi of Bologna wrote that "the singular character of the individual entirely dissuades us from attempting this work [tissue transplantation] on another person."[2] One cannot know what stimulated Tagliacozzi to write these prescient words a full three centuries before the biological basis of individuality was firmly established. Since he himself recorded the successful repair of a lost nose using a pedicle flap autograft from the patient's own arm (a procedure still in use today), it is not unlikely that he attempted similar procedures from allogeneic donors, with unhappy results. In Tagliacozzi's century, medicine was still a curious mixture of primitive science and superstition, and the already long history of attempts at tissue transplantation reflected more the latter qualities than the former. Thus, instances of miraculous transplants were recorded, such as that involving replacement of a leg by Sts. Cosmas and Damian, so well recorded by such famous artists as Fra Angelico and Ambrosius Franken. On the darker side, medieval bestiaries pictured monsters that represented chimerical mixtures of parts of different animal species, and it was suspected that some of them might have been put together by satanical surgeons.

As the centuries passed, medical science slowly replaced medical superstition, and the dream of replacing diseased or missing tissues with healthy ones was advanced with increasing frequency.[3] The ever-daring surgeons attempted skin transplantation for the most part; and while success was not infrequent with autografts, the results were quite contradictory when allografts were employed, and almost uniformly negative with xenografts. It was the ophthalmic surgeons, however, who led the way with successful transplantation of the cornea. In what may have been the first successful penetrating (full thickness) corneal allograft, the Irishman Samuel Bigger reported in 1837 the successful transplantation of an allogeneic cornea into the blind eye of a pet gazelle, an operation that he performed while a prisoner in Egypt.[4] Throughout the nineteenth century, continuing technical improvements and increasingly frequent trials brought a higher success rate among animals, and finally in 1906 the first entirely successful case of a corneal allograft in the human was reported.[5] Therapeutic transplantation of the cornea thenceforth became a more-or-less standard procedure in the practice of ophthalmology, although no theoretical foundation existed that might explain why corneal transplantation should succeed and skin not, or why some corneal grafts were in fact rejected.

Meanwhile, attempts to transplant skin and other tissues continued in both animals and man. In 1902 Alexis Carrel perfected the technique of vascular anastomosis, and beginning in 1905 he reported the experimental transplantation of limbs, kidneys, and other organs.[6] It quickly became apparent that while autografts generally succeed, allografts most often fail. He was forced to conclude that while the technical problems of organ grafting had been solved, "from a biological standpoint no conclusion has thus far been reached, because the interactions of the host and of the new organ are practically unknown." The increasing appreciation that the resistance to foreign grafts is systemic and somehow humoral in nature led to the repeated suggestion by surgeons that an immune response of the "anaphylactic type" was somehow responsible for graft rejection.[7] But despite the demonstration of second-set skin graft rejection in the human as early as 1924,[8] the successful exchange of skin between identical twins in 1927,[9] and the study of parabiotically united animal pairs as early as 1909,[10] no useful generalizations appear to have been drawn by the surgeons that might point the way to further elucidation of mechanisms involved. Thus, save for the ophthalmologists, who continued with their moderately successful practice of corneal allotransplantation, plastic and other surgeons seemed to have concluded by the late 1920s that tissue and organ transplantation was impracticable, a fallen banner that would not be picked up and waved by them for another 20 years.

THE TUMOR RESEARCHERS CONTINUE

It is interesting to compare the relative contributions to the science of transplantation biology made by the surgeons on the one hand and by the tumor workers on the other. Both had eminently practical ends in sight: the surgeons wished to repair defective tissues and malfunctioning organs by replacement; the tumor specialists wanted to cure cancer by specific eradication. But surgeons are an admittedly practical group, and even those among them who engaged in transplantation research were at the same time practicing clinicians (almost the lone exception, Alexis Carrel was a physiologist by training). On the other hand, those investigators interested in tumor biology were for the most part not clinical oncologists but basic scientists attracted to the field from careers in anatomy, experimental pathology, physiology, etc. For them, success lay as much in understanding the basic mechanisms involved as in "solving" the problem. Indeed, their upbringing in the basic sciences had taught them that practical results most often emerge from strong theoretical underpinnings. It was perhaps this more basically scientific approach that enabled the tumor investigators not only to work out in detail the phenomenology and rules governing the transplantation biology of tumors but indeed to contribute more to the understanding of skin and organ transplantation than had the surgeons.

The demonstrations during the last decades of the nineteenth century that immunization might protect against infectious diseases and that antibodies might be employed with sometimes startling therapeutic efficacy caught the attention of the medical world; it was only natural that those interested in cancer should ask whether similar approaches might not also help to solve their problems.[11] However, early efforts at preventive immunization or serum therapy of naturally occurring tumors in man and animals met with almost uniform failure. It was only with the development of transplantable tumor lines in experimental animals[12] that a pathway was opened for the study not only of tumor pathophysiology but of tumor immunology as well. From the very outset of these investigations with transplantable tumors, it was noted that there were very strict limitations on the ability of the tumor transplant to survive in the new host. The experimental work of barely a decade was summarized in 1912 in a remarkable book by Georg Schöne entitled *Heteroplastic and Homoplastic Transplantation*.[13] The importance attached to these studies is attested to by the fact that this summary lists almost 500 references. As Schöne made clear, tumor researchers had already established by 1912 the following general rules governing the acceptance or rejection of tumor grafts (and Schöne's coinage of the term "transplantation immunity" makes it clear what he believes to be the underlying basis for these rules):

1. Transplantation into a foreign species (heteroplastic = xenogeneic) invariably fails.
2. Transplantation into unrelated members of the same species (homoplastic = allogeneic) usually fails.
3. Autografts almost invariably succeed.
4. There is a primary take and then delayed rejection of the first graft in the allogeneic recipient.
5. There is an accelerated rejection of a second graft in a recipient that had previously rejected a graft from the same donor, or of a first graft in a recipient that had been preimmunized with material from the tumor donor.
6. The closer the "blood relationship" between donor and recipient, the more likely is graft success.

Here, in 1912, are the "laws of transplantation" substantially as we understand them today. But Schöne's book does more than summarize a set of observations applicable only to the arcane world of tumor transplantation. He and the other tumor specialists went farther and generalized these observations to encompass the transplantation of skin and organs. The reasons why the tumor investigations made such important contributions to the science of skin and organ transplantation (far beyond that accomplished by the surgeons) are interesting. It was not clear to them at the outset whether there was something unique about tumors that might differentiate them in this sense from other normal tissues; thus, the tumor workers felt obliged to employ skin and other tissues in control experiments. They quickly discovered that the phenomenology of graft rejection was similar in both cases. In fact, skin would presensitize a recipient for "second-set" rejection of a tumor, and vice versa. Furthermore, they observed in the course of these studies of normal tissues that skin grafts fail more consistently than grafts of other organs such as kidney.

In a further review entitled "Tumor Immunity" in 1916 by E. E. Tyzzer,[14] the general findings reported by Schöne were confirmed, and several further important advances were reported. Now the conclusions could be drawn in frank immunological terms: "The degree of immunity which develops thus depends on the foreignness of the immunizing cell with respect to the organism into which it is introduced. The more foreign cells accordingly serve as the more effective and the more closely related cells as the less effective antigens."[15] Moreover, it was now noted that presensitization for "second-set rejection" requires *living* cells; that cytotoxic antibodies cannot be found; that "the delayed reaction of host tissue is difficult to explain except by the hypothesis that an immune body [of some sort] has been produced;" that lymphocytes predominate at the rejection site, i.e., "the reaction is not merely *exudative*, but is *proliferative* as well;" and that there is no tissue specificity, but rather "racial specificity with respect to the genetic origin . . . of the antigens."

With the availability of an inbred strain of mice, the "Japanese waltzing mouse," Tyzzer was able to report a further extension of these studies.[16] Breeding experiments showed that the F_1 hybrid generation obtained by crossing two unrelated strains would accept parental tumors, that the backcross generation (F_1 by tumor donor, i.e., parent–offspring mating) would also accept transplants, but that there was a decreasing incidence of acceptance in further sibling crosses. These results permitted Tyzzer to conclude that "it is quite apparent from these data that susceptibility is not inherited as a single Mendelizing factor. The only hypothesis . . . [nonsusceptibility] is dependent upon the presence of a complex of independently inherited unit factors."[17] Indeed, his data appeared to him to justify the existence of at least 12 to 14 independently inherited factors to explain the ratios of tumor acceptance to tumor rejection.

It was during this period, and partly as a result of the tumor work already described, that the prominent biologist Leo Loeb undertook his long series of investigations into the basis of the individuality of tissues, as exemplified by the results of these transplantation studies. The results of this lifetime of work are well summarized in two major monographs, one, "Transplantation and Individuality," published in 1930, and the other, *The Biological Basis of Individuality*, in 1945.[18] Loeb recognized the genetic basis of individual differences and transplantation incompatibility but would not ascribe the latter to specific immunological mechanisms. Rather, he argued that there exists a specific capability for what one would today call self–nonself discrimination, but at the level of the somatic cell. Thus, a foreign tissue could not make the connections necessary to its physiological survival in the new environment to which it had been transplanted.

Loeb's arguments were forceful and probably exerted a degree of restraint upon truly immunological speculation about transplantation, but evidence continued to mount in favor of an immunological interpretation, especially from studies on the preimmunization of graft recipients. These studies are summarized in a massive review entitled "Immunity to Transplantable Tumors," written by William Woglom in 1929.[19] This review summarized the contributions of no fewer than 600 reports published since the appearance of Schöne's book in 1912. Broad confirmation was reported of the following observations: that *all* tissues would immunize for accelerated graft rejection;[20] that only living tissues would serve—dead cells were ineffective; that passive transfer of tumor immunity could not be achieved with serum (and that newborns of immune mothers were not themselves immune); and that tumor rejection was not accompanied by detectable cytotoxins or other "antitumor" antibodies. It was also shown that transplantation immunity is systemic and not local but that certain sites such as the brain might be exempt from the systemic sensitization and thus able to support the grafted tissues (in current terminology, an immunologically "privileged site"). It had by this time also been shown that while washed erythrocytes would not immunize a recipient for graft rejection, whole blood would, and that the activity resided in the leukocyte moiety.[21]

One of the more fascinating sections of Woglom's review summarized a large number of studies of the cytological changes that accompany tumor graft rejection. It had apparently been Da Fano[22] who first called attention to the fact that the bed of a rejecting tumor allograft characteristically contained large numbers of lymphocytes rather than the polymorphonuclear leukocytes that might have been expected to surround dying cells. As I noted above, Tyzzer commented on the same observations in his 1916 review and emphasized the fact that the lymphoid response was proliferative as well as infiltrative. Tyzzer's attention was undoubtedly drawn to this observation by the work of James Murphy, who contributed to the field a truly impressive series of reports, the first of which appeared in 1912. It was probably his work with Peyton Rous on the histopathology of fowl sarcoma rejection[23] that stimulated Murphy to pursue these studies, which he summarized in extensive detail in a monograph, "The Lymphocyte in Resistance to Tissue Grafting, Malignant Disease, and Tuberculous Infection."[24] Not only did Murphy assign to the lymphocyte the predominant role in the rejection of tumor grafts, but he also tested and confirmed the speculation in an elegant series of experiments. First, he anticipated later studies on the ontogeny of the immune response by showing that a tumor transplanted into the chick embryo might enjoy uninhibited growth until the eighteenth day of embryonic life, when the tumor would undergo spontaneous rejection.[25] To prove that this maturational event involved the lymphocyte, Murphy demonstrated that tumor rejection could be induced in even younger embryos by the co-transplantation of bits of adult spleen or preparations of free "lympho-cytes." In a similar manner, he showed that while a tumor might grow in the "privileged site" of the brain, rejection even in that site could be induced by local inoculation of lymphoid tissue preparations.

To support further his argument on the importance of lymphocytes in graft rejection, Murphy undertook to manipulate both the systemic lymphocyte levels in the grafted host as well as those available at the local site of graft implantation. Thus, he demonstrated that nonspecific stimulation of a lymphocytosis in the host would retard tumor growth and accelerate rejection. On the other hand, lymphopenia should inhibit the rejection of allogeneic tumors. To the latter end, Murphy was able to show that X irradiation of the host, resulting in severe lymphopenia, would inhibit the development of immunity to the graft and delay or even obviate the rejection process. Murphy and Sturm later showed that similar X-ray treatment would depress antibody formation,[26] an obser-vation that had earlier been made by Ludwig Hektoen.[27]

Having implicated the lymphocyte in the rejection of tissue grafts, little more could be said on this subject at that time. The lymphocyte was then a cell of mysterious ancestry and function, and, indeed, even 25 years later Arnold Rich could say little about it. Writing in the context of the pathogenesis of tuberculosis, Rich could say as late as 1951:

> There are numerous reasons . . . for believing that the *lymphocytes* play a role of importance in acquired resistance, though the precise manner in which they act is still obscure, chiefly because so little is known about the function of these cells. The lack of more adequate information regarding the function of the lymphocyte is one of the most lamentable gaps in medical knowledge. Produced in enormous numbers . . . these cells undoubtedly must serve the body in a most important way; and yet little is known of their function.[28]

ENTER THE GENETICISTS

It is testimony to the hope that the study of transplantable tumors might lead to a more general and useful approach to the problems of cancer that for almost 40 years geneticists examined transplantation almost entirely in the context of tumors. One of the first of the young geneticists to enter this field was Clarence C. Little, who very early became interested in the genetic differences that control the response of mice to transplantable tumors. In 1916, he published his first paper in this field with Tyzzer, a follow-up study of Tyzzer's earlier work on the susceptibi-lity to tumors of the Japanese waltzing mouse. Little maintained his interest in tumor genetics even after becoming, at age 33, the president of the University of Maine. While limited in his ability to continue his experimental studies, he maintained an active interest in the field, as is witnessed by a review on the genetics of tissue transplantation written in 1924.[29] As he says, "This paper has its justification in the fact that the subject of the genetics of tissue transplantation is likely to become in the not distant future of far greater general importance . . . There has not been brought to experimental biologists any considerable amount of evidence as regards the type of inheritance found in the case of tissue transplantation." In fact, this paper was a strong criticism of Loeb's genetics and of the basis for Loeb's conclusions on the nature of incompatibility between donor and host (a criticism that many subsequent workers shared in evaluating Loeb's work).

Throughout his career, Little was wedded to the idea that careful study of genetically homogeneous animals would provide one of the more profitable approaches to the problems of cancer, and to this end he founded the Jackson Memorial Laboratory at Bar Harbor, Maine in 1929. "The founding of the fledgling laboratory was to use the mice [inbred strains of which Little and others had developed] in research against that continuing scourge, cancer. In the differences of resistance and susceptibility between the inbred strains, they believed, might lie an answer to cancer's causes."[30] One of the more significant events during the early years of the Jackson Laboratory was the hiring in 1935 of George D. Snell, as committed as was Little to the use of inbred mice for the study of cancer. To this end, Snell "invented" the congenic mouse strain, carefully selected from a parental inbred stock to differ at but a single locus from its congenic cousins. Very quickly, Snell discovered a locus intimately related to the rejection of tumor grafts that he labeled H (for histocompatibility). When Peter Gorer in England discovered a hemagglutinating antibody associated with the rejection of tumor grafts,[31] it appeared that the long-sought-after cytotoxic antibody responsible for tumor rejection might be associated with the blood group antigens. It was soon established that such an antibody response was not a general feature of graft rejection, but not before the antigen involved was named by Gorer antigen II, and it was established that the gene for the production of this antigen was located at Snell's H locus; hence, the term H-2, which would eventually define an entire complex of murine histocompatibility genes.

TRANSPLANTATION RESEARCH IN THE 1930S

Having noted the impressive advances made in the first decades of this century in the understanding of the immunological basis for tissue graft rejection and the "rules of transplantation" that were formulated, one might inquire why so much of this work was forgotten and why Medawar's studies in the 1940s were received as "new" discoveries. In attempting an explanation of these events, one must consider separately the three principal disciplines that had been engaged in research on transplantation up to this time: the surgeons, the tumor specialists, and the geneticists.

Despite the technological improvements introduced by Alexis Carrel and others, surgeons (save for the ophthalmologists with corneal transplantation) had for decades seen all of their attempts at skin and organ transplantation fail in the face of the rejection process. The only method known to suppress the immune response to grafted tissue—that of whole-body X irradiation—had been shown to be at least partially successful in experimental animals, but it was apparently deemed too radical an approach to be employed in man. Thus transplantation, as a clinically useful tool, seemed doomed to disappointment. The ever-practical surgeons therefore "gave up" on the procedure, as is witnessed by the decreasing reports in the literature on work along these lines, starting as early as the late 1920s.

The position of the tumor biologists was in many respects similar to that of the surgeons. Early on, approaches employing transplantable tumors had appeared to offer a fruitful avenue toward the solution of the problem of cancer, and indeed much valuable information was obtained about the immunology and genetics underlying the rejection of tumor grafts. But having worked out the basic phenomenology of the process by the mid-1920s, little further progress was made or appeared likely; consequently a "solution" to the cancer problem began to appear to be beyond reach, at least employing these approaches. One may therefore conclude that, like the surgeons, tumor researchers lost faith in their approach to tumor biology via transplantation, and moved on to other more promising areas.

The shift in the interest of the geneticists was somewhat more subtle than those described earlier. Since they too had entered the field of transplantation in the context of tumor biology, they were undoubtedly affected by the growing disenchantment of the cancer researchers. But something else occurred that merits attention, and this is well reflected in the work of George Snell. At the outset, Snell probably viewed (with Clarence Little) the inbred mouse as the perfect tool to study tumor graft rejection, i.e., as a fruitful approach not only to therapy but to understanding initial susceptibility as well. If the early work to identify the histocompatibility locus in mice was aimed at understanding the immune response to tumor grafts, it quickly lost its oncological and even immunological motivations and became a study in pure genetics—

analyzing the size of the growing histocompatibility complex; assessing the extent of the polymorphism at each locus; and establishing the rules of segregation of these genes in backcrosses.[32] Only later would the studies return to the realm of transplantation biology, when their practical applicability to tissue typing and histocompatibility matching was appreciated.

One may therefore conclude that the science of tissue transplantation had, by the last half of the decade of the 1930s, lost its appeal to those disciplines that had earlier maintained an active interest in and great hopes for this subject. One may also note in passing that despite the significant contributions made during the teens and twenties to the immunology of tissue transplantation, no investigator who might have termed himself an immunologist had been involved in these efforts, and even the text books and reviews of immunology of that period failed to mention the studies of the nature of tumor or other tissue graft rejection.[33] New data, new technologies, and, above all, a new point of view would be required to rekindle the interest of research scientists in the value of transplantation studies.

The Renaissance of Transplantation Biology

Among the many horrors that accompanied World War II, with its more mechanized methods and its incendiary bombings of cities, was a marked increased in the numbers of burn victims seen in both military and civilian hospitals. Such patients would previously have succumbed to such extensive burns, but with the advent of antibiotics to control infection and the use of skin autografts to assist in the healing process, there was now hope for such individuals. Where the burn area was extensive, an adequate source of autograft skin might not be available; thus, while it was generally understood that skin homografts would invariably be rejected, the war provided the impetus to reexamine the question of homograft rejection, in the hopes of developing techniques to circumvent it. It was in this context that zoologist Peter B. Medawar became interested in skin grafting and was assigned by the War Wounds Committee of the British Medical Research Council to explore this question, first in a clinical setting with Thomas Gibson at the Burn Unit of the Glasgow Royal Infirmary and then using experimental animals at his home base at Oxford University.

Medawar's first paper, with Gibson in 1943,[34] revealed that they possessed a thorough knowledge of the earlier work in this field, including that of Schöne, Woglom, Loeb, and others who had used both tumors and normal tissues. They concluded, however, that the question of the mechanism of homograft rejection was still unsettled. They then reported their results in what would become the hallmark of Medawar's future work: an elegantly designed, carefully executed, and lucidly described report. In this paper, Gibson and Medawar described experiments on a single burn victim and demonstrated with serial biopsies that (1) autografts succeed; (2) allografts fail, after an initial take; (3) second-set homografts suffer an accelerated rejection; and (4) there is little evidence of a "local cellular reaction" (a term presumably employed in the original sense of Leo Loeb). The authors then concluded that these data "suggest that the destruction of the foreign epidermis was brought about by a mechanism of active immunization."[35]

These results excited Medawar's scientific interests, and "It did not go unremarked that we were building rather a lot upon the study of the single case, and when I returned to Oxford I felt I should study the whole phenomenon of homograft rejection in laboratory animals to see if this renewed study gave results that would be fully compatible with our hypothesis that the rejection of homografts was an immunologic phenomenon."[36] The results of the extensive experiments in the rabbit that followed were compiled in two reports to the War Wounds Committee and published in the *Journal of Anatomy* in 1944 and 1945.[37] In his studies of graft rejection in the rabbit, Medawar was able to confirm and to extend considerably his earlier work with Gibson. In the course of "the hardest stint of work I have ever undertaken in my life," Medawar carefully studied the pertinent parameters of timing, dosage, specificity, first- and second-set rejection, and the clinical and histological changes that accompany the rejection process. If, in these studies, Medawar had "rediscovered" the laws of transplantation earlier summarized by Schöne in 1912, by Tyzzer in 1916, and by Woglom in 1929, it had been done now with a set of carefully devised and controlled experiments and a mass of supporting data that rendered the conclusions beyond any doubt. More than this, he had now convincingly demonstrated that the rejection process originates systemically and not locally; and his study of the mutual exchange of grafts between a large number of donor–recipient pairs allowed him to conclude that "the homograft reaction is governed by the operation of *at least* 7 antigens freely combined."[38]

After acknowledging with reservation the immunological nature of the homograft rejection reaction, Medawar went on to consider the likely mechanism involved. Given the prevailing view of the importance of circulating antibodies in *any* allergic (or hypersensitivity) event, and the absence in the contemporary literature of almost all reference to the notion of cellular immunity (in even its Metchnikovian sense),

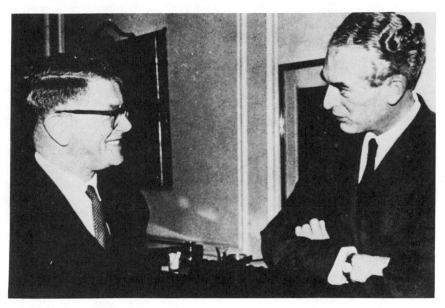

Macfarlane Burnet (left) and **Peter Medawar** (right) (Courtesy University of Wisconsin Library)

Medawar's conclusion is understandable. Even so, one must admire the acuity represented by the caveat that he inserted into his conclusion:

> The inflammation which accompanies the homograft reaction in rabbits is very probably of the anaphylactic type . . . yet, though all of the ingredients of the inflammatory process are present—vascular and lymphatic proliferation, edema, and the mobilization and deployment of mesenchyme cells of every type—the reaction is nevertheless atypical; for the lymphocyte takes the place of the polymorph in the "classical picture". . . . It is as yet impossible to judge of the significance of this difference.[39]

It is curious that in these first reports, and in those transplantation studies that followed during the next decade, Medawar did not review again any of the pertinent earlier transplantation literature, contenting himself with indicating that these had been covered earlier in his paper with Gibson and in another paper published in 1943 in the transiently published *Bulletin of War Medicine*.[40] Not until his Harvey lecture of 1957[41] did he provide a broad history of transplantation studies and pay full attention to the earlier work on tumor transplantation and on skin and tissue grafting and to the studies of Snell and Gorer.

Medawar continued his studies of skin transplantation in a further report in 1946 in the *British Journal of Experimental Pathology*.[42] In this paper, he demonstrated that skin graft rejection is unaccompanied by the formation of isohemagglutinins for the donor's erythrocytes; that immunization with donor red cells confers no appreciable immunity to skin but that immunization with donor *leukocytes* does; and that the intradermal inoculation of leukocytes is 18 times more effective than immunization via the intravenous route. As in his two earlier reports, Medawar is here repeating almost seriatim the decades-earlier work done with tumor grafts. Somewhat surprisingly, he makes no mention of these earlier studies in his discussion of the results, even though he had previously shown a familiarity with this work, much of which had in fact been done in London in the laboratories of the Imperial Cancer Research Fund.

Despite the obvious immunological orientation of these transplantation studies, it would appear from an examination of the indexes of the several journals devoted to immunology and of the meeting programs of organizations such as the American Association of Immunologists, that the studies had not yet captured the attention of the immunological world. There were, however, certain stirrings, both within and outside the field of transplantation that would soon bring transplantation into the immunological fold. Perhaps the most significant event for transplantation was provided by the work of Owen in 1945 on the immunological consequences of natural vascular anastomoses established between nonidentical cattle twins *in utero*.[43] Owen showed by serological tests that these animals are erythrocyte chimeras, i.e., they possess mixtures of their own and of their twin's red cells but fail to produce isoantibodies against the foreign component. Burnet and Fenner called attention to this finding and to its implication for an understanding of the immune response to antigenic stimulus, in their 1949 edition of *The Production of Antibodies*.[44] But it was the demonstration in Medawar's laboratory in 1951 and 1952 that such cattle are unable to reject one another's skin[45] that signaled that here was a finding not only of profound theoretical interest to immunology but of possible practical interest to tissue transplanters as well. It was these findings that focused the attention of Medawar's laboratory on this problem, an emphasis that soon eventuated in the reports of Billingham *et al.* on the experimental production in laboratory animals of the phenomenon of immunological tolerance,[46] akin to that seen by Owen in cattle twins.

Here finally was at least the theoretical promise that the immune response to foreign tissue grafts might be overcome. This observation, together with subsequent demonstrations that the host response might be inhibited by the use of nitrogen mustard or corticosteroid therapies, fostered a renewal of interest by the surgical community in the possibilities of tissue and organ transplantation. For some years thenceforth, it was primarily the surgeons who paid attention to Medawar's work and who organized the national and international symposia that helped to establish the foundations for future work in this field.

Meanwhile, other forces that were at work would help to incorporate transplantation into the mainstream of immunology. Or rather, it might be more accurate to say that it was less a change in the nature of transplantation studies than a shift in the course of immunology itself that caused it to encompass the growing field of transplantation, a shift already discussed in Chapters 7 and 9. Thanks in part to Burnet's clonal selection theory, to the increasing realization that autoimmune diseases are real phenomena of great clinical importance, to the discovery of immunological deficiency diseases, and now to the discovery of immunological tolerance, the entire field of immunology found itself moving away from its former preoccupation with essentially chemical approaches to antibodies and the problems of specificity and toward more biological questions of cellular mechanics and disease pathogenesis. A new generation of immunologists would quickly be attracted to the field, to sort out the biological basis of antibody formation and the molecular and cellular mechanisms responsible for an increasing number of immunogenic inflammatory processes.

Thus, transplantation studies were at once a contributor to the stimulus for this phase-shift in immunological interests and one of the beneficiaries of the new movement. Now a concerted effort could be undertaken to relate transplantation immunity to other immunological phenomena, an undertaking aided immeasurably by the renewal of interest in the implication of delayed-type hypersensitivity as one of the important contributors to immunopathological reactions. Perhaps the key that enabled this door to be opened was provided by the demonstration by Mitchison and by Billingham, Brent, and Medawar in 1954 that transplantation immunity could be adoptively transferred with cells and not with serum from sensitized donors,[47] a finding that immediately put graft rejection into the same category as tuberculin hypersensitivity and contact dermititis.[48] This view was strongly reinforced by the report of Algire and co-workers that grafts implanted within cell-impermeable chambers evaded rejection even in previously sensitized hosts,[49] but that inclusion in the chamber of immune spleen or lymph node cells would result in graft destruction.[50]

Two other observations contributed to the increasing attention drawn to transplantation studies, both from Medawar's laboratory. The first was that graft immunity could be elicited by *non*living cells and even by cell extracts.[51] This discovery was quite important, for it removed from transplantation immunology the somewhat mystical quality that had been associated with the earlier belief in the requirement for *vital* cells, and made graft immunogenicity akin to all of the other more familiar antigen systems. The other significant observation was that of the graft-versus-host reaction.[52] The injection of genetically disparate but immunologically competent cells into a recipient would cause differing forms of host damage, depending upon the recipient. In the chick embryo, splenomegaly and death occur; in the neonatal mouse, "runt disease;" in the F_1 hybrid given parental lymphoid cells, "F_1 hybrid disease;" and in parabiotically attached animals, "parabiosis intoxication." These clinical processes and the mechanisms that underlay them could not fail to excite interest.

As early as his Harvey lecture of 1957, Medawar could give voice to the conceptual change that had taken place in the previous few years:

> The balance of evidence suggests that skin transplant immunity and hypersensitivity reactions of the delayed type are reactions which are fundamentally cellular as opposed to humoral, and which depend upon the activation, deployment, and peripheral engagement of the lymphoid cell— [but he was quick to add wryly that this was] a remark whose euphony will, I hope, distract attention from the fact that we are very ignorant of what these processes are.[53]

A further testimony to the fact that it was about this time that transplantation biology was integrated into the discipline of immunology comes from an analysis of how workers in a field perceive themselves and are perceived by others. Prior to the early 1950s, Medawar and his colleagues directed their work primarily at surgeons and at biologists in general. From the mid-1950s onward, they would increasingly be invited to speak at symposia organized by immunologists and to contribute chapters to immunological publications. Indeed, before this period, neither Medawar nor his colleagues considered themselves to be "immunologists," an appellation to which thereafter they would feel entitled.[54]

The changing character of the developing science of tissue transplantation is perhaps best illustrated by the developments in the field recorded in the periodic symposia on transplantation organized by the New York Academy of Sciences.[55] What had started as an exchange predominantly among surgeons (with, admittedly, strong immunological overtones) gained momentum with the addition of geneticists interested in the basis of histocompatibility differences, serologists interested in histocompatibility testing, and immunologists and immunopathologists interested in underlying mechanisms. The marriage of these different disciplines was celebrated in the establishment in 1967 of the Transplantation Society, and the nuptials were recorded in the proceedings of the First International Congress of the Transplantation Society.[56] As the table of contents of this volume attests, not only were the surgeons, the geneticists, and the immunologists now joined together in a common cause, but even the tumor immunologists had finally been brought back into the fold. Indeed, one can see here the beginnings of a new discipline in its own right, that of "transplantation biology," with an organization, a set of aspirations, and even a language of its own.

Progress in Transplantation Research

The 20 years since the founding of the Transplantation Society have seen remarkable advances in the genetics and in the immunobiology of tissue grafting. The principal components of the major histocompatibility complex and the molecular biology of its constituents have been well worked out, as have been the major aspects of the host response to alloantigens and the underlying mechanisms of allograft rejection. Nevertheless, the *practice* of tissue transplantation remains a curiously pragmatic enterprise, whose newer directions appear to be directed less by theory than by trial-and-error experiments to determine "what works." Indeed, modern transplantation studies have seemingly given up on the possibilities of success with the very tissue that prompted the renaissance in transplantation—the use of allogeneic skin transplants in burn victims—and are now devoted primarily to improvements in the transplantation of kidneys and other organs. This pragmatic approach to transplantation was recognized as long ago as 1977 when Leslie Brent, in his Presidential Address on the tenth anniversary of the Transplantation Society,[57] discussed Roy Calne's feeling that progress in transplantation would come less from basic immunological research than from the search for better immunosuppressive drugs.[58] Brent was, at the time, cautiously optimistic, but he pointed out that the immunological solution of graft rejection might involve "a time-scale of progress that is greater than self-interest and our natural urge for human advance demand." Little that has occurred during the 10 years since Brent made this statement suggests that the time scale has been foreshortened.

THE TISSUES EMPLOYED IN TRANSPLANTATION

It is now generally conceded that corneal transplantation succeeds in general because the avascular nature of the tissue endows the cornea with a degree of immunological privilege, more or less isolating it from both the afferent and efferent arcs of the immune reponse. Skin, on the other hand, by virtue of its rich vascular bed and direct access to lymphatic channels, is highly immunogenic and equally highly susceptible to invasion by those effector cells that mediate the rejection process. Occupying an intermediate position in this hierarchy of immunological susceptibilities are organs such as the kidney and the heart, which can be transplanted in their entirety by the anastomosis of only a few major blood vessels—a connection that serves at least in part to isolate them from the immune response of the host. The validity of this interpretation was elegantly demonstrated by Barker and Billingham,[59] who showed that even skin grafts might enjoy prolonged survival if transplanted onto a raised dermal pedicle connected to the host only by artery and vein, and not by lymphatic channels.

Yet another type of transplant that offers hope of success is exemplified by the transplantation of pancreatic β islet cells, for the production of insulin in diabetic recipients. While the basis for the success of this procedure is not fully understood, it may well be related to the small antigenic mass involved in the transplantation of only modest numbers of such cells. Indeed, Billingham showed many years ago that even epidermal melanocytes may be transplanted successfully onto the skin if small enough numbers are employed.[60] Presumably, the host does not even "see" (in an immunological sense) the small antigenic mass and fails to become sensitized.

Finally, there is yet another type of tissue graft that holds promise of success—that of bone marrow transplantation in the therapy of certain lymphatic leukemias. In this case, substantially the entire immunological apparatus of the recipient is ablated chemotherapeutically and replaced with the immunocytes of the donor. This approach is currently accompanied by techniques that render it possible to induce immunological tolerance of the transplanted cells on the part of any residual immunological competence of the host. However, tolerance of the host is not shared by the donor lymphoid elements, so that systemic graft-versus-host reactions continue to constitute one of the more serious side effects of this approach.

TISSUE TYPING AND DONOR–RECIPIENT MATCHING

There exist within the major histocompatibility complex a number of loci that control the production of those antigens that play a major role in inciting the rejection process and a larger number of loci coding for less important (but nonetheless contributory) histocompatibility antigens.[61] The polymorphism at each of these loci is impressively large; hence, the number of different combinations that may exist within an individual makes it extremely difficult to match a recipient to an optimal donor. Two approaches to donor–recipient histocompatibility matching have been developed, each with its adherents. The first involves the assembling of a large library of antibodies specific for the different antigens that may exist at the important loci. Such tests provide an objective assessment of the antigenic differences between donor and recipient and utilize prior experience to assess the practical importance of a mismatch at a given locus. The second approach is a more fundamental one, in which a one-way mixed lymphocyte reaction between donor and recipient cells is measured. Here, the extent of the response of recipient lymphocytes to the histocompatibility antigens of the donor provides a measure of the likely response to the grafted tissue.

It is clear that the better the histocompatibility match between donor and recipient, the more optimistic will be the prognosis for the grafted organ. Nevertheless, perfect matches (except between identical twins) are difficult to obtain, so nationwide and even worldwide organizations have been established to direct available organs to the most promising (i.e., the most closely matched) recipients.

IMMUNOSUPPRESSIVE THERAPY

Given the availability of donor tissues or organs not perfectly matched to the recipient, a greater or lesser degree of host sensitization with consequent attack on the graft would appear inevitable. The countervailing strategy employed in clinical transplantation studies has sought, therefore, to employ immunosuppressive agents in an attempt to minimize the effects of the rejection process. As I noted earlier, X irradiation of the graft recipient was found to be moderately successful in preventing the rejection of tumor transplants in experimental animals and, despite deleterious side effects, is still occasionally employed as an adjunct to immunosuppressive therapy in man. Advantage has also been taken of the antiinflammatory action of corticosteroids in moderating the rejection process, a form of therapy especially useful when applied locally to interrupt the rejection of a corneal graft. It is not surprising that many of the chemical antimetabolites applied to the problem of graft rejection have emerged from developments in cancer chemotherapy, since the aim in both fields is similar: to destroy or inhibit the tumor cell (or the threatening sensitized lymphocyte) without inflicting too much damage on other host cell types. Thus, such drugs as 6-mercaptopurine, methotrexate, 5-fluorouracil, cyclophosphamide, and many others have been applied to the inhibition of graft rejection with variable results. Even though a number of these drugs have been found to be effective, they are usually accompanied by undesirable and even serious side effects, since efficacy is in general directly related to cytotoxicity. There has been much interest recently in the drug cyclosporine A, claimed to be highly effective in controlling graft rejection with but minimal side effects.[62]

One of the more interesting approaches to immunosuppression in the field of transplantation is based upon an observation in 1937 by Chew and Lawrence that a serum with a powerful antilymphocytic effect *in vivo* can be prepared by immunizing an animal with suspensions of heterologous lymphocytes.[63] Interest in this preparation was revived in the 1960s,[64] and early reports suggested that anti-lymphocyte (or anti-thymocyte) serum might inhibit the rejection process without serious side effects. With the advent of hybridoma techniques for the production of pure and specific monoclonal antibodies, it has become possible to ablate selectively one or another lymphocyte subset in the graft recipient, thus further limiting undesirable damage to the immune apparatus of the host.

The last approach to inhibition of the rejection process that I shall mention is especially interesting, since it corroborates nicely the suggestion mentioned earlier that advances in transplantation biology are based more upon pragmatic observation than upon theoretical prediction. Immunological theory would hold that great care should be taken that the graft recipient not be presensitized to the histocompatibility antigens of the donor. Since blood transfusion is a frequent accompaniment of organ transplantation, the possible consequences of presensitization by transfusion (or that seen in multiparous women) seemed a thing to be feared. In fact, such presensitization appears now to favor graft survival, and indeed donor-specific transfusion appears to be more effective in this sense than that from unrelated donors.[65] It is not yet clear whether the beneficial effects of this treatment are due to the stimulation of suppressor T cells or to the production of suppressive anti-idiotypic antibodies.

THE PROMISE OF IMMUNOLOGICAL TOLERANCE

Peter Medawar has suggested[66] that if the field of transplantation has borrowed most of its working concepts from orthodox immunology, it has in large measure repaid that debt by contributing back to immunology the concept of immunological tolerance. The possibilities inherent in tolerance were already implicit in the work of Owen on cattle chimeras, as pointed out by Burnet and Fenner; and its implications for transplantation research were made abundantly clear when it was demonstrated that these animals were unable to reject each other's skin. The conditions required for the induction of transplantation tolerance were elaborated upon by Billingham and Brent, by Woodruff and Simpson, and most notably by Hašek and his colleagues.[67] The generality of this phenomenon and its broad implications for immunology were first made clear by Hannan and Oyama,[68] who showed that tolerance may also be induced by nonliving antigens, a demonstration that led to extensive experimentation with a variety of simple proteins[69]—this latter study would have important implications in the study of autoimmune diseases (see Chapter 7).

It was the initial hope and expectation that the induction of tolerance of donor histocompatibility antigens in a graft recipient would offer the ultimate solution to the problem of tissue and organ graft survival. However, even though tolerance might be induced readily in the immunologically immature fetus or neonate (depending upon the species), it was found to be far more difficult to induce this state in the immunologically mature adult who might require an organ graft. Again, even though effective tolerance might be attained with simple protein antigens, the difficulties attendant upon attempts to induce tolerance of the large complex of histocompatibility antigen differences between donor and recipient would render the process more formidable. Thus far, immunological tolerance has only proved of practical value in the special case of bone marrow transplants, where some practitioners utilize special preparatory regimens that favor the development of tolerance. Nevertheless, tolerance is still viewed today as the Holy Grail of the transplantationist, as it was 30 years ago.

Immunogenetics

An International Society of Monists was founded in 1906 by Ernst Haeckel and Wilhelm Ostwald, dedicated to the belief in the ultimate unity of all knowledge. At a time when vitalism still infused much of biology and when each discipline followed its own guiding rules and methodology, the view that all sciences would ultimately converge and even merge under the general laws of chemistry and physics seemed somewhat questionable. Nevertheless, the history of much of biological science in the first three-quarters of the twentieth century seems to point precisely at a convergence of disciplines. As Garland Allen has pointed out in *Life Science in the 20th Century*,[70] "embryology, biochemistry, cytology, and genetics began to come together [in the 1920s and 1930s] to form a unified, cellularly and physiologically oriented view of development." Similarly, as this chapter makes abundantly clear, immunology, genetics, biochemistry, and molecular and cellular biology have become so intimately intertwined that in recent years many investigators have been hard put to know how to identify themselves. In the study of blood groups, of histocompatibility relationships between graft donor and recipient, of the basis for the generation of immunological diversity and the formation of the immunoglobulin molecule, and of the mechanisms for disease predisposition and resistance, the overlap between genetics and immunology has become increasingly evident, with each making major contributions to the other's progress.[71]

BLOOD GROUPS

The first report of the existence of naturally occurring isohemagglutinins in man was made by Karl Landsteiner[72]—apparently the result of a chance observation. Ehrlich and Morgenroth had described similar isoantibodies in goats that would lyse the erythrocytes of other goats, this time in animals immunized with red cells in the search for autoantibodies.[73] In a further examination of human sera, Landsteiner was able to describe three erythrocyte groups, each of the first two containing its own red cell antigen, whereas the third group had erythrocytes that contained neither antigen.[74] Based upon these studies, he was able to define "Landsteiner's rule," which held that the serum of any individual would contain hemagglutinins for those erythrocyte antigens *not* present on his own red cells. Subsequently, von Decastello and Stürli in Landsteiner's laboratory discovered a rarer fourth group of individuals, those whose erythrocytes contained both of the antigens present in Landsteiner's groups I and II.[75]

In 1910, von Dungern and Hirszfeld published two landmark papers[76] in which they showed that different blood groups also exist in the canine population. They went on to name the human blood groups A, B, AB, and O, reflecting the presence or absence of the two antigens A and B. Moreover, they showed that these human blood group antigens obey the normal Mendelian rules of inheritance, that A and B are dominant, and that it is possible to measure the frequency of these traits in the population; and they suggested that blood group identification might prove useful in forensics.[77] Very much in line with Ehrlich's chemical interpretation of the complementary structures of antigen and antibody, von Dungern and Hirszfeld implied that A and B antigens were inherited from one's parents as "chemical structures," perhaps the first interpretation of Mendelian inheritance in terms of the formation of specific molecular entities.

These observations on the existence of different blood groups led, in the years that followed, to an impressive burst of research activity made in an effort to understand the origin and implications of this new phenomenon. These studies are well summarized in two massive reviews of the field, the one in 1925 by Lattes[78] and the other in 1926 by Hirszfeld.[79] Of prime importance was the application of blood typing to the problem of blood transfusion, which was made immeasurably safer when donor and recipient could be matched. In addition, blood typing was applied to forensic medicine and especially to the establishment of paternity. Throughout the world, anthropologists studied the incidence of different blood groups in various populations to establish racial interrelationships or to confirm theories of mass migrations. Blood typing was also applied to the study of evolution and species relationships among primates,[80] and even to the confirmation of the existence and nature of interspecies hybrids.[81] Of special interest was the early realization that these genetic markers might be associated with an increased susceptibility or resistance to disease, and numerous investigators sought to correlate differing ABO frequency ratios with both infectious and noninfectious disease processes and especially with different forms of cancer.

In 1927 Landsteiner and Philip Levine discovered the M, N, and P blood groups;[82] and in 1940 Landsteiner and Alexander Wiener discovered the RH system,[83] setting the stage for the eventual solution of the problem of hemolytic disease of the newborn (erythroblastosis fetalis). Since then, numerous other blood group systems have been described (including Lutheran, Kell, Lewis, Duffy, Kidd, Diego, and I), thus expanding the forensic value of blood group identification. In addition, some of these minor blood groups have proved especially important in anthropological studies and have been extremely useful in linkage studies to establish chromosomal mapping.[84]

THE GENETICS OF ATOPIC ALLERGY

The establishment before the First World War of a medical subspecialty devoted to allergic diseases permitted practitioners to see and to compare large numbers of cases, and the impression of a high familial incidence of such diseases was rapidly gained. The first careful study of this situation was published in 1916 by Cooke and Vander Veer,[85] who studied a large series of 621 cases (including identical twins). The high incidence of allergic disease in the children of allergic parents "warrants the conclusion that inheritance is a definite factor in human sensitization." By comparing the allergens to which their patients (and especially the twins) were sensitive, they were able to show that *specific* sensitization is not inherited. "To sum up, then, we must say that the results of a clinical study compel us to conclude that sensitized individuals transmit to their offspring not their own specific sensitization but an unusual capacity for developing bioplastic reactivities to any foreign proteins."[86] Their data permitted them further to conclude that the predisposition for sensitization is inherited as a dominant Mendelian characteristic. In a review of the problem some years later, J. Adkinson modified Cooke and Vander Veer's conclusion[87] and suggested that while inheritance might be dominant in some cases, it appeared to be recessive in the majority. Adkinson also pointed out that "it is the tendency or power to develop asthma . . . which is transmitted, and not the condition itself." The data on the hereditary nature of these allergic diseases appeared so convincing that Coca and Cooke felt justified in suggesting in 1923 that the special term "atopy" be employed to designate those human hypersensitive conditions that are genetically inherited from one's parents.[88]

In a follow-up publication from Cooke's clinic, another series of families with allergic disease was reported.[89] In analyzing their results, Spain and Cooke questioned Adkinson's conclusion on the recessive nature of the transmission of allergic disease and suggested instead that a multifactorial inheritance might explain why all children of atopes are not themselves allergic. Since hay fever and asthma are recognized as the two principal forms of atopic allergy, a comparison of their respective inheritance suggested that while there might be a hereditary connection between the two conditions, it was clear that there was a certain tendency to independent transmission.

THE MAJOR HISTOCOMPATIBILITY COMPLEX (MHC)

I noted earlier that the H-2 region on chromosome 17 of the mouse (and the HLA region on chromosome 6 of the human) were discovered during the search for the basis of histoincompatibility between graft donor and recipient. Since then, these major histocompatibility complexes have been shown to comprise perhaps hundreds of different loci, only some of which encode for the cell surface glycoproteins responsible for allograft rejection. Others code for gene products that play an important role in other facets of immunorecognition and immunoregulation; consequently, the alternative name "major immunogene complex (MIC)" has been suggested as the more appropriate.[90]

Among the many biological functions subserved by the different loci within the MHC, it has recently become apparent that the murine H-2D and H-2K regions (and their human counterparts) have not been conserved in evolution merely to confound the transplantation biologist.

The products of these genes (called class I antigens) contribute also to an MHC-restricted recognition mechanism important for the function of cytotoxic T lymphocytes. The gene products of the multilocus I region (termed class II antigens) appear to be concerned principally with mediating positive or negative cooperative events, maturation signals, and sequential interactions among macrophages, T cells, and B cells. The S region of the murine H-2 complex codes for, among other products, the fourth component of complement, whereas the G region, which comprises almost half of the H-2 complex, is still relatively unexplored territory. In addition to the H-2 complex, there is another set of widely separated DNA sequences known collectively as T (for T cell) regions, which code for a large group of T cell membrane differentiation markers, of undoubted importance to the function of the various T cell subsets.

HLA and Disease Susceptibility. The past 20 years have seen a remarkable burst of activity in the identification of certain HLA haplotypes that appear to predispose to an increased susceptibility to certain diseases. While some of these haplotype–disease associations involve the A, B, and C loci (e.g., A3 and B14 with idiopathic hemochromatosis; B27 with ankylosing spondylitis and Reiter's disease; B47 with congenital adrenal hypoplasia; and CW6 with psoriasis vulgaris), most associations appear to involve the D/DR region genes. Thus, D/DR3 is intimately associated with systemic lupus erythematosus, dermatitis herpetiformis, sicca syndrome, celiac disease, and others; D/DR4 is involved in insulin-dependent diabetes and pemphigus; and D/DR5 with Hashimoto's thyroiditis, pernicious anemia, pauci-articular juvenile rheumatoid arthritis, and other disorders. In general, the mechanisms underlying these disease associations are not well understood, although there are some suggestions that the ABC associations in some way involve cytotoxic T cells, whereas the D/DR associations, so often characterized by autoimmune phenomena, may involve the participation of immune response (Ir) or immune suppression (Is) genes.

Immune Response Genes. One of the first demonstrations that genetic factors may play a role in the capacity to form specific antibodies was that of Scheibel in 1943.[91] Random-bred guinea pigs were separated into good and poor responders to diphtheria toxoid, and selective inbreeding of these two groups over several generations resulted in a positive selection for such high or low responders. The fact that so marked an effect could be had in a small number of generations indicated to Scheibel that there were relatively few genes segregating between the two groups. With the introduction by Sela of the use of antigens composed of polymers of L-amino acids of defined structure,[92] the search for genetic control of the immune response was substantially simplified. Levine *et al.* were able to show in 1963 to 1965[93] that random-bred guinea pigs varied in their response to dinitrophenyl poly-L-lysine (DNP-PLL), and breeding experiments confirmed that a single gene controls the response to the PLL carrier, independent of the hapten to which most of the antibody is directed. The first systematic study of this phenomenon in mice was carried out by McDevitt and Sela,[94] using branched copolymers such as TGAL (tyrosine, glutamic acid, -alanine, -lysine) and similar compounds in which phenylalanine or histidine were used in place of tyrosine. The genes that control the level of response to these different antigens were termed immune response (Ir) genes, and it was shown by McDevitt and Chinitz[95] that the Ir loci are intimately linked to the murine major histocompatibility complex. In 1972, McDevitt *et al.* were able to map the Ir gene controlling responsiveness to TGAL to a new region of the H-2 complex called the I region, located between the K and S regions.

It is not yet clear how Ir genes function. While Ir genes seem to regulate helper T cell recognition and Ia molecules participate in this recognition process, it is not clear that the Ia molecule is itself the product of an Ir gene. Moreover, it must be recognized that Ir gene control is not absolute but merely a regulatory factor controlling the *degree* of the immune response to the given hapten–carrier complex. This view is compatible with a second model of Ir gene function, which postulates that the gene products are primarily expressed on the surface of T cells and are concerned with the production of specific helper and suppressor factors, coded for by loci in the I-A and I-J subregions, respectively. Benacerraf and Germain have concluded that in all likelihood, both of these mechanisms may operate simultaneously as components in the general regulation of immune responses.[96]

NOTES AND REFERENCES

1. P. B. Medawar, *Encounter* **32** (Jan.), No. 1 (1969). [Reprinted in P. B. Medawar, *Pluto's Republic*, p. 30. Oxford University Press, New York, 1982.

2. G. Tagliacozzi, *De Curorum per Insitionem.* Venice, 1597. [English translation by M. T. Gnudi and J. P. Webster in *The Life and Times of Gaspare Tagliacozzi*, p. 185. Reichner, New York, 1950.]

3. See, e.g., D. Hamilton, A history of transplantation. In *Tissue Transplantation* (P. J. Morris, ed.), p. 1. Churchill-Livingstone, Edinburgh, 1982; J. M. Converse and P. R. Casson, The historical background of transplantation. In

Human Transplantation (F. T. Rapaport and J. Dausset, eds.), p. 3. Grune & Stratton, New York, 1968; R. E. Billingham, *J. Invest. Dermatol.* **41**, 165 (1963). See also the numerous references in M. F. A. Woodruff, *The Transplantation of Tissues and Organs.* Thomas, Springfield, Illinois, 1960.

4. S. L. Bigger, An inquiry into the possibility of transplanting the cornea . . . *J. Med. Soc. Dublin* **11**, 408 (1837).

5. E. Zirm, *Albrecht von Graefes Arch. Ophthalmol.* **64**, 580 (1906). Earlier, A. von Hippel [*Albrecht von Graefes Arch. Ophthalmol.* **34**, 108 (1888)] had devised the lamellar corneal graft (which uses only the superficial layers) and had reported successes with homograft material.

6. A. Carrel, *Lyon Med.* **98**, 859 (1902); *J. Exp. Med.* **10**, 98 (1908); *N.Y. Med. J.* **99**, 839 (1914).

7. See, e.g., H. M. Underwood, *J. Am. Med. Assoc.* **63**, 775 (1914); E. Holman, *Surg. Gynecol. Obstet.* **38**, 100 (1924); C. Todd, *Proc. R. Soc. London, Ser. B* **106**, 20 (1930).

8. Holman, ref. 7.

9. K. H. Bauer, *Beitr. Klin. Chir.* **141**, 442 (1927).

10. F. Sauerbruch and M. Heyde, *Z. Exp. Pathol. Ther.* **6**, 33 (1909). There is even the suggestion from these studies that something akin to the graft-versus-host reaction had occurred; see G. Schöne, *Die Heteroplastische und Homöoplastische Transplantation,* pp. 73–74. Springer-Verlag, Berlin, 1912.

11. As early as 1895, there was a flurry of activity involving studies of the possibilities of serotherapy of cancer; investigators in this area included C. Richet and J. Héricourt [*C. R. Hebd. Seances Acad. Sci.* **120**, 948 (1895)].

12. H. Morau, *C. R. Seances Soc. Biol. Ses. Fil.* **3**, 289 (1891).

13. Schöne, ref. 10. Much of the work on immunity to transplantable tumors came principally from E. F. Bashford, in the *Annual Reports of The Imperial Cancer Research Fund,* 1903–1910. A history of the early years and contributions of this organization will be found in J. Austoker, *The History of the Imperial Cancer Research Fund.* Oxford University Press, London (forthcoming).

14. E. E. Tyzzer, *J. Cancer Res.* **1**, 125 (1916).

15. Reference 14, p. 131.

16. See also C. C. Little and E. E. Tyzzer, *J. Med. Res.* **33**, 393 (1916).

17. Reference 14, p. 142.

18. L. Loeb, Transplantation and individuality. *Physiol. Rev.* **10**, 547 (1930); *The Biological Basis of Individuality.* University of Chicago Press, Chicago, Illinois, 1945.

19. W. H. Woglom, *Cancer Rev.* **4**, 129 (1929).

20. E. F. Bashford, *Trans. Int. Congr. Med., 17th, London* Sect. III, Part 2, p. 59 (1913).

21. S. Itami, *J. Cancer Res.* **10**, 128 (1926).

22. C. Da Fano, *Z. Immunitaetsforsch* **5**, 1 (1910); *Sci. Rep. Imp. Cancer Res. Fund* **5**, 57 (1912); cited in Woodruff, ref. 3, p. 69.

23. P. Rous and J. B. Murphy, *J. Exp. Med.* **15**, 270 (1912).

24. J. B. Murphy, *Monogr. Rockefeller Inst. Med. Res.* No. 21 (1926).

25. J. B. Murphy, *J. Exp. Med.* **19**, 181 (1914); **24**, 1 (1916).

26. J. B. Murphy and E. Sturm, *J. Exp. Med.* **41,** 245 (1925).

27. L. Hektoen, *J. Infect. Dis.* **17,** 415 (1915).

28. A. R. Rich, *The Pathogenesis of Tuberculosis,* 2nd Ed., p. 600. Thomas, Springfield, Illinois, 1951.

29. C. C. Little, *J. Cancer Res.* **8,** 75 (1924).

30. J. Holstein, *The First 50 Years at the Jackson Laboratory,* p. x. Jackson Lab., Bar Harbor, Maine, 1979.

31. P. A. Gorer, *J. Pathol. Bacteriol.* **44,** 691 (1937); **47,** 231 (1938).

32. See, e.g., G. D. Snell, Methods for the study of histocompatibility genes. *J. Genet.* **49,** 87 (1948); G. D. Snell, P. Smith, and F. Gabrielson, *J. Natl. Cancer Inst.* **14,** 457 (1953).

33. For example, Hans Zinsser's 1914 book, *Infection and Resistance,* discusses tumors only in the context of the possibility of serological diagnosis, while neither Karsner and Ecker's *Principles of Immunology* of 1921 nor Topley and Wilson's *Principles of Bacteriology and Immunology* of 1936 even lists "tumors" or "transplantation" in their indexes.

34. T. Gibson and P. B. Medawar, *J. Anat.* **77,** 299 (1943).

35. Reference 34, p. 309.

36. P. B. Medawar, *Memoirs of a Thinking Radish,* p. 83. Oxford University Press, London, 1986.

37. P. B. Medawar, *J. Anat.* **78,** 176 (1944); **79,** 157 (1945).

38. Reference 37, 1945, p. 174.

39. Reference 37, 1944, p. 195.

40. P. B. Medawar, *Bull. War Med.* **4,** 1 (1943).

41. P. B. Medawar, *Harvey Lect.* **52,** 144 (1956–1957).

42. P. B. Medawar, *Br. J. Exp. Pathol.* **27,** 15 (1946).

43. R. D. Owen, *Science* **102,** 400 (1945).

44. F. M. Burnet and F. Fenner, *The Production of Antibodies,* 2nd Ed. Macmillan, New York, 1949.

45. D. Anderson, R. E. Billingham, G. H. Lampkin, and P. B. Medawar, *Heredity* **5,** 379 (1951); R. E. Billingham, G. H. Lampkin, P. B. Medawar, and H. L. Williams, *Heredity* **6,** 201 (1952).

46. R. E. Billingham, L. Brent, and P. B. Medawar, *Nature (London)* **172,** 603 (1953).

47. N. A. Mitchison, *Proc. R. Soc. London, Ser. B* **142,** 72 (1954); R. E. Billingham, L. Brent, and P. B. Medawar, *Proc. R. Soc. London, Ser. B* **143,** 43 (1954). It was in this latter paper that the term "adoptive transfer" was coined.

48. Passive transfer of these sensitivity states had previously been demonstrated by K. Landsteiner and M. W. Chase, *Proc. Soc. Exp. Biol. Med.* **49,** 688 (1942); M. W. Chase, *Proc. Soc. Exp. Biol. Med.* **59,** 134 (1945).

49. G. H. Algire, J. M. Weaver, and R. T. Prehn, *J. Natl. Cancer Inst.* **15,** 493 (1954).

50. J. M. Weaver, G. H. Algire, and R. T. Prehn, *J. Natl. Cancer Inst.* **15,** 1737 (1955).

51. R. E. Billingham, L. Brent, and P. B. Medawar *Nature (London)* **178,** 514 (1956).

52. R. E. Billingham, L. Brent, and P. B. Medawar, *Ann. N.Y. Acad. Sci.* **59,** 409 (1955); J. J. Trentin, *Proc. Soc. Exp. Biol. Med.* **92,** 688 (1956); **96,** 139 (1957); M. Simonsen, *Acta Pathol. Microbiol. Scand.* **40,** 480 (1957); R. E. Billingham and L. Brent, *Transplant. Bull.* **4,** 67 (1957). For a broad review of the early work in this field, see S. C. Grebe and J. W. Streilein, *Adv. Immunol.* **22,** 119 (1976).

53. Reference 41, p. 165.

54. R. E. Billingham, personal communication, 1987; confirmed also by L. Brent, personal communication, 1987.

55. *Ann. N.Y. Acad. Sci.* **59,** 277 (1954); **64,** 735 (1957); **73,** 1 (1958); **87,** 1 (1960); **94,** 335 (1962); **120,** 1 (1964).

56. J. Dausset, J. Hamburger, and G. Mathé, eds., *Advances in Transplantation.* Williams & Wilkins, Baltimore, Maryland, 1968.

57. L. Brent, *Transplant. Proc.* **9,** 1343 (1977).

58. R. Calne, Immunological tolerance. *Br. Med. Bull.* **32,** 107 (1977).

59. C. F. Barker and R. E. Billingham in rcf. 56, p. 25.

60. R. E. Billingham and E. Sparrow, *J. Exp. Biol.* **31,** 16 (1954).

61. M. Simonsen [*Transplant. Bull.* **19,** 2765 (1987)] has called attention to the fact that the role of weak, non-MHC antigens has been seriously neglected in recent times.

62. See, e.g., *Transplant. Proc.* **17** (1985), passim.

63. W. B. Chew and H. S. Lawrence, *J. Immunol.* **33,** 301 (1937). See also A. M. Cruikshank, *Br. J. Exp. Pathol.* **22,** 126 (1941).

64. M. F. A. Woodruff and N. A. Anderson, *Nature (London)* **200,** 702 (1963); A. P. Monaco *et al., J. Immunol.* **96,** 229 (1966); R. H. Levey and P. B. Medawar, *Ann. N.Y. Acad. Sci.* **129,** 164 (1966).

65. See, e.g., *Transplant. Proc.* **17,** 2327–2375 (1985).

66. Reference 41, p. 166.

67. R. E. Billingham and L. Brent, *Transplant. Bull.* **4,** 67 (1957); M. F. A. Woodruff and L. O. Simpson, *Br. J. Exp. Pathol.* **36,** 494 (1955). Hašek's many early contributions are summarized by M. Hašek, A. Lengerová, and T. Hraba, *Adv. Immunol.* **1,** 1 (1961).

68. R. Hanan and J. Oyama, *J. Immunol.* **73,** 49 (1954). See also R. E. Billingham, L. Brent, and P. B. Medawar, *Philos. Trans. R. Soc. London, Ser. B* **239,** 357 (1956); M. Simonsen, *Acta Pathol. Microbiol. Scand.* **39,** 21 (1957).

69. R. T. Smith, *Adv. Immunol.* **1,** 67 (1961).

70. G. Allen, *Life Science in the 20th Century,* p. 113. Wiley, New York, 1975.

71. For general reviews of the entire field of immunogenetics, the reader is referred to W. H. Hildemann, E. A. Clark, and R. L. Raison, *Comprehensive Immunogenetics.* Elsevier, New York, 1980; H. H. Fudenberg, J. R. L. Pink, A.-C. Wang, and G. B. Ferrara, *Basic Immunogenetics.* Oxford University Press, New York, 1984.

72. K. Landsteiner, *Zentralbl. Bakteriol. Orig.* **27,** 357 (1900).

73. P. Ehrlich and J. Morgenroth, *Berl. Klin. Wochenschr.* **37,** 453 (1900).

74. K. Landsteiner, *Wein. Klin. Wochenschr.* **14,** 1132 (1901).

75. A. von Decastello and A. Stürli, *Muench. Med. Wochenschr.* **49,** 1090 (1902).

76. F. von Dungern and L. Hirszfeld, *Z. Immunitaetsforsch.* **4,** 531; **6,** 284 (1910).

77. In this latter connection, see also W. L. Moss, *Bull. Johns Hopkins Hosp.* **21,** 63 (1910).

78. L. Lattes, *Die Individualität des Blutes.* Springer-Verlag, Berlin, 1925.

79. L. Hirszfeld, *Ergeb. Hyg. Bakteriol.* **8,** 367 (1926).

80. K. Landsteiner and P. Miller, *J. Exp. Med.* **42,** 863 (1925); *Science* **61,** 492 (1925).

81. K. Landsteiner and J. van der Scheer, *J. Immunol.* **9,** 213, 221 (1924).

82. K. Landsteiner and P. Levine, *Proc. Soc. Exp. Biol. Med.* **24,** 600, 941 (1927).

83. K. Landsteiner and A. S. Wiener, *Proc. Soc. Exp. Biol. Med.* **43,** 223 (1940).

84. See, e.g., A. E. Mourant, *The Distribution of Human Blood Groups.* Blackwell, Oxford, 1964; R. R. Race and R. Sanger, *Blood Groups in Man,* 6th Ed. Davis, Philadelphia, Pennsylvania, 1975.

85. R. A. Cooke and A. Vander Veer, *J. Immunol.* **1,** 201 (1916).

86. Reference 85, p. 215.

87. J. Adkinson, *Genetics* **5,** 363 (1920).

88. A. F. Coca and R. A. Cooke, *J. Immunol.* **8,** 166 (1923).

89. W. C. Spain and R. A. Cooke, *J. Immunol.* **9,** 521 (1924).

90. Hildemann *et al.,* ref. 71.

91. I. F. Scheibel, *Acta Pathol. Microbiol. Scand.* **20,** 464 (1943).

92. E. Katchalski and M. Sela, *Adv. Protein Chem.* **13,** 243 (1958); M. Sela, *Adv. Immunol.* **5,** 29 (1966).

93. B. B. Levine, A. Ojeda, and B. Benacerraf, *J. Exp. Med.* **118,** 953 (1963); *Nature (London)* **200,** 544 (1963); B. B. Levine and B. Benacerraf, *Science* **147,** 517 (1965).

94. H. O. McDevitt and M. Sela, *J. Exp. Med.* **122,** 517 (1965).

95. H. O. McDevitt and A. Chinitz, *Science* **163,** 1207 (1969).

96. B. Benacerraf and R. N. Germain, *Immunol. Rev.* **38,** 70 (1978).

12

Magic Bullets and Poisoned Arrows: The Uses of Antibody

The immune substances . . . in the manner of
magic bullets, seek out the enemy.
—Paul Ehrlich

L OOKING BACK upon the entire century-long panorama of immunological progress, one cannot help but be struck by a curious phenomenon involving that aspect of the sociology of science that deals with the interrelationship among scientific disciplines. In its first 25 years or so, immunology and the theories that propelled it interacted extensively with other sciences. Not only were these theories grounded upon general biological principles derived from other fields, but their implications carried over to scientific disciplines well beyond the boundaries of immunology. Thus, Metchnikoff's phagocytic theory of immunity was based upon the evolution of digestive functions and contributed importantly both to immunology and to the general pathology of inflammation. Ehrlich's side-chain theory of antibody formation was similarly based upon broad general principles of the control of such cell functions as nutrition, intoxication, and drug interaction. His concept of specific cell-surface receptors not only defined the origin and role of antibodies but also assisted in the understanding of many other physiological mechanisms and indeed helped to define the basic principles of scientific pharmacology and chemotherapy. The concepts of immunology and even its vocabulary were widely adopted by the biomedical sciences of the day.

There then came a period of over half a century (between about 1910 and the early 1960s) when immunology ceased to interact appreciably with other specialties. I have elsewhere described this period as the Dark

305

Ages of immunology, and it was characterized by a general preoccupation with more chemically oriented studies. Little attention was paid
by most contemporary investigators to biological or medical problems.
Those theoretical proposals that were made at the time, such as the
several instructive theories of antibody formation, seemed to address
only parochial immunological concerns and offered little of substance to
other disciplines.

The time finally came, however, when immunological theory, and
indeed the entire discipline, emerged from its self-preoccupation and
once again began to exert a far-reaching influence on other biological
and medical disciplines. The clonal selection theory of antibody formation, with its extension to include the interactions among various
lymphocyte subsets, contributed to general concepts of cell differentiation and cell–cell intercommunication. Cellular and molecular theories
of immunoregulation exerted a profound influence far beyond the
borders of immunology. The implications of transplantation immunology and of the concept of immunological tolerance have penetrated to
almost every level of the disciplines of surgery and medicine. Conceptual
and practical developments in the area of immunopharmacology, involving the many cytokines and mediators of anaphylactic events, have
once again brought immunology back to the very center of progress in
the general pathology of inflammation. Finally, the concepts of immunoglobulin isotype maturation, of minigene assemblage of immunoglobulins in the generation of immunological diversity, and of allelic
exclusion, have exerted an important influence on many aspects of
molecular genetics.

But whether immunology at any given time was inward- or outward-
looking, and regardless of the implications of its theoretical constructs
for other fields, it has throughout its history made consistent contributions to other sciences by virtue of a unique technological asset—the
specific antibody. Since the development and application of many of
these techniques were unrelated to the history of immunological *ideas*
described in the foregoing chapters, they may have been neglected.
Nevertheless, each of them represented a forward step in the science of
immunology, and many contributed significantly to other disciplines as
well. This chapter will therefore be devoted to these disparate technologies, in order to examine briefly their roles in immunology itself as well
as the applications to which they have been put in other fields.[1] In
entitling this chapter "The Uses of Antibody," I employ the term
antibody in its widest sense, to include all of the products, interactions,
and ancillary factors that are properly associated with the immune
system.

Immunotherapy

ACTIVE PROPHYLACTIC IMMUNIZATION

The eighteenth-century demonstrations of the efficacy of inoculation and Jennerian vaccination to protect against smallpox were based on pragmatic observation rather than on an understanding of the mechanisms involved. It was only with acceptance of the germ theory of disease and with Louis Pasteur's demonstration of etiological specificity and of the use of attenuated organisms that preventive immunization was able to build upon a firm theoretical base. At the outset, it was thought that only live organisms would suffice to furnish protective immunity, as in the case of Pasteur's demonstrations with fowl cholera, anthrax, and rabies (where the pathogen could not even be isolated and cultured at the time). Then, with the demonstration that dead organisms and even their components might serve, many new approaches to prophylactic immunization were revealed. The discovery that diphtheria and tetanus were mediated by exotoxins permitted these substances to be used *prospectively,* an approach rendered immeasurably more efficient with the development of detoxified antigens, the toxoids.[2] It was observations of this type that paved the way for the development of effective vaccines not only for a variety of bacterial pathogens but also for viral diseases such as measles, mumps, and poliomyelitis.[3]

But not all infectious diseases were amenable to these approaches. Syphilis, trachoma, and essentially all parasitic diseases have remained unapproachable with preventive vaccines. The use of killed organisms or toxoid for cholera and of bacillus Calmette-Guérin for tuberculosis are only partially effective, and the latter has not gained acceptance everywhere. In some diseases such as influenza and trypanosomiasis, the pathogens elude the immunologists' efforts by changing their antigenic coat almost faster than specific vaccines can be developed.

The past few years have witnessed radical changes in the approach to vaccine development. Along with the concept of idiotype–anti-idiotype immunoregulation came the recognition that the anti-idiotype possesses the same three-dimensional combining site as the antigen initially employed to induce the formation of the specific idiotypic antibody. The use of such anti-idiotypes as immunogens, in place of antigens derived from the pathogen itself, is currently being actively explored, with quite promising preliminary results.[4] Yet another new approach to vaccine development has accompanied the current revolution in genetic engineering. Now, those portions of a pathogen's genome that encode for the desired antigen can be excised and reincorporated into the genome of an appropriate carrier (such as a vaccinia virus). Introduced into the vaccine recipient by this route, the antigen will be actively produced within the host during viral replication, thereby rendering immunization much more efficient. Alternatively, those antigens that are difficult to isolate may be produced *in vitro* in large quantities, using cultures of bacteria or yeasts into whose genome the antigen-encoding plasmid has been inserted.

PASSIVE SEROTHERAPY

The discovery of diphtheria and tetanus antitoxins by von Behring and Kitasato in 1890[5] seemed at the time to guarantee victory in the war against infectious diseases. Not only would these antibodies protect prospectively against infection by their respective pathogens, but timely use might even arrest the disease once started. Unfortunately, this approach was limited in the main to those few diseases mediated by exotoxins, so serotherapeutic approaches to most other infectious processes met with little success. Moreover, the readily available horse antitoxins employed to treat diphtheria and tetanus in humans often led to the development of systemic serum sickness, caused by the massive amounts of xenogeneic protein contained in the antitoxin preparation. With the availability of suitable toxoids for preventive immunization and boosting, this form of serotherapy has substantially disappeared in developed nations.

The passive transfer of protective antibody has found two other interesting applications in modern times. In diseases like infectious hepatitis, where an effective vaccine has not yet been developed and where circulating antibody efficiently neutralizes the infecting virus, human immune globulins have been utilized to advantage. The second application of passive antibody depends upon the observations that specific antibody may actually interfere with host sensitization and active antibody formation.[6] This approach has been applied to the prevention of erythroblastosis fetalis, in which the red cells of an Rh positive fetus are hemolyzed *in utero* by anti-Rh antibodies, produced by the Rh-negative mother after stimulation by transplacental passage of fetal erythrocytes. Where such maternal–fetal incompatibility is anticipated, human γ globulin containing antibody against the fetal red cells is given the mother in small amounts, to inhibit her active sensitization by the fetal cells.[7]

In addition to the suppression of specific antibody formation, passively administered antibodies have also been used to suppress the production of entire classes of immunoglobulins, an approach most often employed to study the fundamental mechanisms of the immune response. Thus, since any given B lymphocyte can only employ one of the two allelic genes that govern immunoglobulin formation (a phenomenon called *allelic exclusion*), specific antibody against one or the other allelic gene product administered during the early ontogenetic development of the B cell repertoire will selectively inhibit those cells destined to produce that allotype; consequently only the other is formed.[8] Again, the maturation of an antibody response generally involves the sequential utilization of those genes that encode for the constant region of heavy chains (in the order IgM, IgD, IgG, IgE, and IgA; this phenomenon is called *isotype switching*). The administration of a heterologous antibody against an immunoglobulin isotype, especially during the initial immune responses of experimental neonates, results in suppression of the formation of that isotype and of the others further along in the switching sequence.[9] Along the same lines, entire classes of T lymphocytes may be suppressed by appropriate use of monoclonal antibodies directed against those surface marker antigens that characterize the particular subset.[10]

IMMUNOTOXINS

The term *immunotherapy* was employed as early as 1906 by Paul Ehrlich, not so much to illustrate a successful achievement as to describe the ideal model for his new ventures into chemotherapy. It was already clear by this time that many of the diseases that afflict mankind could not be prevented by immunization or alleviated by serotherapeutic approaches. Specific antibody was to be the model for a new pharmacology, in which a drug would be so endowed with a combining site (haptophore group) that it would, like a magic bullet, unerringly seek out its pathogenic target. Moreover, appropriate chemical manipulation would ideally confer upon the molecule a toxophore group that would, like a poisoned arrow, kill the target organism while sparing the neighboring tissues of the host. Ehrlich's grand goal for the new pharmacology was nothing less than a *therapia magna sterilisans,* the specific chemotherapy of infectious diseases. He recognized, however, that "magic substances like the antibodies, which affect exclusively the harmful agent, will not be so easily found."[11]

Another reason for Ehrlich's shift from immunology to chemotherapy was the disappointment experienced by his and other laboratories in their attempts to apply serotherapy to the problem of cancer. In the mid-1890s, such investigators as Héricourt and Richet in France[12] and Salvati and de Gaetano in Italy[13] had reported on attempts to treat various forms of cancer with antitumor antibodies, along the lines of von Behring's brilliant success with diphtheria and tetanus. This approach excited a great deal of interest and activity, but the bright promise was not fulfilled. Five to ten years later, Ehrlich's Royal Institute for Experimental Therapy in Frankfurt saw the future in drugs rather than in antibodies. This disappointing assessment of the potential of immunotherapy in cancer found confirmation in a major summary of the field in 1908 by Bashford, Murray, and Haaland from the Imperial Cancer Research Fund in London. These authors concluded that "As regards the hope of a practical outcome, we consider that it is not at present to be sought in the direction of a curative serum"[14] Forty-five years later, in a lengthy review of the immunological aspects of cancer, Hauschka could offer little more hope.[15]

Throughout the 50 years of study of the possibilities of immunotherapy of cancer, it had never been clear whether the failure of this approach was due to the inability to raise specific antibodies against *unique* tumor antigens or whether, conversely, such antibodies exist but fail to exert a cytotoxic effect on the tumor targets. To the best of my knowledge, the first person to suggest that the latter alternative could be corrected by the preparation of immunotoxic molecules was David Pressman. Pressman had trained in immunochemistry with Linus Pauling, and in 1946 he established a laboratory at the Sloan-Kettering Institute for Cancer Research to investigate the localization of antitumor and antitissue antibodies, employing the now-popular techniques of radioactive tracers.[16] Here was not only the forerunner of the future use of radiolabeled antibodies in tumor diagnosis (see later), but an approach with important therapeutic potential as well.[17] As Pressman speculated, "it is not impossible that if antibodies can be found which go specifically to a certain tissue, they can be made to carry physiologically active amounts of radioactivity to the tissue. Thus, reliance need not be placed upon the capacity of the antibodies themselves to produce a physiologic effect."[18] Indeed, Pressman's studies led him to conclude that as much as 100 mCi of radioiodine might be carried to the target tissue to effect its local irradiation and destruction.[19] Unfortunately, these efforts were doomed to failure, since despite all efforts to absorb out all cross-reacting antibodies using appropriate tissue extracts, preferential localization of these crude antibody preparations (if indeed they were antitumor) was at best marginal. Too high a portion of the radioactive antibody was found to localize in such undesired targets as the lung, spleen, and kidney.

It was only with the advent of monoclonal antibody techniques that the sharp specificity required of an immunotoxin approach to tumor therapy could be realized.[20] One might now hope to localize more of the immunotoxin in the desired target tissue; and, in addition to radioactive isotopes, toxic substances such as the polypeptide chains of ricin were attached to the monoclonal antibody to form effective immunotoxins.[21] Of course, the ultimate efficacy of this approach depends upon the finding of antigens that are unique to the tumor in question and are not shared by normal tissues. Since such unique antigens may not often exist, one sometimes has to settle for a target antigen that predominates in the tumor but is shared with other tissues. Thus, the immunotoxin approach to the treatment of hepatoma now involves the use of radioactive anti-ferritin,[22] a protein antigen that is not unique to the hepatoma cell but is found in normal hepatic cells as well.

NONSPECIFIC IMMUNOTHERAPY

There is a 2-fold rationale behind the numerous nonspecific approaches to the therapy of various infectious diseases and of cancer. On the one hand, where an organism or a tumor-specific antigen may be only poorly immunogenic, one attempts to enhance the protective immune response engendered in such a system with the use of nonspecific adjuvants, in order to stimulate further one or another of the components of the immune response. Alternatively, where the principal attack is mediated by essentially nonspecific factors (such as by macrophages acting against dermal melanomas or by killer T cells acting against certain solid tumors), the approach is to render these components more plentiful or more active at the desired location. This method is reminiscent of the way that Metchnikoff, over 90 years ago, was able to enhance the destruction of cholera organisms by activating macrophages in peritoneal exudates.

Other approaches to the immunological control of tumors involve efforts aimed at increasing the immunogenicity of tumor cells, employing BCG, neuraminidase treatment, and muramyl dipeptides. Alternatively, attempts have been made to stimulate individual components of the immune response, including thymosin activation of T cells, levamisole activation of T cells and macrophages, interleukin-2 activation of cytotoxic T lymphocytes, or the use of hapten-conjugated tumor cells to enhance helper T cell function. In seeking to foster a greater participation of macrophages and natural killer cells in the destruction of tumors, systemic activation has been attempted with BCG adjuvants and interleukin-2, respectively.[23] To accomplish the same end at the precise site of tumor growth, dermal tumors have been locally infiltrated with bacterial products such as BCG and PPD.[24] The immunogenic inflammation that results at the site brings in activated macrophages and other cells that may contribute incidentally to tumor destruction.

Immunodiagnosis

The active vertebrate immune response to antigenic stimulus is almost invariably accompanied by detectable changes in the blood of the host. Within days, there appear in the circulation new or increased titers of specific antibody and/or specifically sensitized T cells. In either case, the circulating products of the immune response can be utilized to identify the inciting antigen and therefore provide many approaches to the etiological diagnosis of a wide variety of infectious or autoimmune diseases.

SEROLOGICAL TESTS

One of the most widely used of all immunodiagnostic tests was that involving complement fixation, most notably the Wassermann test for syphilis first introduced in 1906.[25] This procedure was based upon two fundamental demonstrations from the laboratory of Jules Bordet: that complement would mediate the hemolysis of antibody-sensitized erythrocytes,[26] and that any antigen–antibody interaction would result in the nonspecific fixation of complement.[27] The presence of antibody in a patient's serum can be detected and even quantitatively measured by mixing it with specific antigen and a measured amount of complement. A positive serology results when the antigen–antibody complex fixes complement, as measured by a reduction in the ability of the residual free complement to hemolyze the test erythrocytes.

It is interesting that while most complement fixation tests do in fact measure the interaction of bacterial or viral antigen with specific antibody, the prototypical serological test—the Wassermann reaction for syphilis—actually utilizes a nontreponemal lipid antigen, cardiolipin, and measures an antibody that is incapable of interacting with the offending pathogen. But whatever its basis, the reaction proved reasonably satisfactory, and its offshoots were widely employed for diagnosis and screening. In addition to numerous modifications of the Wassermann complement fixation test for syphilis, a flocculation test was introduced by Reuben Kahn,[28] involving the formation of visible aggregates of cardiolipin–lecithin mixtures by the serum of syphilitic patients. Perhaps the most specific of the tests for syphilis was the *Treponema pallidum* immobilization test of Nelson and Mayer.[29] Although the treponeme can still not be grown *in vitro*, viable preparations of motile treponemes can be obtained from infected rabbits. Specific antibody in the serum of an infected patient is detected by its ability, with added complement, to inhibit the motility of these treponemes in test suspensions.

Another serological approach to the etiological diagnosis of infection takes advantage of the availability of standardized cultures of various bacterial pathogens. The mixture of a patient's serum with a suspension of the suspected organism results in a visible agglutination of these organisms in the test tube, a reaction permitting identification not only of the genus of the pathogen but often of the species and even the strain as well. In the case of such pathogens as pneumococci, which are surrounded by large polysaccharide capsules, the various types can be differentiated by observing the swelling of the capsule induced by type-specific antibodies.[30]

The etiological diagnosis of autoimmune diseases can similarly be established by examining the sera of affected patients for specific antibodies, whether or not those antibodies are intimately involved in the pathogenesis of the disease in question.[31] Given the availability of an appropriate antigen, any one of a number of tests for antibody may be employed, including complement fixation, precipitin reactions in aqueous solution or in gels, or one of the more sensitive radioimmunoassays currently available (see later). It was such approaches that established the autoimmune nature of Hashimoto's thyroiditis, Sjögren's syndrome, and the presence of anti-immunoglobulins in the serum of rheumatoid patients and of antinuclear antigens in the serum of patients with systemic lupus erythematosus. Similar tests have implicated an autoimmune pathogenesis in diseases such as insulin-dependent diabetes, Addison's disease, and a variety of autoimmune diseases that depend upon the development of autoantibodies directed at physiologically important receptors such as those for acetylcholine, insulin, and thyroid-stimulating hormone.

DERMAL REACTIONS

Ever since the observation by Maurice Arthus in 1903 that antibody-mediated inflammation could be elicited in the skin of sensitized animals upon local introduction of an appropriate antigen,[32] such reactions have been utilized extensively for both diagnostic and pathogenetic purposes. Although the Arthus phenomenon was originally described as "local anaphylaxis," it was later shown to be a mixture of antibody- and cell-mediated mechanisms. Nevertheless, it has served as the founding model for 80 years of study by allergists in both clinic and laboratory.

With the isolation of a variety of pollen and bacterial allergens, the intracutaneous skin test soon became the approach of choice for the etiological diagnosis of hay fever, asthma, and other allergic disorders.[33] It was common practice in allergy clinics to subject the backs of patients to massive arrays of skin tests, utilizing entire libraries of allergenic extracts.

The demonstration by Prausnitz and Küstner in 1921 that skin reactivity could be transferred passively with the serum of sensitized individuals (*reverse passive anaphylaxis*)[34] firmly established this response as an antibody-mediated phenomenon. Now, with the modern knowledge that the antibody involved is a cytophilic IgE that binds to the patient's leukocytes, etiological diagnosis can also be made by exposing these leukocytes *in vitro* to various allergens. A positive response is indicated by the release of histamine from these cells, indicative of a specific IgE–allergen interaction on their surface membranes.[35]

Delayed-Type Skin Tests. The first such test described was that by Robert Koch in 1891.[36] Koch showed that tuberculin, a product of the culture of tubercle bacilli, would elicit a severe local inflammatory reaction in tuberculous patients upon intradermal application. The tuberculin test has proved to be invaluable in the diagnosis of past or present exposure to tubercle bacilli, and it set the stage for the development of numerous other diagnostic skin tests. Thus, luetin, an extract of treponemes, has been used for the diagnosis of syphilis; mallein, an extract of *Pfeifferella mallei* is used for the diagnosis of glanders; lepromin, an extract of Hanson's bacillus, is used for the diagnosis of leprosy; and so on.[37] Similar positive skin tests have been employed to demonstrate immunity to viruses such as measles and mumps.

It had originally been thought that such skin tests, like local anaphylactic reactions, were mediated by circulating antibodies; but differences in their temporal development, cytology, and the frequent inability to find circulating antibodies in such patients soon demanded their reclassification as "delayed" skin reactions.[38] Finally, the demonstrations that delayed skin reactivity to tuberculin and to poison ivy could only be transferred passively with cells[39] helped to rule out the participation of classical antibodies in these reactions and ushered in the new field of cellular immunology.

DIAGNOSTIC ANTIBODY LIBRARIES

The ability of specific antibodies to distinguish among even closely related antigenic structures is limited only by the availability of the appropriate specific antisera. This need has led to the development of entire libraries of immune sera, with a wide variety of applications in the clinical laboratory. For example, the availability of antibodies against the various blood group substances is widely used to type blood donors and recipients in order to avoid incompatible blood transfusion.[40] Again, rapid etiological diagnosis of bacterial infection is made possible by the availability of specific antibodies capable of identifying the genus, species, and even strain of the microorganism. Finally, libraries of antibodies specific for the most important histocompatibility antigens have been widely employed to assure the best possible match of donor and recipient for tissue and organ transplantation.[41]

RADIOIMMUNODIAGNOSIS

The early studies employing radiolabeled antibodies appeared to hold promise not only for the therapy of cancer but for its diagnosis as well. With the development of techniques for computerized axial tomography, this promise is now being realized. For example, the injection of radioiodine-labeled anti-ferritin into patients with hepatoma results in localization of the labeled antibody wherever a ferritin-producing metastasis exists. Such labeled metastases may then be visualized by radioimmunoimaging, in which the site of emission of the gamma rays from the radioiodine can be determined accurately by emission tomography.[42]

Identification, Assay, and Localization

All of the techniques described in this section take advantage of that unique quality of immunological interactions, the fine specificity of antibody for antigen. Some of these approaches yield only qualitative results, whereas others are capable of being quantified to an extraordinary degree. It will be apparent that in almost all instances in which a known antibody is available, this specificity can be employed to test for the corresponding antigen; similarly, when the antigen is known, its antibody can be examined.

IMMUNOPRECIPITATION

Ever since the precipitin reaction was described by Kraus in 1897,[43] the technique has been employed for the qualitative identification of antigens and antibodies, simply by observing the development of turbidity in an aqueous mixture of antiserum and antigen. (A rapid form of this qualitative approach is known as the *ring test*. Here, a dilute solution of antigen is carefully layered over the immune serum in a test tube, and the diffusion of the specific reactants produces a visible immune precipitate at the interface.) The precipitin reaction was adapted in the 1930s by Heidelberger and Kendall[44] to permit the quantitative measurement of antibody and antigen. This determination is accomplished by allowing the precipitate of optimal ratios of antibody to antigen to form under standard conditions, whereupon it is washed extensively and then subjected to nitrogen analysis to determine the amount of reactant present in the test serum.

GEL DIFFUSION ANALYSIS

In the mid-1940s, Jacque Oudin showed[45] that if an antigen is incorporated into an agar gel and antiserum layered over it, diffusion of specific antibody into the gel would result in the formation of discrete lines of precipitate down the length of the gel—in theory, one line per pair of specific interactants. The utility of this one-dimensional approach was enhanced immeasurably by Ouchterlony,[46] who adapted it for two-dimensional double diffusion. Ouchterlony showed that the addition of an antigen and an antibody into adjacent wells bored into a thin layer of agar would permit their diffusion toward each other through the medium. A thin line of immune precipitate forms where the reactants meet, its position depending upon the relative concentrations of antigen and antibody and upon their diffusion rates. Not only was this approach useful in determining the purity of an antigen solution, but it could also establish the partial cross-reaction of two antigens (containing both common and unique epitopes) by the development of precipitin spurs where the respective immune precipitate lines meet in the agar plate.

IMMUNOELECTROPHORESIS

The utility of gel double diffusion was further enhanced by Grabar and Williams,[47] First in separating one of the components (most often the antigen) in one dimension by electrophoresis and then permitting the antiserum to diffuse from the other direction from a long trough cut in the agar. The antigen could now be characterized and mixtures separated by electrical charge as well as by specific antibody, an approach especially useful for the study of the complex mixture of proteins in serum. In addition, the characteristics of different antibodies could now be studied by subjecting an immune serum to electrophoresis and placing the antigen in the lateral well.

RADIOIMMUNOASSAY

This technique, of exquisite sensitivity, was devised by Yalow and Berson[48] primarily for the quantitative assay of peptide hormones. It involves, in its most widely used form, the use of a specific antiserum to measure the competition for the binding sites on antibody of a standard preparation of radioiodine-labeled antigen and a solution of the unknown. The higher the concentration of antigen in the unknown, the more radioactive antigen will be left in the supernatant, to be compared with a reference standard. This valuable technique won for Yalow the Nobel prize for 1977.

ELISA ASSAYS

Except in endocrinological laboratories, the enzyme-linked immunosorbent assay (ELISA) has largely replaced radioimmunoassays for the quantitative determination of antigens, and of antibody as well.[49] The approach is based on the ability to immobilize one of the immunological reagents (antigen or antibody) on the surface of an insoluble carrier, without compromising its activity. The reciprocal reagent is then linked to an enzyme, so that once fixed to the carrier and washed, the amount of enzyme-coupled reagent can be estimated by permitting it to react with a substrate that yields a colored product. The most common approach employs a "sandwich" technique, in which excess antibody (or antigen) is adsorbed to the plastic microplate, washed, and then treated with the test sample. The amount of antigen (or antibody) fixed from that sample is then measured by using enzyme-linked antibody (or antigen). The intensity of the resulting substrate color then provides a precise measure of the amount of reagent in the middle layer of the sandwich. In an indirect adaptation of this method, used in the assay of antibodies, the final step can employ an enzyme-linked antiglobulin specific for the appropriate species, or even labeled anti-immunoglobulin isotypes to measure the isotype composition of the unknown antibody sample.

FLUORESCENCE-ACTIVATED FLOW CYTOMETRY
AND SORTING

The discovery that the several lymphocyte subsets possess distinctive surface membrane differentiation antigens and the subsequent production of monoclonal antibodies against these markers have opened up a new dimension in lymphocyte analysis. Antibodies specific for one or another of the lymphocyte subset markers are labeled with fluorescent dyes and mixed with suspensions of the lymphocytes to be analyzed. These mixtures are then run through a flow cytometer, where those cells rendered fluorescent by combination with labeled antibody are enumerated, using a laser beam with a wavelength appropriate for activation of the fluor employed.[50] Not only can this technique be used for quantitative analysis, but specific subsets may even be sorted in very dilute solutions, by having the laser-activated label trigger the separation of individual microdroplets in which these cells are distributed.[51]

IMMUNOHISTOCHEMISTRY

The first use of a distinctive label on an antibody, in this case to measure an antibody–antigen interaction, was that of Breinl and Haurowitz in 1932.[52] These investigators coupled the arsenic-containing compound atoxyl to antigen and were able to analyze the arsenic content of immune precipitates formed in this system. An analogous approach was employed in 1933 by Heidelberger and Kendall,[53] who attached the colored compound "R salt" to antigen for the quantitative analysis of antigen–antibody precipitates. Marrack utilized the same approach[54] to show that antibodies coupled to R salt would color bacteria that had undergone specific agglutination.

The use of color-labeled antigens to study their distribution *in vivo* was introduced by Florence Sabin in 1939.[55] Wherever the R salt-labeled antigen localized in sufficient quantity, the red color of the dye would show up on histological sections. These studies were confirmed and extended by Smetana in 1947[56] and by Kruse and McMaster in 1949.[57] The localization of antigen using radioactive tracers was first reported by Libby and Madison in 1947 (using radiophosphorus-labeled tobacco mosaic virus).[58]

The use of labeled antibodies to study the *in vivo* distribution of antigens was first explored by Pressman and Keighley in 1948.[59] These investigators used radioiodine-labeled anti-kidney antibodies and were able to show by radioautography that the antigens involved are associated primarily with the glomerulus. However, the most significant developments in the field of immunohistochemistry came from the laboratory of Albert Coons. In 1941, Coons *et al.*[60] reported the use of a fluorescent-labeled anti-type III pneumococcus (coupled with β-anthrylcarbamido groups) and were able to detect the distribution of the specific carbohydrate by examination of histological sections in a fluorescence microscope. The fluorescent antibody technique was substantially improved in 1950 by Coons and Kaplan[61] and thenceforth found broad application in the *in vivo* localization of a wide variety of antigens, both autologous and exogenous. Employing an indirect method, even the site of antibody formation or antibody deposition could be determined. This localization involves treatment of the histological section first with an antigen and then with specific labeled antibody for that antigen. In addition, a more generally applicable "sandwich technique" was also developed; in this procedure a nonlabeled antibody is localized on a section and then the fluorescence picture developed using a single fluorescein-labeled anti-immunoglobulin.

More modern applications of immunohistochemistry have entailed the development of two additional procedures. In the one, by analogy with the ELISA test described earlier, an avidin–biotin immunoperoxidase method is employed. Biotin-linked antibody is localized on a tissue section, and its specific position then established by permitting the avidin–biotin–peroxidase complex to act upon a substrate that forms an insoluble colored deposit wherever the enzyme has been localized.[62] Alternatively, the electron-opaque molecule ferritin can be attached to antibody and the location of specific antigen established by detecting the ferritin label with the electron microscope.[63]

PLAQUING TECHNIQUES

The idea of a technique for detecting and enumerating antibody-forming cells was developed independently by Jerne and Nordin and by Ingraham and Bussard in 1963.[64] This technique involves the distribution of a single-cell suspension of anti-erythrocyte-forming cells in agar, together with the species of erythrocytes employed for immunization. The red cells immediately surrounding a single antibody-forming cell become sensitized by the antibody diffusing out and are hemolyzed with added complement to yield a clear circular "plaque" in the otherwise cloudy suspension. Since the technique is most effective for the detection of IgM antibody-producing cells (because that isotype most efficiently fixes complement), a modification was introduced that facilitates hemolysis by specific IgG antibodies. This method involves the intermediary treatment of the agar plate with anti-IgG antibodies and then complement, to enhance the hemolysis of the IgG-sensitized erythrocytes. The method has also been extended to the study of antibody formation against other antigens, where these can be attached to the surface of erythrocytes to mediate immune hemolysis by their respective antibodies. These approaches have been especially useful to study the distribution and cellular kinetics of the antibody response.

Taxonomy and Anthropology

The demonstration in the 1890s of the specificity of antibodies and that this specificity could be utilized easily and with visible results in bacterial agglutination, the precipitin reaction, and immune hemolysis led rapidly to widespread application of these procedures. It was clear from the early work of Ehrlich and Morgenroth not only that different species can be identified by their response to hemolytic antibodies, but that even closely related species would show cross-reactions among their erythrocyte antigens. Even closely related plants could be identified with the precipitin reaction, utilizing appropriate antisera to test for the degree of cross-reaction shown by their protein antigens.[65] It thus became evident that serological approaches might offer a powerful tool to study the taxonomic relationships among various species, and this approach was undertaken in a major way by G. H. F. Nuttall.

Nuttall's aim was nothing less than to establish a complete evolutionary tree based upon serological studies, but the subtitle of his 1904 book, *Blood Immunity and Blood Relationships*[66] was the more modest "A demonstration of certain blood-relationships amongst animals by means of the precipitin test for blood." In this massive report, 16,000 tests were described, employing a large variety of antisera to compare the blood of many species from lobsters to primates. It was not possible with this technique, and with the limited number of tests made, to establish a clear sequence of evolutionary development, but certain close relationships could be confirmed, such as that between man and the higher primates and between these and lower primates. Many of these relationships found later confirmation with the study of blood group antigens, the best example being the sharing of the Rh antigen by man and other primates.

But the serological approach to animal (and plant) taxonomy was found to be somewhat flawed, for at least two reasons. First, with the crude antisera available, directed against a multiplicity of antigens, the apparent closeness of the relationship between two species would depend upon the relative titers for the many different antigens contained in a given antiserum. Depending upon the specificities involved, one antiserum might show a close relationship while another might suggest a greater disparity between the species tested. Even with the availability of more specific sera, however, the relationship between species might be misinterpreted, depending upon whether the antibody specificity was directed against a more highly evolutionarily conserved protein or against one more subject to the mutational hazards of time. The same variability might result if the specificity were directed against a more highly conserved or less highly conserved region of the same protein. Given these shortcomings, the use of serological approaches to the study of taxonomy has given way to the estimation of amino acid sequence homologies for various proteins. Perhaps the best example of this is the evolutionary tree for vertebrates established by the comparative study of the amino acid sequences of immunoglobulin light and heavy chains.[67]

One of the most useful applications of serology has been to the study of anthropological relationships among the different races of man. This technique is based upon the identification of the numerous blood group systems possessed by the human. Having shown that the inheritance of these blood groups follows fairly simple Mendelian genetic rules,[68] Ludwig Hirszfeld went on to illustrate the broad applicability of blood typing for anthropological study in his 1926 review "Serologic Predispositions and Blood Group Research."[69] It has since become well established that the gene frequencies for one or another blood group vary from one race or subpopulation to another,[70] so comparison of the incidence of the several blood groups among different populations may reveal significant relationships between peoples and provide important information on their mass migrations and intermixing. In a similar fashion, the variable incidence of many of the human lymphocyte antigens among different populations has contributed importantly not only to such anthropological studies but to the epidemiological distribution of certain HLA-related diseases.[71]

Forensic Pathology

Just as the antisera prepared against the serum proteins of different species may be used to determine similarities, so may they be employed to identify the species of origin of a blood by measuring antigenic differences. The possibilities inherent in this approach were recognized and adapted early by forensic laboratories, to distinguish between human and animal bloods in criminal cases or to test for the substitution of an inferior species in meat and meat products.

A more common medicolegal application of serological techniques involves the analysis of the red cell group of blood specimens. As early as 1903, Landsteiner and Richter[72] noted the possible application of blood group differences to forensic practice. Relying only upon the major ABO blood group system, Lattes pointed out in 1915[73] that even if the certain identification of a blood stain with a given individual could not be made, definite exclusion of that individual was possible if his blood group differed from that of the specimen. In 1923, the same author pointed out that similar considerations apply to questions of paternity.[74] Comparison of the blood group of an infant with that of its putative father might yield results only suggestive of paternity if they are compatible, but would definitely rule out that possibility if incompatible. Since spermatozoa also manifest the major blood group antigens on their surface, blood typing has also been applied forensically in cases of rape, with an interpretation of results similar to that employed in the analysis of blood specimens.

If all of the minor blood groups are included in these analyses, then the number of combinations is so large as to provide a red cell identification almost as unique as that of a fingerprint. However, recent advances in molecular biology have demonstrated the uniqueness of an individual's DNA sequence, and this approach is rapidly gaining judicial acceptance for identification purposes. It may soon supplant the forensic applications of serological approaches.

NOTES AND REFERENCES

1. In addition to the specific references detailed below, descriptions of the many techniques described, with their applications, may be found in D. M. Weir, ed., *Handbook of Experimental Immunology*. Mosby, St. Louis, Missouri, 1985; N. R. Rose, H. Friedman, and J. L. Fahey, eds., *Manual of Clinical Laboratory Immunology*, 3rd Ed. Am. Soc. Microbiol., Washington, D.C., 1986.

2. It was Ehrlich in the 1890s who first described toxoids, and Glenny and Ramon 30 years later who showed how they might be prepared efficiently.

3. See, e.g., one of the early editions of Topley and Wilson's *Principles of Bacteriology and Immunity*, 2nd Ed. Williams & Wilkins, Baltimore, Maryland, 1938. See also H. J. Parish, *A History of Immunization*. Livingstone, London, 1968.

4. See, e.g., M. I. Greene and A. Nisonoff, eds., *The Biology of Idiotypes*. Plenum, New York, 1984; H. Köhler, J. Urbain, and P. Cazenave, eds., *Idiotypy in Biology and Medicine*. Academic Press, New York, 1984; *Immunol. Rev.* **90,** (1986).

5. E. von Behring and S. Kitasato, *Dtsch. Med. Wochenschr.* **16,** 1113 (1890).

6. J. W. Uhr and J. B. Baumann, *J. Exp. Med.* **113,** 935, 1961. See also J. W. Uhr and G. Möller, *Adv. Immunol.* **8,** 81 (1968).

7. K. Stern, I. Davidsohn, and L. Masaitis, *Am. J. Clin. Pathol.* **26,** 833 (1956).

8. S. Dray, *Nature (London)* **195,** 677 (1962). See also T. J. Kindt, *Adv. Immunol.* **21,** 35 (1975).

9. P. W. Kincade, A. R. Lawton, D. E. Bockman, and M. D. Cooper, *Proc. Natl. Acad. Sci. U.S.A.* **67,** 1918 (1970).

10. See *Immunol. Rev.* **74,** (1973).

11. This declaration was made by Ehrlich in 1906 at the dedication ceremony marking the opening of the Georg-Speyer-Haus at his Royal Institute for Experimental Therapy in Frankfurt. See *Collected Papers of Paul Ehrlich*, Vol. 3, p. 60. Pergamon, London, 1960.

12. J. Héricourt and C. Richet, *C. R. Hebd. Seances Acad. Sci.* **120,** 948; **121,** 567 (1895); C. Richet and J. Héricourt, *Sem. Med. Paris* **3,** 510 (1895).

13. V. Salvati and L. de Gaetano, *Riforma Med.* **11,** 495, 507 (1895).

14. E. F. Bashford, J. A. Murray, and M. Haaland, *Sci. Rep. Imp. Cancer Res. Fund* **3,** 396 (1908).

15. T. S. Hauschka, *Cancer Res.* **12,** 615 (1953).

16. D. P. Pressman and G. Keighley, *J. Immunol.* **59,** 141 (1948). A long series of papers on this subject by Pressman and co-workers is summarized in D. P. Pressman, *Ann. N.Y. Acad. Sci.* **69,** 644 (1957).

17. Pressman's first published suggestion on the therapeutic possibilities of radiolabeled antibodies is *Conference on Biological Applications of Nuclear Physics* [Brookhaven Nat. Lab., Upton, New York, 1948, see p. 66]. He later expanded on the potential of the technique as follows: "in the case of antitumor antibodies there is the possibility of using such radiolabeled antibodies diagnostically as indicators to determine the location of tumors and their metastases and, perhaps, even therapeutically to carry physiologically active concentrations of radioactivity to the tumor." (Pressman, ref. 16).

18. D. P. Pressman, *J. Allergy* **22,** 387 (1951).

19. Reference 18. The same suggestion was made by W. F. Bale, R. L. Spar, R. L. Goodland, and D. E. Wolfe, [*Proc. Soc. Exp. Biol. Med.* **89,** 564 (1955)] and by J. H. Lawrence and C. A. Tobias [*Cancer Res.* **16,** 185 (1956)] with respect to the carriage of radioactive isotopes to a tumor. Bale and Spar went further [*J. Immunol.* **73,** 125, 134 (1954)] and suggested that even nonradioactive isotopes such as boron-10, with a high absorption cross-section for slow neutrons, might be attached to antibody and localized at a tumor, so that exposure to a high neutron flux would lead to local irradiation of the desired target.

20. R. H. Kennett, K. B. Bechtol, and T. J. McKearn, eds., *Monoclonal Antibodies and Functional Cell Lines: Progress and Applications.* Plenum, New York, 1984.

21. See chapters by E. J. Wawrzynczak and P. E. Thorpe; R. J. Fulton, N. Street, J. W. Uhr, and E. S. Vitetta; and L. L. Houston and S. Ramakrishnan, in *Immunoconjugates* (C.-W. Vogel, ed.). Oxford University Press, New York, 1987.

22. S. E. Order, J. L. Klein, and P. K. Leichner, in *International Symposium on Labeled and Unlabeled Antibodies in Cancer Diagnosis and Therapy,* Natl. Cancer Inst. Monogr. No. 3, 37 (1987).

23. See, e.g., M. A. Chirigos, ed., *Control of Neoplasia by Modulation of the Immune System.* Raven, New York, 1977; E. Mihich, ed., *Immunologic Approaches to Cancer Therapeutics.* Wiley, New York, 1982; S. E. Salmon, ed., *Adjuvant Therapy of Cancer V.* Grune & Stratton, New York, 1987.

24. M. J. Mastrangelo and D. Berd, in Mihich, ed., ref. 23.

25. A. von Wassermann, A. Neisser, C. Bruck, and A. Schucht, *Z. Hyg.* **55,** 451 (1906).

26. J. Bordet *Ann. Inst. Pasteur, Paris* **12,** 688 (1899).

27. J. Bordet and O. Gengou, *Ann. Inst. Pasteur, Paris* **15,** 289 (1901).

28. R. L. Kahn, *Serum Diagnosis of Syphilis by Precipitation . . .* Williams & Wilkins, Baltimore, Maryland, 1925.

29. R. A. Nelson and M. M. Mayer, *J. Exp. Med.* **89,** 369 (1949).

30. This "Quellung reaction" was first described by Neufeld [*Z. Hyg. Infektionskr.* **40,** 54 (1902)].

31. These diagnostic procedures are reviewed in N. R. Rose and I. R. Mackay, eds., *The Autoimmune Diseases.* Academic Press, Orlando, Florida, 1985.

32. M. Arthus, *C. R. Seances Soc. Biol. Ses. Fil.* **55,** 817 (1903).

33. A. F. Coca, M. Walzer, and A. A. Thommen, *Asthma and Hay Fever in Theory and Practice.* Thomas, Springfield, Illinois, 1931.

34. K. Prausnitz and H. Küstner, *Zentralbl. Bakteriol.* **86,** 160 (1921).

35. A. B. Kay, K. F. Austen, and L. M. Lichtenstein eds., *Asthma, Physiology, Pharmacology, and Treatment.* Academic Press, Orlando, Florida, 1984.

36. R. Koch, *Dtsch. Med. Wochenschr.* **16,** 756; **17,** 101, 1189 (1891).

37. These and other such tests are described in Topley and Wilson, ref. 3, passim.

38. See discussion in Chapter 9.

39. K. Landsteiner and M. W. Chase, *Proc. Soc. Exp. Biol. Med.* **49,** 688 (1942); M. W. Chase, *Proc. Soc. Exp. Biol. Med.* **59,** 134 (1945).

40. R. Sanger, *Blood Groups in Man,* 6th Ed. Davis, Philadelphia, Pennsylvania, 1975.

41. See section on Immunogenetics and transplantation immunology, in Rose *et al.,* eds., ref. 1, pp. 822–920.

42. S. W. Burchiel and B. A. Rhodes, eds., *Radioimmunoimaging and Radioimmunotherapy.* Elsevier, New York, 1983. See also Vogel. in ref. 22.

43. R. Kraus, *Wien. Klin. Wochenschr.* **10,** 736 (1897).

44. M. Heidelberger and F. E. Kendall, *J. Exp. Med.* **50,** 809 (1929).

45. J. Oudin, *Ann. Inst. Pasteur, Paris* **75,** 30 (1948).

46. Ö. Ouchterlony, Antigen–antibody reactions in gels. *Acta Pathol. Microbiol. Scand.* **26,** 507 (1949).

47. P. Grabar and C. A. Williams, *Biochim. Biophys. Acta* **10,** 193 (1953). See also P. Grabar and P. Burtin, *Immunoelectrophoretic Analysis.* Elsevier, Amsterdam, 1964.

48. R. S. Yalow and S. A. Berson, *J. Clin. Invest.* **40,** 2190 (1961).

49. S. P. Avrameas, P. Druet, R. Masseyeff, and G. Feldmann, *Immunoenzymatic Techniques.* Elsevier, Amsterdam, 1983.

50. J. A. Steinkamp, Flow cytometry. *Rev. Sci. Instrum.* **55,** 1375 (1984); E. L. Reinherz *et al.,* eds., *Leukocyte Typing,* Vol. II. Springer, New York, 1985.

51. D. R. Parks, L. L. Lanier, and L. A. Herzenberg, in *Handbook of Experimental Immunology* (D. M. Weir, ed.). Mosby, St. Louis, Missouri, 1985.

52. F. Breinl and F. Haurowitz, *Z. Immunitaetsforsch.* **77,** 176 (1932).

53. M. Heidelberger and F. E. Kendall, *J. Exp. Med.* **58,** 137 (1933).

54. J. R. Marrack, *Nature (London)* **133,** 292 (1934).

55. F. R. Sabin, *J. Exp. Med.* **70,** 67 (1939).

56. H. Smetana, *Am. J. Pathol.* **23,** 255 (1947).

57. H. Kruse and P. D. McMaster, *J. Exp. Med.* **90,** 425 (1949).

58. R. L. Libby and C. R. Madison, *J. Immunol.* **55,** 15 (1947).

59. D. P. Pressman and G. Keighley, *J. Immunol.* **59,** 141 (1948).

60. A. H. Coons, H. J. Creech, and R. N. Jones, *Proc. Soc. Exp. Biol. Med.* **47,** 200 (1941); also *J. Immunol.* **45,** 159 (1942).

61. A. H. Coons and M. H. Kaplan, *J. Exp. Med.* **91,** 1 (1950). See also R. C. Nairn, *Fluorescent Protein Tracing*, 4th Ed. Churchill-Livingstone, Edinburgh, 1976.

62. See, e.g., ref. 49. See also L. A. Sternberger, *Immunocytochemistry*, 2nd Ed. Wiley, New York, 1979.

63. Sternberger, ref. 62.

64. N. K. Jerne and A. A. Nordin, *Science* **140,** 405 (1963); J. S. Ingraham, *C. R. Hebd. Seances Acad. Sci.* **256,** 5005 (1963); J. S. Ingraham and A. Bussard, *J. Exp. Med.* **119,** 667 (1964). See also R. I. Mishell and R. W. Dutton, *Science* **153,** 1004 (1966).

65. A. Kowarski, *Dtsch. Med. Wochenschr.* **27,** 442 (1901).

66. G. H. F. Nuttall, *Blood Immunity and Blood Relationships.* Cambridge Univ. Press, Cambridge, England, 1904.

67. W. M. Fitch and E. Margoliash, *Science* **155,** 279 (1967); H. M. Grey, *Adv. Immunol.* **10,** 51 (1969); L. Hood and J. Prahl, *Adv. Immunol.* **14,** 291 (1971).

68. F. von Dungern and L. Hirszfeld, *Z. Immunitaetsforsch.* **4,** 531; **6,** 284 (1910).

69. L. Hirszfeld, *Ergeb. Hyg. Bakteriol.* **8,** 367 (1926).

70. A. E. Mourant, *The Distribution of Human Blood Groups.* Blackwell, Oxford, 1964.

71. R. L. Dawkins *et al.*, eds., HLA and Disease Susceptibility. *Immunol. Rev.* **70,** (1983); J. L. Tiwar and P. I. Terasaki, eds., *HLA and Disease Association.* Springer, New York, 1985.

72. K. Landsteiner and M. Richter, *Z. Medizinalbeamte* **16,** 85 (1903).

73. L. Lattes, *Arch. Antropol. Crim. Psichiatr. Med. Leg.* **36,** 4 (1915); *Arch. Ital. Biol.* **64,** 3 (1915); L. Lattes, *Individuality of the Blood.* Oxford University Press, London, 1932 [Engl. trans.].

74. L. Lattes, *Riforma Med.* **39,** 169 (1923). The history of the numerous applications of blood grouping is discussed by W. H. Schneider, *Bull. Hist. Med.* **57,** 545 (1983).

Appendix A

The Calendar of Immunological Progress

Epochs in Immunology

Most fields of science, even those born in the present century, go through periods of high excitement and productivity interspersed by periods of relative inactivity. The active periods, and the renaissance that may follow a period of doldrums, are often stimulated by a single individual—an Aristotle, a Newton, or an Einstein—with a startling new observation or with a theoretical construct that opens up new vistas. Similarly, the quiet periods in the life of a science (its "Dark Ages") usually occur when the old theories and the old observations have been substantially milked dry of their useful consequences; much of the activity in the field is devoted to repeating and refining the already well-worked phenomenologies while awaiting the spark that will ignite a renaissance. As the foregoing pages have made abundantly clear, the field of immunology has witnessed three such epochs in the first hundred years of its existence.

THE GOLDEN AGE OF BACTERIOLOGY

Immunology was born of the dramatic success of Louis Pasteur's germ theory of disease, with the significant assistance of Robert Koch. With the realization that each infectious disease has a specific and identifiable etiology, a happy laboratory accident permitted Pasteur (he of the prepared mind) to discover that specific acquired immunity can be induced by the use of bacterial cultures whose virulence had been attenuated. This task was accomplished in 1880, to protect chickens against the *choléra des poules,* and was quickly followed by similar observations on anthrax, rabies, and numerous other diseases for which the agents responsible were being reported with ever-increasing frequency. Here were the methodology and the rationale that made a science of immunology and were able, at last, to explain the 80-year-old observation of Edward Jenner.

With the discovery by von Behring and Kitasato that active *and even passive* immunity could be induced, to protect against diphtheria and tetanus toxins, it appeared for a time that no infectious disease could resist the armamentarium of the new immunology—prophylactic vaccination and therapeutic serum treatment. It seemed that all that was required was to identify the pathogen using Koch's postulates, attenuate it, and vaccinate—or, alternatively, identify its toxin and manufacture (in horses) its antidote. The euphoria was great, as was the activity in every laboratory, each anxious to be the first to claim a cure for one or another of the many diseases that had plagued mankind up to that point but would soon be erased with these new approaches. And indeed, many were the accomplishments of this Golden Age. The plague bacillus was identified and a reasonable vaccine produced. The cholera organism was identified and a useful vaccine appeared imminent. It seemed only a matter of time before those great scourges of mankind—tuberculosis, leprosy, typhus, typhoid fever, syphilis—would be brought under control.

This hubris lasted less than a quarter-century. Despite the ready availability of well-characterized etiological agents, prophylactic immunization just did not seem to function as expected in some diseases, for example, tuberculosis. Again, it became apparent that even though one could kill cholera vibrios *in vitro* and *in vivo* with appropriate antisera, these same antisera did not seem to protect against the gastrointestinal ravages of the clinical disease. In other instances such as syphilis, the pathogen was identified but could not be grown in culture, and efforts at preventive vaccination came to naught. In numerous other diseases (later shown to be caused by various viruses and rickettsiae), the nature of the agents themselves remained a mystery. Rabies proved to be the exception and not the rule. Thus it was that by the first decade of this century the easy victories over disease belonged mostly to the past, and the more difficult problems of tuberculosis, syphilis, yellow fever, trypanosomiasis, and a host of others began to appear insurmountable.

The once-promising young field of immunology now appeared unlikely to satisfy all that had been expected of it.

THE DARK AGES OF IMMUNOCHEMISTRY

It is perhaps too harsh a verdict to call the 50-odd years between about 1910 and 1960 the Dark Ages. Work continued in immunology, and some of it proved to be extremely useful. But it was activity of a different sort than that witnessed earlier. As pointed out in various chapters of this book, the immunological concerns with disease that typified the bacteriological era slowed and became more sporadic. Improvements were made in the use of diphtheria toxoid and in the quantitative measurement of toxins and antitoxins. It required 25 years to develop a vaccine against yellow fever and some 30 years to work out the problems of preventive immunization against pneumococcal pneumonia, an advance perhaps unfortunately aborted by the advent of antibiotics.

It was during this period that immunology passed from the hands of the bacteriologist into those of the chemist. The humoral theory of immunity, involving molecules and stereochemical structures, had replaced Metchnikoff's essentially biological theory of cellular (phagocytic) immunity. The emphasis was now on the study of antibodies and antigens, their specificities, and the modes of their interactions. While impressive progress was made in this area by Karl Landsteiner and others, it appeared slow and incremental and brought with it few important generalizations. Others devoted themselves to the problem of quantitation of the precipitin and the agglutinin reactions, to complement fixation and immune hemolysis, and to improvements in the various serodiagnostic tests then available. Since the mainstream of immunology was now dominated by chemical approaches, it is no wonder that the theories of antibody formation then extant had the antigen chemically instruct the formation of the antibody combining site. In addition, the immunological leaders of the day appeared content to leave the more biologically oriented aspects of immunology to others; allergy was left to the clinicians, and any excursions into questions of immunopathology were left to experimental pathologists and little remarked in the mainstream of immunology.

Perhaps the best way to characterize this era in immunology, and contemporary perceptions of it, is by citing the actions and the words of Dr. Gerald Webb, one of the founders and the first president of the American Association of Immunologists. Shortly after the start of the great depression in the early 1930s, Dr. Webb resigned his membership in the Immunology Society. This was admittedly due in part to financial problems, but also "he had lost interest because he could not see that it [the Society] was doing much to advance its science."[1]

THE RENAISSANCE OF IMMUNOBIOLOGY

The 10 years following the Second World War saw a number of reports, mostly by outsiders, that would soon unsettle the reigning paradigm of immunology. These were predominantly biological observations that were difficult to integrate into the old way of thinking. Peter Medawar showed that the rejection of skin grafts is due to a genetically controlled immunological mechanism, unlike the standard antigen–antibody interaction then in vogue; Ray Owen reported on the existence of cattle chimeras, which led to Burnet's prediction and Billingham, Brent, and Medawar's confirmation of the existence of immunological tolerance, a notion incompatible with previous theory; Ogden Bruton reported on agammaglobulinemia in children, a discovery that opened up new avenues for immunological research.

None of these phenomena could be easily integrated into previous notions of the structure and functions of the immune apparatus, and they cried out for a new conceptual synthesis. This was quickly forthcoming, in Niels Jerne's natural selection theory of antibody formation and in Macfarlane Burnet's clonal selection theory of antibody formation. Taken together, these new phenomena and new concepts led to a radical shift in the direction of immunology, away from the old chemical pursuits and toward more biological directions. As a result, cellular immunology, immunopathology, autoimmunity, immunogenetics, and many other biological avenues began to flourish, after 50 years of relative neglect. This is not to say that immunochemistry dropped out of the picture; on the contrary, work on the structure of the immunoglobulin molecule and the molecular basis of immunological specificity attest to the great progress in this area. But these advances depended less on following the old pathways than on participation in the modern revolution in molecular biology.

REFERENCE

1. Helen Clapesattle, *Dr. Webb of Colorado Springs*, p. 401. Associated Univ. Press, Boulder, Colorado, 1984.

Seminal Discoveries

1714 Report to Royal Society on oriental practice of variolation for smallpox—Emanuele Timoni [*Philos. Trans. R. Soc. London* **29,** 72]

1721 First immunological clinical trial, for smallpox variolation—Sir Hans Sloane [*Philos. Trans. R. Soc. London* **49,** 516 (1756)]

1798 Cowpox vaccination—Edward Jenner [*An Inquiry . . .* Sampson Low, London]

1880 First modern controlled experiment in immunology—Louis Pasteur [*C. R. Hebd. Seances Acad. Sci.* **90,** 239, 952]

1884 Phagocytic theory of immunity—Elie Metchnikoff [*Virchows Arch.* **96,** 177]

1888 Isolation of diphtheria toxin—Emile Roux and Alexandre Yersin [*Ann. Inst. Pasteur, Paris* **2,** 629]

1888 "Natural" immunity—George Nuttall [*Z. Hyg.* **4,** 353]

1889 Discovery of complement (alexin)—Hans Buchner [*Zentralbl. Bakteriol.* **6,** 561]

1890 Antitoxic antibodies and passive transfer—Emil von Behring and Shibusaburo Kitasato [*Dtsch. Med. Wochenschr.* **16,** 1113]

1891 Koch phenomenon and tuberculin skin test—Robert Koch [*Dtsch. Med. Wochenschr.* **17,** 101]

1891 Immunity to plant toxins ricin and abrin—Paul Ehrlich [*Dtsch. Med. Wochenschr.* **17,** 976, 1218]

1895 Immune bacteriolysis, "Pfeiffer phenomenon"—Richard Pfeiffer [*Z. Hyg.* **18,** 1]

1896 Bacterial agglutination—Max von Gruber and Herbert E. Durham [*Muench. Med. Wochenschr.* **43,** 285]

1897 Quantitative titration of diphtheria toxin and antitoxin—Paul Ehrlich [*Klin. Jahrb.* **6,** 299]

1897 Side-chain theory of antibody formation—Paul Ehrlich [*Klin. Jahrb.* **6,** 299]

1897 Precipitin reaction—Rudolph Kraus [*Wien. Klin. Wochenschr.* **10,** 736]

1898 Immune hemolysis—S. Belfanti and T. Carbone [*G. R. Acad. Torino* **46,** 321]; Jules Bordet [*Ann. Inst. Pasteur, Paris* **12,** 688 (1899)]

1899 Anti-tissue (anti-sperm) antibodies—Karl Landsteiner [*Zentralbl. Backteriol.* **16**, 13]

1900 Blood groups (ABO)—Karl Landsteiner [*Zentralbl. Backteriol. Orig.* **27**, 357]

1901 Complement fixation—Jules Bordet and Octave Gengou [*Ann. Inst. Pasteur, Paris* **15**, 289]

1902 Danysz phenomenon—Jean Danysz [*Ann. Inst. Pasteur, Paris* **16**, 331]

1902 Anaphylaxis—Paul Portier and Charles Richet [*C. R. Seances Soc. Biol. Ses Fil.* **54**, 170]

1903 The Arthus reaction—Maurice Arthus [*C. R. Seances Soc. Biol. Ses Fil.* **55**, 817]

1903 Opsonins—Almroth Wright and S. R. Douglas [*Proc. R. Soc. London, Ser. B* **72**, 364]

1903 Organ specificity of antigens—Paul Uhlenhuth [in *Festschrift zum 60 Geburtstag von Robert Koch.* Fischer, Jena]

1904 First autoimmune disease, paroxysmal cold hemoglobinuria—Julius Donath and Karl Landsteiner [*Muench. Med. Wochenschr.* **51**, 1590]

1906 Specificity of chemically treated antigens—Friedrich Obermayer and Ernst P. Pick [*Wien. Klin. Wochenschr.* **19**, 327]

1906 Serodiagnosis of syphilis—A. von Wassermann, A. Neisser, C. Bruck, and A. Schucht [*Z. Hyg.* **55**, 451]

1906 Serum sickness—Clemens von Pirquet and Bela Schick [*Die Serumkrankheit.* Deuticke, Vienna]

1907 Defines "immunochemistry"—Svante Arrhenius [*Immunochemistry.* Macmillan, New York]

1910 Autoantigenicity of lens protein—F. F. Krusius [*Arch. Augenheilkd.* **67**, 6]

1920 Hapten inhibition—Karl Landsteiner [*Biochem. Z.* **104**, 280]

1921 Passive transfer of allergy—Carl Prausnitz and Heinz Küstner [*Zentralbl. Bakteriol.* **86**, 160]

1923 Pneumococcal polysaccharides—Michael Heidelberger and Oswald T. Avery [*J. Exp. Med.* **38**, 73]

1926 MNP blood groups—Karl Landsteiner and Philip Levine [*Proc. Soc. Exp. Biol. Med.* **24**, 600, 941]

1929 Quantitative precipitin reaction—Michael Heidelberger and Forrest E. Kendall [*J. Exp. Med.* **50,** 809]

1929 Delayed hypersensitivity to simple proteins—Louis Dienes and E. W. Schoenheit [*Am. Rev. Tuberc.* **20,** 92]

1930 Instruction theory of antibody formation—F. Breinl and Felix Haurowitz [*Z. Physiol. Chem.* **192,** 45]

1934 "Jones–Mote phenomenon"—T. D. Jones and J. R. Mote [*N. Engl. J. Med.* **210,** 120]

1937 Histocompatibility complex—Peter A. Gorer [*J. Pathol. Bacteriol.* **44,** 691]; George D. Snell [*J. Genet.* **49,** 87 (1948)]

1939 Antibodies as globulins—Arne Tiselius and Elvin A. Kabat [*J. Exp. Med.* **69,** 119]

1940 Rh blood group system—Karl Landsteiner and Alexander Wiener [*Proc. Soc. Exp. Biol. Med.* **43,** 223]

1942 Passive cell transfer of delayed hypersensitivity—Karl Landsteiner and Merrill W. Chase [*Proc. Soc. Exp. Biol. Med.* **49,** 688]

1942 Freund's adjuvant—Jules Freund and K. McDermott [*Proc. Soc. Exp. Biol. Med.* **49,** 548]

1944 Transplantation immunology—Peter B. Medawar [*J. Anat.* **78,** 176]

1945 Chimerism in cattle—Ray D. Owen [*Science* **102,** 400]

1948 Agar gel immunodiffusion—Örjan Ouchterlony [*Acta Pathol. Microbiol. Scand.* **25,** 186]

1950 Enzymatic cleavage of antibody molecule—Rodney R. Porter [*Biochem. J.* **46,** 479]

1952 Agammaglobulinemia—Ogden C. Bruton [*Pediatrics* **9,** 722]

1953 Immunoelectrophoresis—Pierre Grabar and Curtis Williams [*Biochim. Biophys. Acta* **10,** 193; **17,** 65 (1955)]

1953 Immunological tolerance—Rupert E. Billingham, Leslie Brent, and Peter B. Medawar [*Nature (London)* **172,** 603]

1954 Transfer factor—H. Sherwood Lawrence [*J. Clin. Invest.* **33,** 951]

1955 Natural selection theory of antibody formation—Niels K. Jerne [*Proc. Natl. Acad. Sci. USA* **41,** 849]

1955 Fluorescent antibody immunohistochemistry—Albert Coons, E. H. Leduc, and J. M. Connolly [*J. Exp. Med.* **102,** 49]

1956 Bursa of Fabricius—Bruce Glick, T. S. Chang, and R. G. Jaap [*Poult. Sci.* **35,** 224]

1956 Size of antibody combining site—Elvin Kabat [*J. Immunol.* **77,** 377 (1956); **97,** 1 (1966)]

1957 Interferon—Alik Isaacs and Jean Lindenmann [*Proc. R. Soc. London Ser. B* **147,** 258]

1957 Clonal selection theory of antibody formation—F. Macfarlane Burnet [*Aust. J. Sci.* **20,** 67]

1959 IgA—Joseph F. Heremans, M. T. Heremans, and H. W. Schultze [*Clin. Chim. Acta* **4,** 96]

1960 Radioimmunoassay—Rosalyn S. Yalow and S. A. Berson [*J. Clin. Invest.* **39,** 1157]

1961 Role of the thymus—Jacques F. A. P. Miller [*Lancet* **ii,** 748]

1961 Immunoglobulin light and heavy chains—Gerald Edelman and M. D. Poulik [*J. Exp. Med.* **113,** 861]

1963 Hemolytic plaque assay—Niels K. Jerne and Albert A. Nordin [*Science* **140,** 405]

1963 Idiotypes—Henry G. Kunkel, M. Mannik, and R. Williams [*Science* **140,** 1218]; Jacques Oudin and M. Michel [*C. R. Hebd. Seances Acad. Sci.* **257,** 805]; Philip G. H. Gell and Andrew Kelus [*Nature (London)* **201,** 687 (1964)]

1966 Lymphokines (MIF)—Barry R. Bloom and B. Bennet [*Science* **153,** 80]; John R. David [*Proc. Natl. Acad. Sci. USA* **56,** 72]

1966 T cell subsets—Henry N. Claman, E. A. Chaperon, and R. F. Triplett [*Proc. Soc. Exp. Biol. Med.* **122,** 1167]; G. F. Mitchell and J. F. A. P. Miller [*J. Exp. Med.* **128,** 801, 821 (1968)]

1966 IgE—Kimishige Ishizaka and Teruko Ishizaka [*J. Immunol.* **97,** 75, 840; *J. Allergy* **37,** 165, 336]

1969 Helper T cells—N. Avrion Mitchinson [in *Immunological Tolerance,* p. 149. Academic Press, New York]

1970 Hypervariable regions of Ig—T. T. Wu and Elvin A. Kabat [*J. Exp. Med.* **132,** 211]

1970 Immunoglobulin domains—Gerald Edelman [*Biochemistry* **9,** 3197]

1970 Suppressor T cells—Richard K. Gershon and K. Kondo [*Immunology* **18,** 723]

1974 Idiotype networks—Niels K. Jerne [*Ann. Immunol. (Paris)* **125C,** 373]

1975 Hybridomas—Georges Köhler and Cesar Milstein [*Nature (London)* **256,** 495]

Important Books in Immunology, 1892–1968

These titles provide a good indication of the changing directions and new developments in the field. After 1968, the volume became overwhelming.

1892 *Die Blutserumtherapie,* Emil von Behring. Thieme, Leipzig

1892 *Lecons sur la Pathologie Comparée de l'Inflammation* Elie I. Metchnikoff. Masson, Paris

1895 *Immunity: Protective Inoculations in Infectious Diseases and Serum-Therapy,* George M. Sternberg. William & Wood, New York

1901 *L'Immunité dans les Maladies Infectieuses,* Elie Metchnikoff. Masson, Paris

1902 *Immunität und Immunisierung. Eine medicinisch-historische Studie,* Ludwig Hopf. Franz Pietzcker, Tübingen

1902 *Ehrlichs Seitenkettentheorie and Ihre Anwendung auf die künstlichen Immunisierungsprozesse,* Ludwig Aschoff. Fischer, Jena

1903 *Die Antikörper,* Emil von Dungern. Fischer, Jena

1904 *Immune Sera, Hemolysins, Cytotoxins, and Precipitins,* August von Wasserman. John Wiley, New York

1904 *Toxine und Antitoxine,* Karl Oppenheimer. Fischer, Jena

1904 *Gesammelte Arbeiten zur Immunitätsforschung,* Paul Ehrlich. August Hirschwald, Berlin. [English edition: Wiley, New York, 1906]

1904 *Blood Immunity and Blood Relationship,* George H. F. Nuttall. Cambridge University Press, Cambridge, England.

1904 *Die Ehrlich'sche Seitenkettentheorie und ihre Bedeutung für die medizinischen Wissenschaften,* Paul Römer. Alfred Hölder, Wien

1906 *Das Heufieber,* Alfred Wolff-Eisner. Munich, 1906.

1906 *Die Serumkrankheit,* Clemens von Pirquet and Bela Schick. Deuticke, Vienna

1907 *Immunochemistry,* Svante A. Arrhenius. Macmillan, New York

1909 *Handbuch der Technik und Methodik der Immunitätsforschung,* R. Kraus and C. Levaditi, eds. Fischer, Jena

1909 *Studies in Immunity,* Robert Muir. Henry Frowde, London

1909 *Die Serodiagnose der Syphilis,* Carl Bruck. Springer-Verlag, Berlin

1909 *Die Krise in der Immunitätsforschung,* E. Sauerbeck. Klinkhardt, Leipzig

1909 *Studies in Immunity, Jules Bordet (Collected Papers)*, translated by Frederick P. Gay. Wiley, New York

1909 *Studies on Immunization and Their Application to the Treatment of Bacterial Infection*, Almroth E. Wright. Constable, London

1910 *Klinische Immunitätslehre und Serodiagnostik*, Alfred Wolff-Eisner. Fischer, Jena

1911 *Allergie*, Clemens von Pirquet. Am. Med. Assoc., Chicago, Illinois

1914 *Handbuch der Immunitätsforschung und Experimentellen Therapie*, R. Kraus and C. Levaditi, eds. Fischer, Jena

1914 *Infection and Resistance*, Hans Zinsser. Macmillan, New York

1914 *Die Anaphylaxie in der Augenheilkunde*, Aurel von Szily. Enke, Stuttgart

1917 *Anaphylaxie et Antianaphylaxie: Bases Experimentales*, Alexandre Besredka. Masson, Paris

1920 *Traité de l'Immunité dans les Maladies Infectieuses*, Jules Bordet. Masson, Paris

1921 *De l'anaphylaxie à l'immunité*, Maurice Arthus. Masson, Paris

1921 *Studien über die Überempfindlichkeit*, Carl Prausnitz and Heinz Küstner. Fischer, Jena

1924 *Immunity in Natural Infectious Diseases*, Felix D'Hérelle. Williams & Wilkins, Baltimore, Maryland

1924 *The Chemical Aspects of Immunity*, H. Gideon Wells. Chem. Catalog Co., New York

1927 *La Vaccination Préventive contre la Tuberculose par le 'B.C.G.,'* Albert Calmette, C. Guérin, A. Bouquet, and L. Négre. Masson, Paris

1928 *Etudes sur l'Immunité dans les Maladies Infectieuses*, Alexandre Besredka. Masson, Paris

1928 *Konstitutionsserologie und Blutgruppenforschung*, Ludwig Herszfeld. Springer-Verlag, Berlin

1929 *The Immunology of Parasitic Infections*, William H. Taliaferro. Century; New York

1930 *Le Choc Anaphylactique et la Principe de la Désensibilisation*, Alexandre Besredka. Masson, Paris

1931 *Asthma and Hay Fever in Theory and Practice*, A. F. Coca, M. Walzer, and A. A. Thommen. Thomas, Springfield, Illinois

1933 *Die Spezifizität der Serologischen Reaktionen*, Karl Landsteiner. Springer-Verlag, Berlin

1933 *Allergy and Immunity in Ophthalmology,* Alan C. Woods. Johns Hopkins University Press, Baltimore, Maryland

1934 *The Chemistry of Antigens and Antibodies,* John R. Marrack. HM Stationery Off, London

1936 *The Principles of Bacteriology and Immunology,* 2nd Ed., W. W. C. Topley and G. S. Wilson. W. Wood, Baltimore, Maryland

1936 *Tissue Immunity,* Reuben L. Kahn. Thomas, Springfield, Illinois

1936 *The Specificity of Serological Reactions* (English revised edition), K. Landsteiner. Thomas, Springfield, Illinois

1937 *Les Immunités Locales,* Alexandre Besredka. Masson, Paris

1937 *The Phenomenon of Local Tissue Reactivity and its Immunological and Clinical Significance,* Gregory Schwartzman. Oxford University Press, London

1938 *The History of Bacteriology,* William Bulloch. Oxford University Press, London

1941 *The Production of Antibodies. A Review and a Theoretical Discussion,* F. M. Burnet, M. Freeman, A. V. Jackson, and D. Lush. Macmillan, New York

1943 *Fundamentals of Immunology,* William C. Boyd. Interscience, New York

1943 *Allergy, Anaphylaxis and Immunotherapy,* Bret Ratner. Williams & Wilkins, Baltimore, Maryland

1944 *The Pathogenesis of Tuberculosis,* Arnold Rich. Thomas, Springfield, Illinois

1945 *Immunocatalysis,* M. G. Sevag. Thomas, Springfield, Illinois

1948 *Antibody Production in Relation to the Development of Plasma Cells* (Suppl. 204 to *Acta Med. Scand.*), Astrid Fagraeus. Esselte Aktiebolag, Stockholm

1948 *Experimental Immunochemistry,* Elvin A. Kabat and Manfred M. Mayer. Thomas, Springfield, Illinois

1949 *The Production of Antibodies,* 2nd Ed. F. M. Burnet and F. Fenner. Macmillan, New York

1951 *Antibodies and Embryos,* F. W. R. Brambell, W. A. Hemmings, and M. Henderson. Constable, London

1951 *Blood Transfusion in Clinical Medicine,* P. L. Mollison. Blackwell, Oxford

1951 *A Study of Avidity Based on Rabbit Skin Responses to Diphtheria*

Toxin–Antitoxin Mixtures, Niels K. Jerne. Munksgaard, Copenhagen

1953 *Immunity, Hypersensitivity, Serology,* Sidney Raffel. Appleton, New York

1954 The Relation of Immunology to Tissue Homotransplantation. *Ann. N.Y. Acad. Sci.* **59,** 277–465

1956 *Blood Group Substances: Their Chemistry and Immunochemistry,* Elvin A. Kabat. Academic Press, New York

1956 *Immunohématologie Biologique et Clinique,* Jean Dausset. Flammarion, Paris

1957 *Collected Papers of Paul Ehrlich,* Vol. 2. Pergamon, New York

1957 *Immunpathologie in Klinik und Forschung, und das Problem der Autoantikörper,* P. Miescher and K. O. Vorlaender, eds., Thieme, Stuttgart

1958 *First International Symposium on Immunopathology,* Pierre Grabar and Peter Miescher, eds. Schwabe, Basel

1959 *Mechanisms of Hypersensitivity* (Henry Ford Hospital International Symposium), J. H. Shaffer, G. A. LoGrippo, and M. W. Chase, eds. Little, Brown, Boston, Massachusetts

1959 *Experimental Allergic Encephalomyelitis* (Suppl. to Vol. 14, *Int. Arch. Allergy Appl. Immunol.*), Byron H. Waksman. Karger, Basel

1959 *The Clonal Selection Theory of Acquired Immunity,* F. Macfarlane Burnet. Cambridge University Press, London

1959 *Cellular and Humoral Aspects of Hypersensitive States,* H. Sherwood Lawrence, ed. Hoeber, New York

1960 *Mechanisms of Antibody Formation,* M. Holub and L. Jarŏsková, eds. Czech. Acad. Sci., Prague

1960 *Analyse immuno-électrophorétique,* P. Grabar and P. Burtin. Masson, Paris

1960 *The Transplantation of Tissues and Organs,* Michael F. A. Woodruff. Thomas, Springfield, Illinois

1960 *Cellular Aspects of Immunity* (Ciba Symposium), G. E. W. Wolstenholme and M. O'Connor, eds. Little, Brown, Boston, Massachusetts

1962 "Tumor Immunity," D. B. Amos, ed. *Ann. N.Y. Acad. Sci.* **101**

1962 *Mechanisms of Immunological Tolerance,* M. Hašek and A. Lengerová, eds. Czech. Acad. Sci., Prague

1962 *Introduction to Immunochemical Specificity,* William C. Boyd. Interscience, New York

1963 *Clinical Aspects of Immunology,* P. G. H. Gell and R. R. A. Coombs, eds. Blackwell, Oxford

1963 *Autoimmune Diseases,* F. Macfarlane Burnet and I. R. Mackay. Thomas, Springfield, Illinois

1963 *Immunology for Students of Medicine,* J. H. Humphrey and R. G. White. Davis, Philadelphia, Pennsylvania

1964 *The Thymus in Immunobiology,* Robert A. Good and Ann B. Gabrielson, eds. Hoeber, New York

1965 *Autoimmunity and Disease,* L. E. Glynn and E. L. Holborow. Davis, Philadelphia, Pennsylvania

1965 *Immunologic Diseases,* Max Samter, ed. Little, Brown, Boston, Massachusetts

1965 *Molecular and Cellular Basis of Antibody Formation,* J. Šterzl, ed. Czech. Acad. Sci., Prague

1965 *Complement* (Ciba Symposium), G. E. W. Wolstenholme and J. Knight, eds. Little, Brown, Boston, Massachusetts

1966 *Immunotolerance to Simple Chemicals,* Alain de Weck and J. R. Frey. Elsevier, New York

1966 *Phylogeny of Immunity,* R. T. Smith, P. Miescher, and R. A. Good, eds. University of Florida Press, Gainesville

1966 *The Thymus* (Ciba Symposium), G. E. W. Wolstenholme and R. Porter, eds. Little, Brown, Boston, Massachusetts

1967 *Delayed Hypersensitivity,* J. L. Turk. North-Holland Publ., Amsterdam

1967 *Gamma Globulin Structure and Control of Biosynthesis* (Proceedings of the Third Nobel Symposium), J. Killander, ed. Almqvist & Wiksell, Stockholm

1967 "Antibodies," Cold Spring Harbor Symposium on Quantitative Biology. Cold Spring Harbor Lab., Cold Spring Harbor, New York

1967 *Natural and Acquired Immunological Unresponsiveness,* William O. Weigle. World Publ., Cleveland, Ohio

1967 *Germinal Centers in Immune Responses,* H. Cottier, N. Odartchenko, R. Schindler, and C. C. Congdon, eds. Springer, New York

1967 *The Gamma Globulins,* Charles A. Janeway ed. Little, Brown, Boston, Massachusetts

1968 *The Structural Basis of Antibody Specificity*, David Pressman and Alan Grossberg. Benjamin, New York

1968 *Structural Concepts in Immunology and Immunochemistry*, Elvin A. Kabat. Rinehart & Winston, New York

1968 *Handbook of Immunodiffusion and Immunoelectrophoresis*, Ö. Ouchterlony. Science Publ., Ann Arbor, Michigan

1968 *Monoclonal and Polyclonal Hypergammaglobulinemia*, Jan G. Waldenström. Vanderbilt University Press, Nashville, Tennessee

1968 *Immunologic Deficiency Diseases in Man*, D. Bergsma, ed. Nat. Found., New York

Appendix B

Nobel Prize Highlights in Immunology

1901. The first Nobel prize in medicine was awarded to **EMIL VON BEHRING** [1854–1917]. von Behring studied under Robert Koch at Koch's Institute in Berlin. Following Löffler's isolation of the diphtheria bacillus in 1883 and the identification of diphtheria exotoxin by Roux and Yersin in 1888, von Behring with his colleagues Kitasato and Wernicke showed in 1890–1892 that diphtheria and tetanus immunity were due to the formation of circulating antitoxins. He showed that passive administration of antitoxin serum to diseased patients might effect a cure, thus opening the way for serum immunotherapy in a number of diseases. His citation read: "For his work on serum therapy, especially its application against diphtheria, by which he has opened a new road in the domain of medical science and thereby placed in the hands of the physician a victorious weapon against illness and death."

1905. To **ROBERT KOCH** [1843–1910], "for his investigations and discoveries in regard to tuberculosis." Koch had been a small-town physician in Germany, when his private investigations on the life cycle of the anthrax bacillus and the etiology of anthrax excited the medical profession in 1876. He was given first a laboratory and then an institute in Berlin, and it was there, with the help of a distinguished series of students, that he made bacteriology a true science, by his development of stringent bacterial isolation and culture techniques and by his emphasis on the famous Koch postulates for proof of etiology. Koch devoted

341

himself to the study of a number of different diseases, but it was his identification of the tubercle bacillus and of tuberculin and his continuing devotion to the study of tuberculosis that earned him the Nobel prize. Both the immunodiagnostic tuberculin reaction and the "Koch phenomenon," involving the excessive dermal reaction to tubercle bacilli in the skin of sensitized animals, played a major role in the later elucidation of the mechanisms of cellular immunity.

1908. The prize this year was shared by **ELIE METCHNIKOFF** [1845–1916] and **PAUL EHRLICH** [1854–1915], "in recognition for their work on immunity." Metchnikoff was born in the Russian Ukraine and studied zoology with an emphasis on comparative embryology. In 1884, working in a marine biology laboratory in Italy, he made the initial observations on the phagocytic cells of starfish larvae that provided the basis for his cellular (phagocytic) theory of immunity. When Metchnikoff left Russia for political reasons, Pasteur offered him a position at his new institute in Paris, where Metchnikoff devoted the rest of his life to an impressive series of investigations in support of his phagocytic theory and to its vigorous defense from the many attacks by those who favored the view that immunity was based upon humoral (i.e., antibody–complement) mechanisms.

Paul Ehrlich was born in Germany, studied medicine, and early became interested in the staining reactions of cells in tissues, devising some of the most useful stains for the tubercle bacillus and for blood leukocytes. In 1890 he became an assistant to Koch at the Institute for Infectious Diseases, where he commenced his immunological studies. Following early work on the antibody response to the plant toxins abrin and ricin, Ehrlich made his most notable early contribution to immunology in 1897, with the publication of his paper describing the first practical method for standardization of diphtheria toxin and antitoxin preparations. This same publication contained also the outline of his famous side-chain theory of antibody formation, which greatly influenced immunological theories for several decades. With Julius Morgenroth, he published an important series of papers on the mechanism of immune hemolysis. Shortly after the turn of the century, Ehrlich gave up most of his activities in immunology to pursue his interests in the chemical treatment of disease, making important discoveries in the treatment of trypanosomiasis and of syphilis (Salvarsan—the "magic bullet") and helping to found scientific pharmacology.

1913. To **CHARLES RICHET** [1850–1935], "for his work on anaphylaxis." Richet was a Parisian who studied medicine and became especially interested in physiology. It was these interests that led him to study the physiological effects on mammals of marine invertebrate poisons, while cruising on the yacht of the Prince of Monaco. With his colleague Paul Portier, he discovered the phenomenon of anaphylaxis, a response dependent not upon the toxic properties of the substance injected but only upon its function as an antigen in the previously sensitized animal. In so doing, he opened up a new and at the time surprising vista in medicine, by showing that the "protective" mechanisms of immunity might function also to cause disease. The later demonstration of the relationship between experimental anaphylaxis and other more familiar human allergies made this observation clinically as well as theoretically important to immunology.

1919. To **JULES BORDET** [1870–1961], "for his studies in regard to immunity." Bordet was a Belgian physician who went to study with Metchnikoff at the Pasteur Institute in Paris at the age of 24. He made important early contributions to an understanding of the mechanism of complement-mediated bacteriolysis, and in 1899 he discovered the phenomenon of specific hemolysis. Shortly thereafter, in collaboration with his assistant and brother-in-law, Octave Gengou, Bordet described the phenomenon of complement fixation and its diagnostic possibilities. This soon developed into a powerful tool in the diagnosis of infectious diseases, most notably in the hands of August von Wassermann and his colleagues, in their complement-fixation test for syphilis. Bordet made many other important contributions to immunology and is also known for his famous debates with Ehrlich on the nature of antigen–antibody–complement interactions.

1930. To **KARL LANDSTEINER** [1868–1943], "for his discovery of the human blood groups." Landsteiner was a Viennese pathologist who developed a keen interest in structural organic chemistry before embarking on a career in immunology. From the very outset, Landsteiner seemed always to choose important areas in which to work or to make important those subjects to which he turned his attention. In early studies of anti-erythrocyte antibodies, he described in 1901 the set of human isoagglutinins that now comprise the ABO system of blood groups. In 1926 Landsteiner and Philip Levine discovered the MNP system, and with Albert Wiener in 1940 the Rh system of blood groups. He was the first to demonstrate that poliomyelitis could be produced in nonhuman primates, and one of the first to make the same observation for syphilis. During the First World War, he became interested in the antibody response to chemically defined haptens and over the next quarter-century, primarily at the Rockefeller Institute in New York, he contributed impressively to an understanding of the chemical basis for antigen–antibody interactions, as summarized in his famous book *The Specificity of Serological Reactions*. While acknowledging the importance of his discovery of blood groups, Landsteiner is said to have felt that his Nobel prize should have been awarded for his work on antibody–hapten interactions.

1951. To **MAX THEILER** [1899–1972], "for his development of vaccines against yellow fever." Theiler was a South African who studied medicine in Britain and then moved to the United States in 1922, first to the School of Tropical Medicine at Harvard and then to the Rockefeller Institute in New York. It was he who showed that yellow fever was caused by a filterable virus, and his description of the mouse protection test (in which serum antibody mixed with the virus protects a mouse from the lethal effects of intracerebral inoculation) provided a very important tool for epidemiological and other studies of yellow fever. In the late 1930s he succeeded in developing attenuated strains of yellow fever virus by serial passage *in vitro* in mouse and chick embryo tissue cultures. By these means, strains were developed that retained their immunogenicity but were devoid of pathogenicity, the basis of the currently effective yellow fever vaccines.

1957. To **DANIEL BOVET** [1907–   ], Swiss physiologist and pharmacologist, "for his development of antihistamines in the treatment of allergy." The discovery of the Schultz–Dale phenomenon, in which a strip of sensitized uterine tissue could be caused to contract under the action of antigen, provided a useful *in vitro* model for allergic reactions and for the clarification of the physiological mechanisms involved. This discovery led to the finding that histamine is the most significant agent released in anaphylaxis; histamine is released along with serotonin and other active substances. Bovet must have been exposed to immunology and allergy while working under Emile Roux at the Pasteur Institute in Paris; and he published extensively on the response of the autonomic nervous system to various chemicals. It was this work that led him to a study of agents that might counter the effects of histamine, and from this latter study emerged the drugs that were to prove so useful in the treatment of asthma and hay fever. Even had he not become famous for his work on antihistamines, his South American adventures with curare and its mode of action, and his development of curare-like relaxants, tranquilizing drugs, and anesthetics would have given him a secure place in the annals of medicine.

1960. To **F. MACFARLANE BURNET** [1899–1985] and **PETER B. MEDAWAR** [1915–1987], "for the discovery of acquired immunological tolerance." The Second World War stimulated basic research in a number of sciences, among them the search to improve the survivability of skin and other tissue grafts on burn and wound victims and to explain their rejection. Medawar, a Briton who had trained in zoology and pathology at Oxford, was interested in tissue repair and, thus, in problems of tissue transplantation. His initial work established conclusively that the rejection of foreign skin grafts followed all of the rules of immunological specificity and was in fact based upon the same mechanisms responsible for protection against bacterial and viral infections. The followup work that he and a series of distinguished students (most notably Rupert Billingham and Leslie Brent) undertook firmly established transplantation immunobiology as an important subdiscipline, yielding many later dividends in the field of clinical organ transplantation. In 1945–1947, Ray Owen reported the curious observation that dizygotic cattle twins which had shared the same circulatory system *in utero* had become blood-cell chimeras, unable to respond immunologically to each other's antigens. This observation was seized upon by the Australian physician-virologist Macfarlane Burnet, not only a productive investigator but also a wide-ranging theoretician. Burnet had published in 1941 a stimulating book, *The Production of Antibodies* and was now preparing a revision of this book with his colleague Frank Fenner. The new book (1949) not only proposed a novel indirect template theory of antibody formation but also provided a theoretical explanation for Owen's findings. Burnet and Fenner suggested that immunological responses arise fairly late in embryonic life and involve a cataloguing by a system of "self-markers" of those antigens then present, to which the host thenceforth would be tolerant and unable to respond immunologically. Any antigens not so catalogued would be "non-self" and could later stimulate an active immune response. The suggestion was made that any antigen introduced during this critical period would be adopted as self, would induce tolerance, and thus would be unable later to activate the immunological apparatus. These concepts were further developed by Burnet in his clonal selection theory of antibody formation. Burnet and Fenner's suggestion on tolerance was put to the test by Medawar and his colleagues, and in 1953 they provided ample confirmation of the Burnet–Fenner hypothesis, using inbred strains of mice, a phenomenon to which Medawar gave the name acquired immunological tolerance.

1972. To **RODNEY R. PORTER** [1917–1985] of Oxford University and **GERALD M. EDELMAN** [1929–   ] of the Rockefeller University, for their work on the chemical structure of antibodies. The demonstration by A. Tiselius and E. A. Kabat that antibodies are high-molecular-weight gamma globulins made it clear that it would be extremely difficult to define chemically the basis for either their primary immunological specificity or for their secondary biological functions. Porter undertook to cleave the antibody molecule with enzymes in an attempt to obtain smaller, active fragments, and he succeeded in 1958 in accounting for the entire molecule in terms of papain cleavage into two identical Fab fragments and a third Fc fragment; the former contained the antibody-binding sites, while the latter was responsible for the secondary biological activity of antibodies. Edelman then showed that homogeneous myeloma globulin could be reductively cleaved into its component polypeptide chains, comprising both light (L) and heavy (H) chains. He also showed that the L chains of different guinea pig antibodies had different electrophoretic mobility patterns and further that the Bence-Jones protein of multiple myeloma was similar to the L chains of antibody. Porter and his colleagues next demonstrated that the immunoglobulin molecule was composed of two light and two heavy chains, a finding leading to the now-accepted model for IgG. The isolation of immunoglobulin chains and fragments permitted an approach to their primary amino acid sequencing, and this was hotly pursued in the laboratories of Porter, Edelman, and many other investigators. From this work emerged an understanding of the existence of both variable and constant regions on the L and H chains and the ability to compare primary sequences among different antibody specificities, different isotypes, and even different species. Finally, in 1969, Edelman and his co-workers succeeded in working out the primary sequence of an entire immunoglobulin molecule, helping to define not only the location of the active site but also the location of the "domains" responsible for the secondary biological activities of antibodies.

1977. To **ROSALYN YALOW** [1921–], "for the development of radio immunoassays of peptide hormones," (shared with **ROGER GUILLEMIN** and **ANDREW SCHALLY**, "for their discoveries concerning the peptide hormone production of the brain"). Beginning in the early 1950s, Yalow and her long-term collaborator Solomon Berson investigated the causes of insulin resistance in diabetes. They discovered that diabetics treated with insulin formed antibodies specific for this insulin, but their initial attempt to publish this important observation was rejected, in the belief that so small a molecule was incapable of being immunogenic. Berson (who died in 1972) and Yalow then showed that the addition of increasing amounts of unlabeled insulin to an immune complex of anti-insulin and its radiolabeled antigen resulted in a measurable displacement of the labeled insulin. This discovery formed the basis of the first radioimmunoassay of a hormone, a test capable of estimating nanogram or even picogram quantities. Since then, this assay system has been applied to other hormones and biologically active substances and has become a valuable tool for much basic and clinical research. It was this technique that contributed importantly to the isolation and characterization of hypothalamic hormones by Guillemin and Schally.

1980. To **BARUJ BENACERRAF** [1920–], **JEAN DAUSSET** [1916–], and **GEORGE SNELL** [1903–], "for their work on genetically determined structures of the cell surface that regulate immunologic reactions." The demonstration that the ability of mice to reject tumors was genetically determined stimulated geneticist Snell to search for methods to study the genes responsible for this phenomenon. This study led Snell in the mid-1930s "to invent the idea of congenic mice," animals that are bred to be genetically identical except at a single locus or genetic region. In collaboration with Peter Gorer, Snell identified a locus important for allograft rejection, designated H(histocompatibility)-2 and subsequently shown to be a complex of many closely linked genes with many different alleles occurring at each locus. The work of many investigators has since contributed to a better understanding of the composition and many of the functions of this complicated stretch of DNA, now called the major histocompatibility complex (MHC). In the 1950s, Jean Dausset of France found isoantibodies against leukocyte antigens in the blood of transfusion recipients, a finding that helped to demonstrate the analogy between the H-2 complex of the mouse and the human leukocyte antigen (HLA) system in man and provided a powerful tool to define individual HLA antigens. In 1965 Dausset and his co-workers described a system of about 10 human antigens encoded for in the histocompatibility complex, containing "sub-loci" each of which specified a limited number of antigenic alleles. It was this approach that finally opened the way for the definition and genetic location of those major and minor antigens responsible for histoincompatibility. But the importance of the genes in the HLA and H-2 complexes had thus far been restricted to the somewhat unphysiological practices of tissue and blood transplantation. It remained for Benacerraf and his co-workers to demonstrate that many of the genes located within the MHC may also control active immune responses to various antigenic stimuli. Utilizing simple antigens such as synthetic polypeptides, Benacerraf, McDevitt, and others found that the ability of an animal to respond immunologically to a given antigen was controlled by specific genes—called Ir (for immune response) genes—that were subsequently shown by others to reside within the I region of the MHC. Since then, work in Benacerraf's and in many other laboratories has shown the importance of I region

A History of Immunology

genes in controlling the intercommunication among immunocytes responsible for the regulation of the immune response and the importance of some MHC genes in predisposing for certain chronic diseases.

1984. The prize this year was shared by **CESAR MILSTEIN** [1927–] and **GEORGES F. KÖHLER** [1946–] for development of the technique of monoclonal antibody formation and **NIELS K. JERNE** [1912–] for his theoretical contributions that have shaped our concept of the immune system. Henry Kunkel and co-workers showed in 1955 that myeloma tumors produced monoclonal antibodies, and Michael Potter showed in 1962 that such plasma cell tumors could be induced in mice; other investigators were able to adapt such tumors to grow indefinitely in culture. In 1974, Köhler started a postdoctoral fellowship in Milstein's laboratory in Cambridge, and the two undertook to immortalize antibody-forming cells by fusing them with myelomas, in order to study the genetic basis of antibody diversity. It was hoped that the tumor cell would endow the otherwise short-lived antibody-forming cell with the capacity for long-term survival in the resulting hybrid (called a hybridoma). The key to success in this venture was the development of a selective technique to recover only fused cells, employing a mutant myeloma cell line deficient in the enzyme hypoxanthine phosphoribosyltransferase. Without this enzyme, the cells would die in a medium containing hypoxanthine, aminopterine, and thymidine (HAT), but the hybrid cells would survive and could be selected, since the normal antibody-forming cell component of the hybrid would contribute the enzyme required. Isolation of a hybridoma clone would thus yield large quantities of monoclonal antibodies specific for a single antigenic determinant. The availability of such pure reagents has provided one of the most powerful tools of the current revolution in molecular biology and has opened up new avenues of investigation in many basic and clinical sciences.

Niels Jerne's contributions to immunology are almost too numerous to record, and his influence on the field impossible to exaggerate. While still a student, Jerne made important observations on the avidity of antibodies and on the changing quality of antibodies in response to successive booster immunizations. In 1963 Jerne and Albert Nordin described the hemolytic plaque assay method for enumerating antibody-forming cells, a technique that would receive broad application in studies of the cellular events underlying the antibody response. But it was Jerne's theoretical contributions that helped to bring immunology and immunologists to their current important position in the biomedical sciences. In 1955 Jerne was the first modern scientist to challenge the then-current instructive theories of antibody formation, by proposing a selective theory in which antigen functions to *select* specifically from a *preexisting* repertoire of antibody-forming capabilities. While the particulars of Jerne's hypothesis might require correction, his theory served as the critical stimulus to Macfarlane Burnet's clonal selection theory of antibody formation. In 1971 Jerne made another conceptual leap to explain the development of the repertoire of T cell specificities. He postulated that the principal driving force stimulating lymphocytes to divide and mutate at a high rate in the thymus is the individual's major histocompatibility complex antigens. Once again, a Jerne formulation served as an important stimulus to experimental and conceptual progress in the field. The third and perhaps the most profound of Jerne's theories was his idiotype network theory of 1974. Jacques Oudin, Henry Kunkel, and Philip Gell had previously shown that the antibody-combining site possesses unique antigenic determinants (idiotypes). Jerne's proposal was that the balanced production of a cascading network of idiotypes and anti-idiotypes might constitute one of the principal regulatory mechanisms governing the immune response. This theory, eminently testable, has profound implications for the physiology of the immune system and for its regulation of such pathological states as autoimmunity.

1987. To **SUSUMU TONEGAWA** [1939–   ], for his work on the molecular biology of immunoglobulin genes, demonstrating how antibody diversity is generated. It had always been difficult to believe that all of the genes required to generate the remarkable diversity of antibodies could be present in the germ line; thus, most investigators favored a somatic mutation theory acting upon only a very limited number of germ-line genes. In 1965, Dreyer and Bennett proposed that less DNA might be required if multiple variable region genes could combine with a single constant region gene for a given isotype (the two gene-one polypeptide theory). This speculation was confirmed in 1976 by Tonegawa and Hozumi, by showing that C region and V region genes were separate in embryonic DNA. Tonegawa, Gilbert, and Maxam then showed that combination of these two genes in differentiated cells still involves their separation by a noncoding DNA sequence (an "intron"). It was further found by Tonegawa, and also by Philip Leder and his colleagues, that the variable region polypeptide chain contains more amino acids than is encoded in the V region DNA of the light chain, a result suggesting that yet another DNA segment might be needed to encode the complete variable region. Tonegawa and his colleagues soon located the missing DNA segment, which was designated J (for joining). Thus, the combination of a single constant region segment with one of several J segments and one of many V region segments would suffice to generate a wide range of different light chains. In studying the assembly of the genes for the heavy chains of antibody, it was found by both Tonegawa and Leroy Hood that now three separate DNA segments must be joined to complete the sequence for the heavy chain variable region. In addition to the V and J segments, a third group of DNA segments termed D (for diversity) was involved. In addition to the ability to choose among multiple V, D, and J elements, additional variability is introduced into the heavy chain by permitting splicing in the middle of a triplet codon, an insertion resulting in a translation shift. The demonstration by Hood and others that mutations in these gene segments could also occur appeared finally to complete the picture of how the immense repertoire of antibody specificities is generated. Tonegawa's work, and that of others, has had important implications in other areas, including the structure and formation of T cell receptors and the DNA rearrangements that might be responsible for lymphomas and leukemias.

Appendix C

BIOGRAPHICAL DICTIONARY

This list has been restricted to those who contributed significantly to the development of immunology prior to the early 1960s.

AKROYD, John Fletcher   MB, Bristol, 1938; D.Sc., London, 1956. Worked at St. Mary's Hosp., London. Described autoimmune thrombocytopenic (Sedormid) purpura. Book: *Symposium on Immunological Methods.* London, 1964.

ARRHENIUS, Svante   [1859–1927]. Born at Vik (Uppsala). Studied physics at Uppsala. Director, Nobel Inst. Physical Chemistry, 1905. Theory of electrolyte dissociation; suggested reversibility of antigen–antibody complexes; coined the term "immunochemistry." Nobel prize for chemistry, 1903. Book: *Immunochemistry.* Macmillan, New York, 1907. Biogr.: E. H. Riesenfeld, *Svante Arrhenius.* Akad. Verlagsges., Leipzig, 1931; *Dict. Sci. Biogr.* **1,** 296 (1970). Obit.: *J. Chem. Soc.* **1,** 1380 (1928).

ARTHUS, Nicolas Maurice   [1862–1945]. Born at Angers. Taught physiology, Fribourg, 1895; Univ. Lausanne, 1907; Int. Pasteur, Lille, 1920; Univ. Marseilles. Studied physiological effects of venoms; discovered local anaphylactic reaction (Arthus phenomenon), 1903. Book: *De*

This biographical dictionary has been assembled with the generous assistance of Mrs. Dorothy Whitcomb and Terrence Fischer of the Health Sciences Library, University of Wisconsin, Madison.

l'Anaphylaxie à l'Immunité. Masson, Paris, 1921. Obit.: *Bull. Acad. Med. Paris* **129**, 374 (1945).

ASCHOFF, Ludwig [1866–1942]. Born at Berlin. Educated at Bonn, Berlin, and Strassburg. Prof. pathology, Freiburg. Developed concept of reticuloendothelial system. Book: *Ehrlichs Seitenkettentheorie* . . . Fischer, Jena, 1902. Obit.: *J. Pathol. Bacteriol.* **55**, 229 (1943).

ASKONAS, Birgitta A. [1923–]. Ph.D., Cambridge. Natl. Inst. Med. Research, 1953; Head, Immunology Division, 1976. Many contributions to mechanism of antibody formation, immunoregulation, viral immunology.

BAIL, Oscar [1869–1927]. Born at Tillisch, Germany. Studied medicine in Vienna. Prof. hygiene, German Univ. of Prague. Advanced theory of aggressins and early instructive theory of antibody formation. Obit.: *Z. Immunitaetsforsch.* **55**, i–iv (1928).

BEHRING, Emil Adolph von [1854–1917]. Born at Deutsch-Eylau. Studied medicine in Berlin. Entered Army Medical Corps; assistant in Koch's Institute, 1889; Prof. hygiene, Halle, 1894; Prof. Marburg from 1895. Established Behringwerke, commercial firm for production of antitoxins. Discovered diphtheria and tetanus antitoxins with Kitasato, 1890. Nobel prize, 1901; ennobled, 1901. Books: *Die Blutserumtherapie.* Thieme, Leipzig, 1902; *Gesammelte Abhandlungen.* Marcus & Webers, Bonn, 1915. Biogr.: H. Zeiss and R. Bieling, *Behring, Gestalt und Werk.* Schultz, Berlin, 1940; P. Schaaf, *Emil von Behring zum Gedächtnis . . .,* Marburg, 1942; *Dict. Sci. Biogr.* **1**, 574 (1970). Obit.: *Berl. Klin. Wochenschr.* **54**, 471 (1917).

BENACERRAF, Baruj [1920–]. Born at Caracas. Studied at New York, Virginia, and Paris (with Halpern). Prof. pathology, N.Y.U., 1958; Chief, Immunology Lab., N.I.H., 1968; Prof. pathology, Harvard, 1970. Numerous contributions, including carrier effect in delayed hypersensitivity; lymphocyte subsets; Ir genes and immunogenetics of MHC. Nobel prize, 1980. Book: *Textbook of Immunology* (with Unanue). Williams & Wilkins, Baltimore, Maryland, 1979.

BESREDKA, Alexandre [1870–1940]. Born at Odessa. M.D., Paris, 1897. Worked at Pasteur Institute under Metchnikoff. Studied anaphylaxis and anti-anaphylaxis; concept of local immunity. Books: *Anaphylaxie et Antianaphylaxie,* 1918; *Histoire d'une Idée: L'Oeuvre de Metchnikoff,* 1921; *Etudes sur l'Immunité dans les Maladies Infectieuses,* 1928. Obit.: *Rev. Pathol. Comp.* **40**, 112 (1940).

BILLINGHAM, Rupert Everett [1921–]. Born at Warminster, Wilts., England. Educated at Oxford. University College, London (with Medawar), 1951; Wistar Inst., Philadelphia, 1957; Chairman, Dept. Cell Biol., Univ. Texas, Dallas, 1971. Many contributions to transplantation biology; established (with Medawar and Brent) immunological tolerance; privileged sites for transplantation; maternal–fetal immunological relationships. Books: *Immunobiology of Transplantation*, 1971; *Immunobiology of Mammalian Reproduction*, 1976.

BORDET, Jules Jean Baptiste Vincent [1870–1961]. Born at Soignies, Belgium. Studied medicine, Univ. Brussels. Préparateur in Metchnikoff's laboratory, 1894–1901; founded Institut Pasteur of Brussels, 1901; Prof. bacteriology in Brussels, 1907. Discovered immune hemolysis, 1899; complement fixation with Gengou, 1901; disputed with Ehrlich about nature and mode of action of antibodies and complement. Nobel prize, 1919. Book: *Traité de l'Immunité dans les Maladies infectieuses*, 1920. Biogr.: P. De Kruif, "Men Against Death." Harcourt, Brace, New York, 1932; *Dict. Sci. Biogr.* **2,** 300 (1970); see "Volume Jubilaire de Jules Bordet," *Ann. Inst. Pasteur, Paris* **79** (1950). Obit.: *Ann. Inst. Pasteur, Paris* **101,** 1 (1961).

BOVET, Daniel [1907–]. Born at Neuchatel. D.Sc., Univ. Geneva, 1929. Worked at Inst. Pasteur, 1929; organized Lab. of Therapeutic Chemistry, Inst. Superiore de Sanitá, Rome, 1948. Studied pharmacology of nervous system, action of curare, therapy of allergies, and other topics. Nobel prize, 1957. Books: *Structure Chimique et Activité Pharmacodynamique des Médicaments du Système Nerveux Végetatif*, 1948; *Curare and Curare-Like Agents*, 1959.

BOYD, William Clouser [1903–1982]. Born at Dearborn, Missouri. Educated at Harvard and Boston Univ. Prof. immunochemistry, Boston Univ. Worked in blood groups; lectins; physical anthropology. Books: *Fundamentals of Immunology*, 1943; *Genetics and the Races of Man*, 1950; *Introduction to Immunochemical Specificity*, 1962.

BRAMBELL, Francis William Rogers [1901–1970]. Born at Sandy Cove, Ireland. Educated at Dublin and London. Prof. zoology, Bangor, Wales. Studied transfer of antibodies from mother to fetus. Books: *Development of Sex in Vertebrates*, 1930; *Antibodies and Embryos*, 1951. Biogr.: *Biogr. Mem. Fellows R. Soc.* **19,** 129 (1973). Obit.: *Nature (London)* **228,** 694 (1970).

BRENT, Leslie [1925–]. Born at Köslin, Germany. Ph.D., London, 1954. Worked with Medawar and Billingham, Univ. College,

London, 1954; Nat. Inst. Med. Res., 1962; Prof. zoology, Univ. Southampton, 1965; Prof. immunology, St. Mary's, 1969. Many contributions to transplantation biology; established immunological tolerance (with Medawar and Billingham); graft-vs-host disease; histocompatibility antigens; immunogenetics.

BRUCK, Carl [1879–1944]. Born at Glatz, Germany. Studied at Munich and Berlin. Breslau Univ., 1908; Director, Dept. Dermatology, Altona City Hosp. Worked in syphilology; developed complement fixation test for syphilis (with Wassermann and Neisser). Obit.: *Arch. Dermatol. Syphilol.* **73**, 426 (1950).

BRUTON, Ogden Carr [1908–   ]. Born at Mt. Gilead, N. Carolina. M.D., Vanderbilt Univ., 1933. U.S. Army pediatrician. Described first case of human agammaglobulinemia.

BUCHNER, Hans [1850–1902]. Born at Munich. Bacteriologist and immunologist. Educated in Munich and Leipzig. Military surgeon, ultimately Surgeon General. Prof. hygiene, Munich, 1894. Discovered complement and studied bactericidal action of normal serum; leading proponent of humoral theory of immunity. Obit.: *Muench. Med. Wochenschr.* **49**, 844 (1902).

BURNET, Frank Macfarlane [1899–1985]. Born at Traralgon, Victoria, Australia. M.D., Melbourne, 1923. Director, Walter and Eliza Hall Inst., 1944. Important contributions to virology; theoretical immunology; clonal selection theory of antibody formation; immunological tolerance. Nobel prize, 1960. Books: *Production of Antibodies* (with Fenner), 1949; *Natural History of Infectious Diseases*, 1953; *Clonal Selection Theory of Antibody Formation*, 1959; *Autoimmune Diseases* (with Mackay), 1963; *Cellular Immunology*, 1969. Autobiogr.: *Changing Patterns*, 1969. Obit.: *Nature (London)* **317**, 108 (1985).

BUSSARD, Alain [1917–   ]. Born at Paris. Director, Cellular Immunology Lab., Inst. Pasteur, Paris. Many contributions to immunological tolerance; molecular immunology; nature of antigenicity. Books: *La Tolérance Acquise et la Tolérance Naturelle à l'Egard de Substances Antigèniques Définies.* CNRS, Paris, 1963; *Antigènicité.* Flammarion, Paris, 1963.

CALMETTE, Albert [1863–1933]. Born at Nice. Educated at Clermont-Ferrand and Paris. Surgeon in naval and colonial service. Founded Institut Pasteur in Saigon. Subdirector, Institut Pasteur, Paris. With Guérin, discovered BCG, and worked on snake venoms and plague serum. Biogr.: Noel Bernard, *La Vie et l'Oeuvre d'Albert Calmette.* Paris, 1961. Obit.: *Ann. Inst. Pasteur, Paris* **51**, 559 (1933).

CAMPBELL, Dan H. [1907–1974]. Born at Fremont, Ohio. Ph.D., Univ. Chicago, 1935. Worked at Cal. Inst. Technol. with Pauling. Many contributions to immunochemistry and antibody specificity; studied persistence of antigen. Book: *Methods in Immunology*, 1963. Obit.: *Immunochemistry* **12**, 439 (1975).

CANTACUZENE, Jean [1863–1934]. Born at Bucharest. M.D., Paris, 1894. Student of Metchnikoff at Pasteur Inst.; Prof. exper. med., Bucharest, 1902. Worked on role of phagocytes in immunity. Biogr.: *Homage à la Mémoire du Prof. Cantacuzène*. Paris, 1934. Obit.: *Bull. Acad. Med. Paris* **111**, 884 (1934).

CHASE, Merrill [1905–]. Born at Providence, Rhode Island. Ph.D., Brown Univ. Assistant to Landsteiner and then Prof., Rockefeller Inst., 1965. Many contributions to delayed hypersensitivity and contact dermatitis; first passive transfer of tuberculin and contact hypersensitivity; mechanism of action of adjuvants; quantitative methods.

COCA, Arthur Fernandez [1875–1959]. Born at Philadelphia. M.D., Univ. Penn.; studied at Heidelberg. Cornell, 1910; Prof., Columbia, 1932; Lederle Labs., 1931–1948. Many contributions to allergy with Robert A. Cooke; classification of human allergies; named atopic antibodies; isolation and use of allergens. Books: *Essentials of Immunology for Medical Students*, 1925; *Asthma and Hay Fever in Theory and Practice* (with Walzer and Thommen), 1931. Founding editor, *J. Immunol.* 1916–1947. Obit.: *J. Am. Med. Assoc.* **172**, 835 (1959).

COHN, Ferdinand Julius [1828–1898]. Born at Breslau. Educated at Breslau and Berlin. Prof. botany, Breslau. Leading botanist; argued for constancy of bacterial species; supported Pasteur against spontaneous generation; "discovered" Koch. Biogr.: Pauline Cohn, *Blätter der Erinnerung*. Breslau, 1901; *Dict. Sci. Biogr.* **3**, 336 (1971). Obit.: *Muench. Med. Wochenschr.* **45**, 1005 (1898).

COHNHEIM, Julius [1839–1884]. Born at Demmin, Pomerania. Prof. in Kiel, 1868; Breslau, 1872; Leipzig, 1878. Eminent pathologist; proposed vascular theory of inflammation. Book: *Lectures on General Pathology*. New Sydenham Soc., London, 1889. Obit.: *Gesammelte Abh., Berlin* pp. vii–li (1885).

COOKE, Robert Anderson [1880–1960]. Born at Holmdel, New Jersey. M.D., Columbia, 1904. Prof. allergy and immunology, Cornell, 1920. Classification of human allergies; developed skin test and desensitization methods; helped found allergy societies. Obit.: *Ann. Allergy* **21**, 107 (1963).

COOMBS, Robin Royston Amos [1921–]. Ph.D., Cambridge. 1947. Prof. pathology, Cambridge Univ. Developed Coombs test for autoimmune hemolytic anemia; many contributions to immunohematology, immunopathology, and serology. Books: *The Serology of Conglutination and Its Relation to Disease,* 1961; *Clinical Aspects of Immunology* (with Gell), 1963.

COONS, Albert Hewett [1912–1978]. Born at Gloversville, New York. M.D., Harvard, 1937. Prof. Harvard Univ. Developed fluorescent antibody immunohistochemistry. Lasker medal, 1959; Ehrlich prize, 1961; Behring prize, 1966. Obit.: *J. Histochem. Cytochem.* **27,** 1117 (1979). See also *Ann. N.Y. Acad. Sci.* **420,** 6 (1983).

DALE, Henry Hallett [1875–1968]. Born at London. M.D., 1909; studied with Starling and Ehrlich. Natl. Inst. Med. Res., 1914–1942; Prof. chemistry, Davy-Faraday Lab., 1942. Discovered histamine; Schultz–Dale test for anaphylaxis; important contributions to chemical transmission of nerve impulses. Nobel prize, 1935. Biogr.: See *Ciba Foundation Symposium on Histamine: Festschrift in Honour of Sir Henry Dale,* Boston, 1956; *Dict. Sci. Biogr.* **15,** 104 (1978). Obit.: *Br. Med. J.* **iii,** 318 (1968).

DAMESHEK, William [1900–1969]. Born at Voronezh, Russia. M.D., Harvard, 1923. Prof. hematology, Tufts Univ., Boston. Leading hematologist; described autoimmune hemolytic anemias; agranulocytosis. Editor-in-Chief of *Blood.* Biogr.: See issue in honor of Dameshek's 60th birthday. *Blood* **15,** May (1960). Obit.: *Blood* **35,** 1 (1970).

DANYSZ, Jan (Jean) [1860–1928]. Born in Poland. Worked at Institut Pasteur, Paris. Discovered Danysz phenomenon of neutralization of diphtheria toxin; discovered virus for destroying rodents; later worked on chemotherapy. Obit.: *Bull. Inst. Pasteur* **26,** 97 (1928).

DAUSSET, Jean Baptiste Gabriel [1916–]. Born at Toulouse. M.D., Paris. Director, Natl. Blood Transfusion Center, 1950; Director, Immunogenetics and Transplantation, Inst. Natl. Santé, 1968. Many contributions to immunogenetics and transplantation; major histocompatibility complex. Nobel prize, 1980. Books: *Immunohématologie, Biologique et Clinique,* 1956; *HLA and Disease* (with Sveljgaard), 1977.

DIENES, Louis Ladislaus [1885–1974]. Born at Tokay, Hungary, M.D., Budapest, 1908; studied in France and Germany. Director, von Ruck Research Lab. Tuberculosis, 1921; bacteriologist, Mass. General Hosp., 1930. Studied bacterial allergy; pleuropneumonia-like organisms; demonstrated production of tuberculin-type hypersensitivity to bland proteins. See Festschrift: *Symposium on Mycoplasma and L Forms of Bacteria, in Honor of Louis Dienes.* Gordon & Breach, New York, 1971. Obit.: *J. Infect. Dis.* **130**, 89 (1974).

DIXON, Frank James [1920–]. Born at St. Paul, Minnesota. M.D., Univ. Minn., 1944. Washington Univ., 1948; Univ. Pittsburgh, 1951; Director, Scripps Inst. Res. Foundation, La Jolla, 1974. Many contributions to antibody formation; immunopathology; pathogenesis of immune complex diseases.

DOERR, Robert [1871–1950]. Born at Tesco, Hungary. M.D., Vienna, 1897. Worked with Paltauf at Vienna Univ.; Director, Hygienic Inst. Basel, 1919. Worked on viral immunology, experimental anaphylaxis, and human allergies. Biogr.: See Festschrift on 70th birthday, *Schweiz. Z. Pathol. Bakteriol.* **4** (1941). Obit.: *Wien. Klin. Wochenschr.* **64**, 129 (1952).

DONATH, Julius [1870–1950]. M.D., Vienna, 1895; assistant to Nothnagel, 1898. Dept. Head, Vienna Merchants' Hospital, 1910–1938; Israelite Comm. Hospital, Vienna, 1938. Described (with Landsteiner) the first autoimmune disease, paroxysmal cold hemoglobinuria, 1904. Biogr.: See Speiser and Smekal's *Karl Landsteiner,* p. 126. Brüder Hollinek, Vienna, 1975.

DONIACH, Deborah [1912–]. M.B., London, 1945. Prof. clinical immunology, Middlesex Hosp. First demonstrated (with Roitt and others) autoantibodies in Hashimoto's disease; many contributions to study of autoimmune thyroid and liver diseases.

DOUGLAS, Stewart Ranken [1871–1936]. Born at Coulston Grange, Caterham. M.B., St. Barts, London; Indian Medical Service (Army); worked under Wright at St. Mary's, London. Director, Bacteriology Dept., Natl. Inst. Med. Res., London. Discovered and developed (with Wright) opsonins and related serotherapy. Obit.: *Lancet* **1**, 229 (1936).

DUCLAUX, Emile [1840–1904]. Born at Aurillac, France. Ecole Normale, Paris; préparateur under Pasteur. Prof. biological chemistry, Sorbonne; succeeded Pasteur as Director, Pasteur Inst. Assisted Pasteur in many immunological discoveries. Biogr.: *Dict. Sci. Biogr.* **4**, 210 (1971). Obit.: *Ann. Inst. Pasteur, Paris* **18**, 273, 337 (1904).

DUNGERN, Emil Freiherr von [1867–1961]. M.D., Munich, 1892; studied also in Freiburg and Pasteur Inst., Paris. Head, Biochem. Dept., Heidelberg Inst. Cancer Res. 1906; Director, Hamburg/Eppendorff

Cancer Inst., 1913. Discovered (with Hirszfeld) heredity of blood groups; defined fourth group as AB and Landsteiner's third group as O.

DURHAM, Herbert Edward   [1866–1945]. Born at London. Educated at Cambridge, Guy's Hospital; worked with von Gruber in Vienna. Discovered (with Gruber) bacterial agglutination; later worked on yellow fever and beriberi. Obit.: *Lancet* **ii,** 654 (1945).

EDELMAN, Gerald Maurice   [1929–   ]. Born at New York. M.D., Penn., Ph.D., Rockefeller Inst. with Kunkel, Prof. Rockefeller Inst., 1966. Immunoglobulin chains; domains; total amino acid sequence of Ig; role of cell adhesion molecules; neurobiology. Nobel prize, 1972.

EHRICH, William Ernst   [1900–1967]. Born at Dahmen, Germany. M.D., Rostock, 1924. Studied pathology at Rockefeller Inst, 1926; privatdozent Rostock, 1931; Univ. Penn., 1936. Worked on antibody formation; lymphoid tissue responses; renal diseases. Obit.: *Verh. Dtsch. Ges. Pathol.* **54,** 589 (1970).

EHRLICH, Paul   [1854–1915]. Born at Strehlen, Silesia. Educated at Breslau and Strassburg. Assistant in Frerich's Clinic, 1878; assistant in Koch's Inst., 1890; Director, Inst. für Serumprufung, Steglitz, 1896; Director, Inst. für exper. Therapie, Frankfurt am Main, 1899. Developed histological stains; many contributions to hematology; side-chain theory of antibody formation; developed assays for diphtheria toxin and antitoxin; mechanism of immune hemolysis; developed chemotherapeutic theory and practice; important early contributions to cancer research. Nobel prize, 1908. Books: *Collected Studies on Immunity,* 1906; *Collected Papers of Paul Ehrlich,* 3 vols., 1957. Biogr.: Martha Marquardt, *Paul Ehrlich als Mensch und Arbeiter.* Berlin, 1924; *Dict. Sci. Biogr.* **4,** 295 (1971); (and many others). Obit.: See centenary tribute, *Bull. N.Y. Acad. Med.* **30,** 968 (1954).

EISEN, Herman Nathaniel   [1918–   ]. Born at New York. M.D., N.Y. Univ. Columbia Univ. P & S, 1944; Prof. Washington Univ., 1955; Prof. MIT, 1973. Developed equilibrium dialysis (with Karush); many contributions to mechanism of contact dermatitis; antigen recognition; antibody structure and function; cytotoxic T cells.

ELSCHNIG, Anton Phillip   [1863–1939]. M.D., Graz. Univ. Vienna, 1895; Prof. Ophthalmology, German Univ. Prague, 1907. Advanced theory of autoimmune pathogenesis of sympathetic ophthalmia; one of leading ophthalmologists of his day. Obit.: *Am. J. Ophthalmol.* **23,** 214 (1940).

FAGRAEUS-WALLBOM, Astrid Elsa [1913–]. Ph.D., Stockholm, 1948. Chief, Virus Dept., Natl. Bacteriol. Lab., 1962; Prof. Immunology, Karolinska Inst., 1965. First clear demonstration (in her doctoral thesis) that antibodies are produced in plasma cells; worked in clinical immunology; cell membrane antigens. Book: *Antibody Production in Relation to the Development of Plasma Cells.* Stockholm, 1948.

FENNER, Frank John [1914–]. Born at Ballaret, Australia. Studied at Adelaide Univ. and Hall Inst. with Burnet. Director, John Curtin School Med. Res., 1967; Director, Center for Resource and Environmental Systems, 1973. Worked in virology; host–parasite interactions. Book: *The Production of Antibodies*, 2nd Ed. (with Burnet). Melbourne, 1949.

FORSSMAN, Magnus John Karl August [1868–1947]. Born at Kalmar, Sweden. Educated at Lund and Stockholm. Prof., Lund. Discovered heterophile antigen (named Forssman antigen). Monographs: Die heterogenetischen Antigene, besonders die sog. Forssman Antigene und ihre Antikörper. *In* Kolle and Wassermann's *Handbuch der pathogenen Mikroorganismen*, Vol. 3, pp. 469–526, 1928; "Heterogenetic Antigens and Antibodies," *Acta Pathol. Microbiol. Scand., Suppl.* No. 16. Obit.: *Acta Pathol. Microbiol. Scand.* **25,** 513 (1948).

FRACASTORO, Girolamo [1478–1553]. Born at Verona. Studied at Padova. Physician, astronomer, geographer, poet, and humanist. Advanced theory of contagion; early theory of acquired immunity; gave syphilis its name. Books: *Syphilis sive Morbus Gallicus*, 1530; *De Sympathia et Antipathia Rerum* and *De Contagione*, 1546. Biogr.: *Dict. Sci. Biogr.* **5,** 104 (1972). See also *Ann. Med. Hist.* **1,** 1 (1917).

FREUND, Jules [1890–1960]. Born at Budapest. M.D., Budapest, 1913. Prof. Preventive Med., Budapest, 1917; Henry Phipps Inst., Penn., 1926; Cornell, 1932; Bureau of Labs., N.Y., 1938; NIH, 1957. Studied allergic encephalomyelitis; antibody formation; developed Freund's adjuvant. Lasker award, 1959. Obit.: *Lancet* **1,** 1031 (1960).

FRIEDBERGER, Ernst [1875–1932]. Born at Giessen. Educated in Berlin, Giessen, Munich, and Würzburg. Taught at Univ. Königsberg, 1903; Berlin Univ., 1913; Director, Prussian Res. Inst. for Hygiene and Immunology, 1926. Many contributions to allergy research. Obit.: *Z. Immunitaetsforsch.* **73,** i (1932).

GAFFKY, Georg Theodore August [1850–1918]. Born at Hanover. Educated in Army Medical Dept., Berlin; assistant to Koch. Prof.

Hygiene, Giessen, 1888; Head, German Plague Comm., India, 1897; Director, Inst. für Infektionskrankheiten, Berlin. First to cultivate typhoid bacillus; fought Pasteur about anthrax (with Koch). Biogr.: *Dict. Sci. Biogr.* **5**, 219 (1972). Obit.: *Berl. Klin. Wochenschr.* **55**, 1062 (1918).

GAY, Frederick Parker [1874–1939]. Born at Boston. M.D., Johns Hopkins; worked under Bordet in Paris. Prof. bacteriology, Columbia Univ., 1923. Studied immune hemolysis and anaphylaxis; translated and popularized Bordet. Book: *Agents of Disease and Host Resistance*. London, 1935. Obit.: *Science* **90**, 290 (1939).

GELL, Philip George Houthem [1914–]. M.B., Cambridge, 1940. Prof. exper. pathology, Birmingham. Studied histopathology and specificity of delayed hypersensitivity; described carrier effect (with Benacerraf); codiscoverer of idiotypy; viral immunology. Book: *Clinical Aspects of Immunology* (with Coombs), 1962.

GENGOU, Octave [1875–1959]. Worked with Bordet in Paris. Studied immune hemolysis; discovered (with Bordet) complement fixation test. Obit.: *Mem. Acad. R. Belg.* **7**, 79 (1969).

GLICK, Bruce [1927–]. Born at Pittsburgh. Ph.D., Ohio State, 1955. Prof., Mississippi State Univ. Discovered role of thymus in antibody formation (while a graduate student).

GOOD, Robert Alan [1922–]. Born at Crosby, Minnesota. M.D., Univ. Minnesota. Prof. microbiology and pediatrics, Minnesota; Director of Research, Sloan-Kettering Inst., NY, 1973; Prof., Univ. Oklahoma, 1982; Chairman, Pediatrics, Univ. S. Florida, 1985. Studied ontogeny and phylogeny of immune response; role of thymus and bursa of Fabricius; clinical and experimental immunodeficiency diseases. Books: *The Thymus in Immunobiology*, 1964; *Phylogeny of Immunity*, 1966; edited many others.

GORER, Peter Alfred [1907–1961]. Born at London. M.D., Guy's Hosp., 1932; studied with J.B.S. Haldane, Univ. College, London. Prof. pathology, Guy's Hospital. Important contributions to transplantation genetics; discovered antigen II associated with tumor rejection; identified (with Snell) the mouse H2 complex. Biogr.: See P. B. Medawar and T. Lehner, eds., *The Gorer Symposium*. Blackwell, Oxford, 1985. Obit.: *Biogr. Mem. Fellows R. Soc.* **7**, 95 (1961); *Lancet* **ii**, 1120 (1961).

GOWANS, James [1924–]. Born at Sheffield, England. M.B., London, 1947; Ph.D., Oxford, 1953. Director, MRC Cell. Immunobiology Unit, Oxford, 1963; Secretary, Medical Research Council U.K.,

1977. Major contributions to knowledge of recirculation and function of lymphocytes.

GRABAR, Pierre   [1898–1986]. Born at Kiev. Educated at Strassburg and Paris. Chef de Service, Pasteur Inst., 1938; Director, Natl. Center for Scientific Research, Paris, 1961. Studied antigen–antibody reactions; developed immunoelectrophoresis (with Williams); "carrier" theory of antibody function. Book: *Analyse Immuno-électrophoretique* (with Burtin), 1960. Obit.: *Bull. Acad. Natl. Med. (Paris)* **170,** 635 (1986).

GRUBER, Max von   [1853–1927]. Born at Vienna. Educated at Univ. of Vienna. Prof., Graz, 1884; Vienna, 1887; Munich, 1902. Studied antigen–antibody reactions; serology; discovered bacterial agglutination (with Durham); fought with Ehrlich on nature of specificity and of antigen–antibody reaction. Biogr.: *Dict. Sci. Biogr.* **5,** 563 (1972). Obit.: *Wien. Klin. Wochenschr.* **40,** 1304 (1927).

HAFFKINE, Waldemar   [1860–1930]. Born at Odessa. Educated at Odessa Univ.; assistant in Pasteur Inst., Paris, 1888. Founded Government Research Lab. (now Haffkine Inst.) in Bombay. Developed and introduced prophylactic immunization for cholera and plague. Biogr.: *Dict. Sci. Biogr.* **6,** 11 (1972). Obit.: *Br. Med. J.* **ii,** 801 (1930).

HARRIS, Tzvee Nicholas   [1912–   ]. Born in Russia. M.D., Univ. Penn. Prof. pediatrics, Univ. Penn. Studied antibody formation; role of lymphocytes; transplantation biology.

HAŠEK, Milan   [1925–1985]. Born at Prague. Ph.D., Prague Univ., 1955. Chairman, Dept. exper. biol. genetics, (later an Inst. of Czech Academy of Sciences), 1961. Developed technique of chick embryo parabiosis; demonstrated immunological tolerance; many contributions to transplantation biology. Obit.: *Immunogenetics* **21,** 105 (1985).

HAUROWITZ, Felix   [1896–1988]. Born at Prague. Educated at German Univ., Prague. Worked on protein chemistry with Breinl at Prague; Univ. Istambul, 1939; Prof. biochemistry, Indiana Univ., 1958. Leading protein chemist; worked on hemoglobin chemistry; immunochemistry; proposed (with Breinl) instruction theory of antibody formation, 1930. Books: *Chemistry and Biology of Proteins.* Academic Press, New York, 1950; *Immunochemistry and the Biosynthesis of Antibodies.* Wiley (Interscience), New York, 1968.

HEIDELBERGER, Michael   [1888–   ]. Born at New York. Ph.D., Columbia Univ. and Federal Polytechnic Inst., Zurich. Rockefeller Inst, 1912; Columbia P & S, 1927; Rutgers Univ. Inst. of Microbiology, 1955;

N.Y. Univ., 1964. Isolation and immunochemistry of pneumococcal polysaccharides; quantitative immunochemistry. Lasker award; National Medal for Science; Behring award; Pasteur medal (Sweden); Légion d'Honneur. Autobiogr.: Reminiscences: A Pure Organic Chemist's Downward Path. *Annu. Rev. Microbiol.* **31,** 1 (1977); *Annu. Rev. Biochem.* **48,** 1 (1979); *Immunol. Rev.* **82,** 7 (1984); **83,** 5 (1985). Biogr.: *Hosp. Pract.* Oct., 214–230 (1983).

HEKTOEN, Ludvig [1863–1951]. Born at Westby, Wisconsin. Studied at Chicago, Uppsala, Prague, and Berlin. Prof. pathology, Univ. Chicago, 1901; Director, McCormick Inst. Infect. Diseases, Chicago. Studied immunochemistry of thyroid and other tissue proteins; mechanisms of immunity. Biogr.: *Dict. Sci. Biogr.* **6,** 232 (1972). Obit.: *Arch. Pathol.* **52,** 390 (1951).

HEREMANS, Joseph F. [1927–1975]. M.D., Louvain, 1952; Ph.D., 1960. Worked with Grabar, Kunkel, and Waldenstrom. Prof. internal med. and immunochemistry, Louvain, 1965. Played a major role in isolation and characterization of IgA; studied secretory immune system. Book: *Molecular Biology of Human Proteins* (with Schultze), 1966. Obit.: *Eur. J. Immunol.* **6,** 1 (1976).

HERICOURT, Jules [1850–1933]. Worked with Richet on serotherapy of cancer; anaphylaxis. Book: *La Sérotherapie: Historique, Etat Actuelle.* Rueff, Paris, 1899.

HUMPHREY, John Herbert [1916–1987]. Born at W. Byfleet, England. Studied at Cambridge and Univ. College Medical School, London. Lister Inst. Preventive Med., 1941; Middlesex Hospital, 1942; Med. Res. Council, 1946; Natl. Inst. Med. Res., 1949; Prof. Royal Postgrad. School of Medicine, 1976. Numerous contributions to antibody formation, immunochemistry, immunopathology. Book: *Immunology for Students of Medicine* (with White), 1963.

JENNER, Edward [1749–1823]. Born at Berkeley, Gloucestershire. Apprenticed in surgery, 1762; studied under John Hunter, 1770; M.D., St. Andrew's, 1792. Practiced medicine privately; many studies in zoology and animal behavior; discovered application of cowpox (vaccinia) virus for preventive vaccination for smallpox. Books: *Inquiry into the Cause and Effects of the Variolae Vaccinae,* 1798; *On the Influence of Artificial Eruptions in Certain Diseases,* 1822. Biogr.: John Baron, *The Life of Edward Jenner,* 1827; William LeFanu, *Biobibliography of Edward Jenner.* Harvey & Blythe, London, 1951; *Dict. Sci. Biogr.* **7,** 95 (1973).

JERNE, Niels Kaj [1911–   ]. Born at London. Studied at Leiden and Copenhagen. Danish State Serum Inst., 1943; W.H.O., Geneva, 1956; Prof. pathology, Univ. Pittsburg, 1962; Goethe Univ., Frankfurt, 1966; Director, Basel Inst. for Immunology, 1969. Studied antibody formation and avidity; natural selection theory of antibody formation, 1955; hemolytic plaque assay for antibody, 1963; idiotype network theory, 1974. Nobel prize, 1984.

KABAT, Elvin Abraham [1914–   ]. Born at New York. Ph.D., Columbia P & S (with Heidelberger); studied with Tiselius at Uppsala. Instructor in pathology, Cornell, 1938; Prof. microbiology, Columbia, 1941. Separated globulins by electrophoresis (with Tiselius); demonstrated 7 S and 19 S γ globulins; studied anti-carbohydrate antibodies; size of antibody combining site; demonstrated (with Wu) hypervariable regions on Ig chains; proposed minigene hypothesis. Books: *Experimental Immunochemistry* (with Mayer), 1948; *Blood Group Substances: Their Chemistry and Immunochemistry*, 1956; *Structural Concepts in Immunology and Immunochemistry*, 1968. Autobiogr.: *Annu. Rev. Immunol.* **1,** 1 (1983). Biogr.: See Schlossman and Benacerraf, *Mol. Immunol.* **21,** 1009 (1984).

KAHN, Reuben Leon [1887–?]. Born at Swir (Kovno), Lithuania. Studied at Valparaiso; D.Sc., N.Y. Univ., 1916. Michigan Dept. Health, 1920; Prof. bacteriology, Univ. Michigan, 1928; Prof. serology, 1951; Prof. microbiology, Howard Univ., 1968. Many contributions to serology of syphilis; Kahn test. Biogr.: *J. Natl. Med. Assoc.* **63,** 388 (1971).

KALLOS, Paul [1902–   ]. Born at Budapest. M.D., Peso, 1929. Lab. Chief, Tuberculosis San., 1924; Research Assoc., Leipzig, 1929, Nürnburg, 1931, Uppsala, 1934; Director, Immunol. Res., Wenner-Gren Inst., Stockholm, 1937. Worked on allergy and tuberculosis. Edited many journals and publications on allergy.

KARUSH, Fred [1914–   ]. Born at Chicago. Ph.D., Chicago, 1938. Chemist, Dupont, 1944; Univ. Penn., 1950, Prof. immunochemistry, 1957. Studied protein interactions; thermodynamics of antigen–antibody interactions; developed (with Eisen) equilibrium dialysis; many contributions to molecular immunology.

KITASATO, Shibasaburo [1852–1931]. Born at Oguni, Kumamoto, Japan. Studied at Imperial Univ., Tokyo; with Koch at Koch's Inst., Berlin, 1885. Founded Inst. for Infectious Diseases (later Kitasato Inst.), Tokyo. Discovered (with Behring) tetanus antitoxin, 1890; discovered plague bacillus (independently of Yersin), 1894. Ennobled to rank of Baron. Biogr.: M. Miyajima, *Robert Koch and Shibasaburo Kitasato*.

Sonor, Geneva, 1931; *Dict. Sci. Biogr.* **7,** 391 (1973). Obit.: *J. Pathol. Bacteriol.* **34,** 597 (1931).

KOCH, Heinrich Hermann Robert   [1843–1910]. Born at Clausthal, Germany. M.D., Göttingen, 1866. Practiced medicine; Kreisphysikus, Wollstein, 1872; founded School of Bacteriology at Gesundheitsamt, Berlin; Director, Inst. für Infectionskrankheiten (Koch's Inst.), Berlin. Working alone as district physician, discovered tubercle bacillus, 1882; developed technique for pure culture of bacteria; discovered cholera vibrio; fought with Pasteur about anthrax; discovered tuberculin. Nobel prize, 1905. Biogr.: Bruno Heymann, *Robert Koch.* Leipzig, 1932; *Dict. Sci. Biogr.* **7,** 420 (1973). Obit.: *Br. Med. J.* **1,** 1386 (1910).

KRAUS, Rudolph   [1868–1932]. Born at Jungbunzlau, Bohmen. M.D., German Univ., Prague, 1893. Assistant to Paltauf in Vienna; Director, Bacteriologic Inst., Buenos Aires; State Serum Inst., São Paulo; State Serotherapeutic Inst., Vienna. Discovered precipitin reaction; edited (with Uhlenhuth and then Levaditi) *Handbuch der Immunitätsforschung und experimentelle Therapie,* 1907, 1914. Biogr.: *Wien. Med. Wochenschr.* **118,** 869 (1968). Obit.: *Z. Immunitaetsforsch.* **76,** i (1932).

KUNKEL, Henry George   [1916–1983]. Born at New York. M.D., Johns Hopkins, 1942. Prof. medicine, Rockefeller Inst. Many contributions to basic and clinical immunology, including myeloma proteins as immunoglobulins; structure and genetics of Ig; human allotypy; discovered idiotypy (independently of Oudin and Gell); rheumatoid facor as autoantibody; discovered IgA. Lasker award; Gairdner award. Obit.: *J. Exp. Med.* **161,** 869 (1985).

LANDSTEINER, Karl   [1868–1943]. Born at Vienna. M.D., Vienna; assistant to Gruber. Worked in pathological anatomy and experimental pathology, Vienna; Ziekenhuis, The Hague, 1919; Prof., Rockefeller Inst., 1922. Discovered ABO and other blood groups; discovered Rh factor; argued nature and origin of antibodies with Ehrlich; demonstrated poliomyelitis infection in monkeys; perfected the use of artificial haptens for the study of antibody specificity. Nobel prize, 1930. Book: *Die Spezifizität der serologischen Reaktionen,* 1933 [English editions: 1936, 1945]. Biogr.: P. Speiser and F. G. Smekal, *Karl Landsteiner.* Vienna, 1975; *Dict. Sci. Biogr.* **7,** 622 (1973). Obit.: *J. Immunol.* **48,** 1 (1944).

LAWRENCE, Henry Sherwood   [1916–]. Born at New York. M.D., New York Univ., 1943. Head, Infectious Dis. and Immunology Unit, N.Y. Univ., 1959; Prof. medicine, 1961. Discovered transfer factor; studied contact dermatitis and delayed hypersensitivity. Book: *Cellular and Humoral Aspects of Delayed Hypersensitivity States,* 1959.

LEDERBERG, Joshua [1925–]. Born at Montclair, New Jersey, Ph.D., Yale (with Tatum), 1947. Univ. Wisconsin, 1947; Stanford Univ., 1954; President, Rockefeller Univ. Showed sexual reproduction in bacteria (with Tatum); demonstrated transduction of genetic material in bacteria; contributed to formulation of clonal selection theory of antibody formation. Nobel prize, 1958.

LEPOW, Irwin Howard [1923–1984]. Born at New York. Ph.D., Case Western Reserve, 1951; M.D., 1958; studied with Pillemer. Case Western Reserve, 1951; Chairman, pathology, Univ. Conn. 1967; President, Sterling Winthrop Res. Inst., 1978. Studied properdin; complement; mechanisms of immunological injury.

LEVADITI, Constantin [1874–1953]. Born in Romania. Educated in Paris. Pasteur Inst., Paris, 1901; Prof., 1924. Many contributions to syphilology and immunology; stain for *T. pallidum;* worked with Landsteiner on polio and scarlet fever; edited (with Kraus) *Handbuch der Immunitätsforschung und experimentelle Therapie,* 1914. Biogr.: *Dict. Sci. Biogr.* **8,** 273 (1973). Obit.: *Ann. Inst. Pasteur, Paris* **85,** 535 (1953).

LEVINE, Philip [1900–]. Born at Kletsk, Russia. M.D., Cornell, 1923. Rockefeller Inst., 1925; Univ. Wisconsin, 1932; Beth Israel Hosp., Newark, 1935; Ortho Res. Foundation, 1944. Discovered (with Landsteiner) M. N, and P blood groups; many contributions to blood groups and immunohematology. See tribute to Dr. Philip Levine, *Am. J. Clin. Pathol.* **74,** 368 (1980).

LINDENMANN, Jean [1924–]. Born at Zagreb. Educated at Zürich. Univ. Florida, 1962; Zurich Univ., 1964. Discovered interferon (with Isaacs); advanced early network theory of idiotype–anti-idiotype; viral immunology; history of immunology.

MACKANESS, George Bellamy [1922–]. Born at Sydney. M.D., Univ. Sydney, 1945; Ph.D., Oxford, 1953. Austr. Natl. Univ., 1954; Univ. Adelaide, 1962; Director, Trudeau Inst., 1965; President, Squibb Inst. Med. Res., 1976. Studied role of macrophages in cellular immunity; tumor immunology.

MACKAY, Ian Reay [1922–]. M.D., Univ. Melbourne. Walter and Eliza Hall Inst., 1955; Chairman, Clinical Res. Unit. Work on autoimmune diseases; immunopathology; clinical immunology. Books: *Autoimmune Diseases* (with Burnet), 1963; *The Human Thymus,* 1969; *The Autoimmune Diseases* (with Rose), 1985.

MADSEN, Thorvald [1870–1957]. Born at Frederickberg, Denmark. Educated Copenhagen Univ., 1893; worked with Ehrlich in

Frankfurt and at Pasteur Inst., Paris. Director, Statens Serum Inst., Copenhagen, 1902; President, Hygienic Commission, League of Nations, 1921–1940. Studied diphtheria toxin–antitoxin interactions and assay; advanced (with Arrhenius) theory of reversibility of antigen–antibody binding. See *Liber Gratulorius in Honorem Thorvald Madsen.* Munksgaard, Copenhagen, 1930. Obit.: *Br. Med. J.* **1,** 1010 (1957).

MANWARING, Wilfred Hamilton [1871–1960]. Born at Ashland, Virginia. M.D., Hopkins, 1904; studied at Berlin, Frankfurt, and London. Asst. in pathology, Univ. Chicago, 1904; Univ. Indiana, 1905; Rockefeller Inst., 1910; Prof. bacteriology and exper. pathology, Stanford, 1913. Studied antibody formation; allergy; fought against Ehrlich's theories; attempted to revive antigen-incorporation theory of antibody formation.

MARQUARDT, Martha [1875–1956]. Long-time secretary to Ehrlich; helped to preserve Ehrlich papers; published biography *Paul Ehrlich als Mensch und Arbeiter,* 1924 [English editions: 1949, 1951]. Obit.: *Br. Med. J.* **ii,** 181, 307 (1956).

MARRACK, John Richardson [1899–1976]. M.B., Cambridge, 1912; M.D., 1923. Prof. chemical pathology, Cambridge, London Hospital; Univ. Texas, Houston (after retirement). Proposed bivalency of antibody; lattice theory of antigen–antibody complex formation; used colored dyes to label antibodies, 1934. Book: *The Chemistry of Antigens and Antibodies,* 1934. Obit.: *Lancet* **ii,** 378 (1976).

MASUGI, Matazo [1896–1947]. M.D., Univ. Tokyo, 1921; studied with Aschoff and Rössle in Germany. Prof. pathology, Chiba Med. College, 1927. Described relationship between monocyte and histiocyte; produced experimental immunogenic kidney disease (Masugi nephritis). Obit.: *Acta Pediatr. Jpn.* **68,** 587 (1964).

MATHE, Georges [1922–   ]. Born at Lermages, France. Educated Univ. Paris. Univ. Paris, 1952; Prof., Cancer Research, 1956; Head, Dept. Hematology, Gustav-Roussy, 1961; Director, Inst. Cancerologie et Immunogenetique, 1965. Many contributions to cancer immunology and immunotherapy; bone marrow transplantation.

MATHER, Cotton [1663–1728]. Born at Boston. M.A, Harvard, 1681. New England divine. Promoted inoculation against smallpox; advanced theory of acquired immunity, 1724. Book: *The Angel of Bethesda,* 1724. FRS. Biogr.: I. Bernard Cohen, *Cotton Mather and American Science and Medicine,* 2 vols. 1980.

MAYER, Manfred Martin [1916–1984]. Born at Frankfurt, Germany. Ph.D., Columbia, 1942. Assistant to Heidelberger, Columbia; Prof. immunology, Johns Hopkins, 1946. Isolated and characterized complement components; mechanism of complement action; discovered *T. pallidum* immobilization test for syphilis (with Nelson); lymphotoxins. Book: *Experimental Immunochemistry* (with Kabat), 1948. Obit.: *J. Immunol.* **134,** 655 (1985).

MEDAWAR, Peter Brian [1915–1987]. Born at Rio de Janeiro. Ph.D., Oxford, 1935. Lecturer zoology, Oxford, 1938; Prof. zoology, Univ. Birmingham, 1947; Prof., Univ. College London, 1951; Director, Med. Res. Council, 1962; Clin. Res. Ctr., Northwick Park, 1971. Founded modern transplantation immunobiology; proved immunological tolerance (with Billingham and Brent); developed anti-lymphocyte serum. Copley medal, Royal Soc.; Nobel prize, 1960. Books: *The Life Science* (with J. S. Medawar), 1977; *Advice to a Young Scientist,* 1979; *Aristotle to Zoos,* 1983 (and others). Autobiogr.: *Memoir of a Thinking Radish.* Oxford Univ. Press, London, 1986. Festschrift, 65th birthday. *Cell. Immunol.* **62,** 231 (1981). Obit.: *Lancet* Oct. 17, p. 923 (1987).

MELTZER, Samuel James [1851–1920]. Born at Ponovyezh, Russia. M.D., Univ. Berlin, 1882; worked with Welch at Bellevue. Head of physiology, Rockefeller Inst., 1904. Identified asthma as manifestation of anaphylaxis. Biogr.: *J. Allergy* **35,** 215 (1964); *Dict. Sci. Biogr.* **9,** 265 (1974). Obit.: *Proc. Soc. Exp. Biol. Med.* **18,** Suppl. (1921).

METALNIKOFF, Sergei [1870–1946]. Worked with Metchnikoff at Pasteur Inst., Paris; Prof. zoology, St. Petersburg; returned to France, 1919. Studied autoanti-sperm antibodies; neurological aspects of immune response. Book: *Role du Système Nerveuse et des Facteurs Biologiques et Psychiques dans l'Immunité.* Masson, Paris, 1934. Obit.: *Ann. Inst. Pasteur, Paris* **72,** 860 (1946).

METCHNIKOFF, Elie (Ilya) [1845–1916]. Born at Ivanovska, Ukraine. Ph.D., Univ. Odessa; studied with Siebold, Leukhart, and Kovalevsky. Prof. zoology, Univ. Odessa, 1867; Chef de Service, Pasteur Inst. Paris, 1888. Discovered defensive role of phagocytes; advanced phagocytic (cellular) theory of immunity; many contributions to bacteriology and immunology. Nobel prize, 1908. Books: *Leçons sur la Pathologie de l'Inflammation,* 1892; *L'Immunité dans les Maladies Infectieuses,* 1901; *Etudes sur la Nature Humaine,* 1903 (and others). Biogr.: Olga Metchnikoff, *Elie Metchnikoff: Life and Work,* English edition, 1921; *Dict. Sci. Biogr.* **9,** 331 (1974). Obit.: *Bull. Med. Paris* **30,** 385 (1916).

MIESCHER, Peter A. [1923–   ]. Born at Zürich. M.D., Lausanne and Zürich, 1948; D.Sc., Basel, 1950. Head, Immunopathology Res., Basel, 1954; Prof. medicine (hematology), 1960. Studied detection of antibodies to nucleoprotein; mechanisms of damage in immunological diseases; role of RE system. Books: *Immunpathologie in Klinik und Forschung* (with Vorlaender), 1957; *First International Symposium on Immunopathology* (with Grabar), 1958.

MILGROM, Felix [1919–   ]. Born at Rohatyn, Poland. M.D., Wroclaw, 1947. Director, Inst. Immunology Exper. Therapy, Polish Acad. Sci., 1954; Silesian Med. School, 1954., Prof. microbiology, SUNY, Buffalo, 1967. Studied serology of syphilis and rheumatoid arthritis; first proposed (with Dubiski) that rheumatoid factor is autoantibody.

MITCHISON, Nicholas Avrion [1928–   ]. Ph.D., Oxford, 1952. Lecturer zoology, Edinburgh; Natl. Inst. Med. Res., London; University College, London. Demonstrated passive cell transfer of transplant immunity; studied antibody response to defined haptens; proposed two-cell cooperation for antibody formation; discovered low-zone tolerance; tumor immunology.

MONTAGU, Lady Mary Wortley [1689–1762]. Born at London. Woman of Belles Lettres. Wife of British Ambassador to the Porte (Istanbul), 1718, where she observed Turkish practice of inoculation against smallpox. On return to England, helped to popularize the practice. Book: *Letters*, 1777. Biogr.: Robert Halsband, *The Life of Lady Mary Wortley Montagu*. Clarendon, Oxford, 1956.

MORGENROTH, Julius [1871–1924]. Born at Bamberg, Germany. Studied with Weigert in Frankfurt. Worked with Ehrlich in Steglitz and Frankfurt; Chemotherapeutic Dept., Koch's Inst., Berlin. Published (with Ehrlich) classical series of papers on immune hemolysis. Obit.: *Dtsch. Med. Wochenschr.* **51**, 159 (1925).

MORO, Ernst [1874–1951]. Born at Laibach. Studied at Graz; worked at the Kinderklinik with Escherich. Pediatrics at Munich 1906; Heidelberg, 1911; Director, Universitäts Kinderklinik. Developed percutaneous tuberculin test (Moro reaction). Biogr.: *Pediatrics* **29**, 643 (1962). Obit.: *Z. Kinderheilkd.* **70**, 323 (1952).

MOURANT, Arthur Ernest [1904–   ]. Born in Jersey. M.B., St. Bart's, London. Cambridge Univ., 1945; Blood Group Ref. Lab., 1946; Director, Serological Population Genetics Lab., 1965; St. Bart's, 1965. Developed Coombs test (with Coombs and Race); many contributions to blood group genetics and anthropology.

MUIR, Robert [1864–1959]. Born at Balfron, Scotland. M.D., Edinburgh, 1890. Head, Pathology Dept., Glasgow. Studied antibody formation; toxin–antitoxin reactions. Books: *Manual of Bacteriology* (with Ritchie), 1897; *Studies in Immunity*, 1909. Festschrift on 70th Birthday. *J. Pathol. Bacteriol.* **39**, 1 (1934). Obit.: *Biogr. Mem. R. Soc.* **5**, 149 (1959); *Br. Med. J.* **1**, 976 (1959).

NEISSER, Albert Ludwig Sigesmund [1855–1916]. Born at Schweidnitz, Germany. M.D., Breslau. Director, Dermatologic Inst., 1882. Studied leprosy; discovered gonococcus organism; devised (with Wasserman and Bruck) complement fixation test for syphilis; leading syphilologist. Biogr.: *Dict. Sci. Biogr.* **10**, 17 (1974). Obit.: *Br. Med. J.* **ii**, 410 (1916).

NISONOFF, Alfred [1923–]. Born at New York. Ph.D., Johns Hopkins, 1951. Head, Dept. Biochemistry, Univ. Illinois Coll. Med., 1969; Brandeis Univ., 1975. Studied enzymatic cleavage of antibody; biosynthesis and genetic control of Ig; idiotypy; properties of antibodies active in allergy. Book: *The Antibody Molecule* (with Hopper and Spring), 1975.

NOSSAL, Gustav Joseph Victor [1931–]. Born at Bad Ischl, Austria. M.B., Sydney, 1955; Ph.D., Melbourne, 1960; studied with Burnet and Lederberg. Director, Walter and Eliza Hall Inst., Melbourne. Major contributions to antibody formation; one cell-one antibody; isotype switching; immunological tolerance; cell–cell interactions. Books: *Antibodies and Immunity*, 1969; *Antigens, Lymphoid Cells, and the Immune Response* (with Ada), 1971.

NOWELL, Peter C. [1928–]. Born at Philadelphia. M.D., Univ. Penn. Head, Pathology Dept., Penn, 1967. Discovered role of phytohemagglutinin in stimulating division of lymphocytes; worked on bone marrow transplantation; discovered "Philadelphia chromosome" (with Hungerford).

NUTTALL, George Henry Falkiner [1862–1937]. Born at San Francisco. Educated in U.S., France, Germany, and Switzerland. Lecturer bacteriology, Cambridge Univ., 1900; Quick Prof. biology, 1906; founded Molteno Inst. of Biology and Parasitology, 1921. First to describe natural bactericidal action of blood; major studies in application of serology to forensics and evolution; studied arthropod-borne diseases; founded *J. Hyg.* (1901); *J. Parasitol.* (1908). Book: *Blood Immunity and Blood Relationships*, 1904. Obit.: *J. Pathol. Bacteriol.* **46**, 389 (1938).

OBERMAYER, Friedrich [1861–1925]. Born at Vienna. M.D., Univ. Vienna. Worked at Inst. Medicinal Chemistry. First demonstrated the nature of antibody response to chemically treated proteins (with Pick), leading to future studies of hapten–antihapten interactions and valuable specificity data. Obit.: *Wien. Klin. Wochenschr.* **38**, 542 (1925).

OSTROMUISLENSKY, Ivan Ivanovich [1880–1939]. Born at Moscow. Ph.D., Zürich, 1902; M.D., 1906. Asst. Prof. chemistry, Moscow; Prof., Nizhny Novgorod; private res. lab., 1911; Scientific Inst., Moscow, 1916; U.S. Rubber Co., 1922; Ardol Rossium Labs., 1932. Proposed instruction theory of antibody formation, 1915; claimed *in vitro* synthesis of antibody.

OUCHTERLONY, Örjan Thomas Gunnersson [1914–   ]. Studied at Karolinska Inst. Prof. bacteriology, Univ. Götheburg. Developed technique of two-dimensional double diffusion analysis of antigens and antibodies in gels. Book: *Handbook of Immunodiffusion and Immunoelectrophoresis,* 1968.

OUDIN, Jacques [1908–1986]. Director, Analytical Immunology Dept., Pasteur Inst., Paris. Developed agar single diffusion technique for antigen–antibody reactions, 1946; independently discovered idiotypy (with Michel), 1963.

OWEN, Ray David [1915–   ]. Born at Genesee, Wisconsin. Ph.D., Wisconsin, 1941. Univ. Wisconsin, 1940; California Inst. Technol., 1947. Worked in immunogenetics, tissue transplantation, serology; discovered erythrocyte mosaicism of cattle chimeras, leading to Burnet's concept of tolerance.

PAPPENHEIMER, Alwin Max Jr. [1908–   ]. Born at Cedarhurst, New York. Ph.D., Harvard, 1932; studied with Dale. Faculty, Univ. Penn., 1939; Prof., New York Univ., 1941; Harvard, 1958. Studied diphtheria toxin–antitoxin reactions; antibody formation; devised (with Uhr and Salvin) method for delayed hypersensitivity to simple proteins. Book: *Nature and Significance of the Antibody Response,* 1953. Biogr.: *Cell. Immunol.* **66**, 1 (1982).

PASTEUR, Louis [1822–1895]. Born at Dôle, France. Educated at Ecole Normale, Paris. Lycée Prof., Dijon, 1848; Prof. chemistry, Strassburg, 1852; Dean of Faculty, Lille, 1854; Sorbonne, 1867; founded Inst. Pasteur, 1888. Crystallized D- and L-tartaric acid; studied mechanism of fermentation and diseases of wine and beer; diseases of silkworms; experimentally disproved spontaneous generation; discovered attenuation of pathogens and their use in preventive immunization (fowl cholera, anthrax, rabies, swine erysipelas, etc.). FRS, Copley medal, Rumford medal, and many other awards. Books: *Les Maladies des Vers à Soie*, 1865; *Etudes sur le Vin*, 1866; *Etudes sur la Bière*, 1876; *Oeuvres*, 1922–1939. Biogr.: Valléry Radot, *La Vie de Pasteur*, 1900; René Dubos, *Louis Pasteur, Freelance of Science*, Little, Brown, Boston, Massachusetts, 1950; *Dict. Sci. Biogr.* **10,** 350 (1974), and many others. Obit.: *Nature (London)* **52,** 576 (1895).

PAULING, Linus [1901–]. Born at Portland, Oregon. Ph.D., Cal. Inst. Technol., 1925. Cal. Tech., 1927; Univ. California San Diego, 1967; Stanford Univ., 1969. Studied the chemical bond; structure of crystals and molecules; proposed instructive theory of antibody formation; structure of proteins and DNA; discovered (with Itano) molecular defect in hemoglobin S (sickling); studied (with Pressman) thermodynamics of antibody–hapten interactions; orthomolecular medicine. Nobel prize for chemistry, 1954; Nobel peace prize, 1963. Books: *The Nature of the Chemical Bond*, 1939; *No More War*, 1958.

PFEIFFER, Richard Friedrich Johannes [1858–1928]. Born at Zduny, Posen. Educated at Schweidnitz, Berlin. Military doctor at Koch's Inst., 1887; Prof. hygiene, Königsburg, 1899; Breslau, 1909. Discovered influenza bacillus; specific lysis of typhoid and cholera organisms (Pfeiffer phenomenon); developed immunization against typhoid fever; many other contributions to bacteriology and serology. Obit.: *Zentralbl. Backteriol.* **1,** 106 (1928); *Muench. Med. Wochenschr.* **75,** 524 (1928).

PICK, Ernst Peter [1872–1960]. Born at Jaromer, Bohemia. M.D., Prague, 1896; worked with Obermayer. Prof., Vienna, 1924; Prof. pharmacology, Columbia Univ., 1938. Studied experimental pathology; biochemistry of antigens; published extensive review of the chemistry of antigens (1912) that stimulated the study of hapten-coupled antigens. Biogr.: See "Festnummer gewidmet Ernst Peter Pick . . . ," *Wien. Klin. Wochenschr.* **64,** Nos. 35/36 (1952). Obit.: *Wien. Klin. Wochenschr.* **72,** 109 (1960).

PIRQUET von Cesenatico, Clemens Peter Freiherr von [1874–1929]. Born at Vienna. M.D., Vienna. Assistant to Escherich, Clinic for Children's Diseases; Prof. pediatrics, Johns Hopkins, 1908; Breslau, 1910; Director, Universitäts Kinderklinik, Vienna, 1911. Defined pathogenesis of serum sickness; introduced term "allergy"; introduced skin test for tuberculosis (Pirquet reaction); studied nutrition in children. Books: *Die Serumkrankheit* (with Schick), 1905; *Klinische Studien über Vakzination und Vakzinale Allergie*, 1907; *Allergy*, 1911. Biogr.: R. Wagner, *Clemens von Pirquet: His Life and Work*, 1968. See also *Ann. Allergy* **31,** 467 (1973); Obit.: *Am. J. Dis. Child.* **17,** 838 (1929).

PORTER, Rodney Robert [1917–1985]. Studied at Cambridge. Natl. Inst. Med. Res., Mill Hill, 1949; St. Mary's Hosp., 1960; Oxford, 1967. Split immunoglobulin with enzymes into Fab and Fc; proposed four-chain structure of Ab; studied order of complement genes in MHC, C4 polymorphism. Nobel prize, 1972; Royal Soc. Medal, 1973; many other awards. Book: *Defense and Recognition*, 1973. Obit.: *Nature (London)* **317**, 383 (1985).

PORTIER, Paul Jules [1866–1962]. Born at Bar-sur-Seine. M.D., Sorbonne, 1897. Physiologist; assistant to Richet. Asst. physiology, Sorbonne, 1901; Prof., Inst. Océanographique, Paris, 1906. Discovered anaphylaxis (with Richet), 1903. Biogr.: B. Masse, *Paul Jules Portier: sa Vie et son Oeuvre*, 1969; *Dict. Sci. Biogr.* **11**, 101 (1975). See also *J. Allergy Clin. Immunol.* **75**, 485 (1985). Obit.: *Bull. Acad. Natl. Med. (Paris)* **146**, 246 (1962).

PRAUSNITZ-GILES, Carl [1876–1963]. Born at Hamburg. M.D., Leipzig, Kiel, and Breslau, 1903. Asst. to Dunbar at State Inst. Hygiene, 1903; Royal Inst. Public Health, London, 1905; State Inst. Hygiene, Breslau, 1910; Dept. Bacteriology, Breslau, 1917; fled Germany, 1933; practiced medicine, Isle of Wight (as Giles). Worked on cholera; allergies; discovered (with Küstner) passive transfer of allergy with serum, 1921. Obit.: *Int. Arch. Allergy Appl. Immunol.* **23**, 281 (1963); *Lancet* **1**, 1058 (1963).

PRESSMAN, David P. [1916–1980]. Born at Detroit. Ph.D., California Inst. Technol.; studied with Pauling. Chief, Immunochemistry, Sloan-Kettering Inst. Cancer Res., N.Y., 1947; Roswell Park Inst., Buffalo, 1954; Assoc. Director, 1967. Studied antibody specificity; chemical nature of antibody combining site; first used radioactive antibodies for tumor localization to develop immunotoxins. Book: *The Structural Basis of Antibody Specificity* (with Grossberg), 1968. Obit.: (Issue dedicated to Pressman). *Transplant. Proc.* **12**, 366 (1980).

PUTNAM, Frank W. [1917–]. Born at New Britain, Connecticut. Ph.D., Univ. Minnesota, 1942. Duke Univ., 1942; Univ. Chicago, 1947; Univ. Florida, 1955; Indiana Univ., 1965. Studied structure of plasma proteins and enzymes; denaturation of proteins; protein synthesis; contributed importantly to structure of immunoglobulin.

RAFFEL, Sidney [1911–]. Born at Baltimore. D.Sc., 1933; M.D., Stanford, 1943. Prof. medical microbiology, Stanford, 1943. Studied immunology of tuberculosis; delayed hypersensitivity. Book: *Immunity*, 1953. Autobiogr.: *Annu. Rev. Microbiol.* **36**, 1 (1982).

RAMON, Gaston [1886–1963]. Born at Bellechaume, France. D.V.M., Alfort, 1911. Inst. Pasteur (Garches), 1911; Asst. Director, Inst. Pasteur, 1933; Head, Bureau Epizootic Diseases, Paris, 1949. Discovered flocculation assay for diphtheria toxin; produced anatoxins with formol and heat; studied adjuvant action of alum, etc.; many contributions to diphtheria toxin–antitoxin interactions. Autobiogr.: *Quarante Années de Recherches et de Travaux,* 1957. Biogr.: *Dict. Sci. Biogr.* **11,** 271 (1975). Obit.: *Bull. Acad. Natl. Med. (Paris)* **147,** 610 (1963).

RHAZES (Abu Bakr Muhammad ibn Zakariya) [ca. 865–932?]. Born at Rayy, Persia. Educated in medicine. Chief physician, Rayy, Baghdad. Held to be greatest physician of Islamic world; celebrated alchemist and philosopher; differentiated smallpox and measles; advanced theory of acquired immunity. Books: *Treatise on the Smallpox and Measles.* Sydenham Soc., London, 1848. Biogr.: *Dict. Sci. Biogr.* **11,** 323 (1975).

RICH, Arnold Rice [1893–1968]. Born at Birmingham, Alabama. M.D., Johns Hopkins, 1919. Dept. pathology, Johns Hopkins, 1919; Chairman, 1947. Leading authority on pathogenesis of tuberculosis, its immunity and hypersensitivity; demonstrated (with Lewis) migration inhibition by antigen, 1932. Gairdner Award, 1959; many other honors. Book: *The Pathogenesis of Tuberculosis,* 1944. Obit.: *Arch. Pathol.* **86,** 453 (1968).

RICHET, Charles Robert [1850–1935]. Born at Paris, M.D., 1869; D.Sc., 1878. Prof. physiology, Paris, 1887. Studied physiology of toxins; thermoregulation in animals; discovered anaphylaxis (with Portier). Nobel prize, 1913. Book: *L'anaphylaxie,* 1911. Autobiogr.: *Souvenirs d'un Physiologiste,* 1933. Obit.: *Bull. Acad. Natl. Med. (Paris)* **115,** 51 (1936).

ROITT, Ivan Maurice [1927–   ]. D.Sc., Oxford. Prof. and Head, Immunology and Rheumatology Research, Middlesex Hospital, London, 1953. Discovered (with Doniach) autoimmune nature of Hashimoto's disease; many contributions to thyroid and other autoimmune diseases. Books: *Essential Immunology,* 1971; *Immunology* (with Brostoff and Male), 1985.

RÖMER, Paul [1873–1937]. Born at Neundorf, Anhalt. Educated at Jena, Greifswald, and Halle. Worked at Ophthalmology Dept., Würzburg, 1902; Greifswald, 1907; Bonn, 1921. Many contributions to ocular anaphylaxis; advanced theory of autoimmune pathogenesis of sympathetic ophthalmia. Book: *Lehrbuch der Augenheilkunde,* Berlin, 1910. Biogr.: *Biogr. Lexikon* **7,** 1311 (1929).

ROSE, Noel Richard [1927–]. Born at Stamford, Conn. Ph.D., Penn., 1951; M.D., Buffalo, 1964. First produced (with Witebsky) experimental autoimmune thyroiditis; many contributions to pathogenesis of autoimmune diseases. Books: *Methods in Immunodiagnosis,* 1973; *Principles of Immunology,* 1973; *Manual of Clinical Immunology,* 1976; *The Autoimmune Diseases* (with Mackay), 1985.

ROSENAU, Milton Joseph [1869–1946]. Born at Philadelphia. M.D., Penn., 1889; studied at Hygienic Inst., Berlin; Inst. Pasteur, Paris. U.S. Marine Hospital Service, 1890; Prof. preventive med., Harvard, 1909; Director Div. Public Health, Univ. N. Carolina, 1936; Dean, 1939. Research in bacteriology and hygiene; leading early contributor to mechanism of anaphylaxis. Obit.: *J. Am. Med. Assoc.* **130,** 1185 (1946).

ROUX, Pierre Paul Emile [1853–1933]. Born at Confolens, France. M.D., Clermont-Ferrand and Paris. Préparateur to Pasteur, 1878; Chef de Service, Inst. Pasteur, 1885; Subdirector, 1893; Director, 1904. Worked with Pasteur on anthrax and rabies vaccinations; isolated diphtheria toxin; many contributions to diphtheria and tetanus immunity. Copley medal, 1913. Biogr.: Mary Cressac, *Le Dr. Roux, mon Oncle,* 1950; *Dict. Sci. Biogr.* **11,** 569 (1975). Obit.: *J. Pathol. Bacteriol.* **38,** 99 (1934).

ROWLEY, Donald Adams [1923–]. Born at Owatona, Minnesota. M.D., Univ. Chicago, 1950. NIH, 1951; Univ. Chicago, 1954; Director, La Rabida Children's Hosp., 1977. Studied regulation of immune response; enhancement and suppression by antigen and antibody.

SABIN, Albert Bruce [1906–]. Born at Bialystok, Russia. M.D., New York Univ. Res. Assoc., N.Y. Univ., 1926; Rockefeller Inst., 1935; Prof. pediatrics, 1939; President, Weizmann Inst., 1970; Univ. S. Carolina, 1974. Research on neurotropic viruses, oncogenic viruses; perfected oral polio vaccine; Lasker award, 1965; many other honors.

SACHS, Hans [1877–1945]. Born at Kattowitz, Silesia. Educated at Freiburg, Breslau, and Berlin. Worked with Ehrlich at Frankfurt; Director, Inst. für experimentelle Krebsforschung, Heidelberg, 1920. Numcrous contributions to immune hemolysis, complement research, and anti-tissue antibodies; long-time defender of Ehrlich's theories. Book: *Methoden in Hämolyseforschung* (with Klopstock), 1928. Biogr.: *Biogr. Lexikon* **7,** 1349 (1929). Obit.: *Nature (London)* **155,** 600 (1945).

SALK, Jonas [1914–]. Born at New York. M.D., New York Univ., 1939. Univ. Michigan, 1947; Univ. Pittsburgh, 1947; founding director, Salk Inst., La Jolla, 1963. Developed killed virus vaccine for polio. Lasker award, 1956; Koch medal, 1963.

SALVIN, Samuel Bernard [1915–]. Born at Boston. Ph.D., Harvard, 1941. Instructor, Harvard, 1941; Rocky Mountain Lab, NIAID, 1946; Ciba Corp., 1965; Univ. Pittsburgh, 1967. Studied antibody formation; delayed hypersensitivity; lymphokines; developed (with Uhr and Pappenheimer) method to induce delayed hypersensitivity to simple proteins.

SAMTER, Max [1908–]. Born at Berlin. M.D., Berlin, 1933. Univ. Illinois, 1946; senior consultant, Max Samter Inst. Allergy Clin. Immunol. Studied role of eosinophiles in allergy; drug reactions; bronchial asthma.

SCHICK, Bela [1877–1967]. Born at Boglar, Hungary. M.D., Graz. Univ. Vienna Children's Dept., 1902; Director Pediatrics, Mt. Sinai Hosp., New York, 1923. Defined serum sickness (with von Pirquet), 1905; developed Schick test for diphtheria, 1913. Book: *Die Serumkrankheit* (with Pirquet), 1905. Festschrift on 80th birthday, *in Current Problems in Allergy and Immunology*, 1959. Biogr.: *Ann. Allergy* **38**, 1 (1977). Obit.: *Ann. Allergy* **26**, 625 (1968).

SELA, Michael [1924–]. Born at Tomaszow, Poland. Ph.D., Hebrew Univ. and Univ. Geneva. Head, Dept. chem. immunology, Weizmann Inst., 1963; Dean, 1970; President, 1975. Introduced use of synthetic amino acid polymers for study of antibody formation and specificity; many contributions to immunochemistry; synthetic vaccines. Otto Warburg medal. Books: *Topics in Basic Immunology* (with Prywes), 1969; *The Antigens*, 1973.

SEVAG, Menasseh Giragos [1897–1967]. Born at Sis, Armenia. Ph.D., Columbia Univ., 1929. Inst. Robert Koch, 1932; research biochemist, Schering-Kahlbaum, 1935; Univ. Penn., 1936. Research in chemotherapy, bacterial physiology; advanced instruction theory of antibody formation involving immunocatalysis. Book: *Immunocatalysis*, 1945.

SHERMAN, William Bowen [1907–]. Born at Providence, Rhode Island. M.D., Columbia Univ., 1931. Columbia Univ., 1935; Director, Inst. Allergy, Roosevelt Hosp., New York, 1960. Many contributions to mechanisms, diagnosis, and treatment of allergic diseases.

SHULMAN, Sidney [1923–   ]. Born at Baltimore. Ph.D., Univ. Wisconsin, 1949. Prof. immunochemistry and biophysics, SUNY, Buffalo, 1958; Chairman Microbiology, N.Y. Med. Coll., 1968. Studied tissue proteins; autoantibodies; cryobiology; immunology of reproduction.

SHWARTZMAN, Gregory [1896–1965]. Born at Odessa. M.D., Brussels, 1920. Prof. microbiology, N.Y. Med. Coll., 1923; Head, Dept. Microbiology, Mt. Sinai Hosp., N.Y., 1926; Prof., Columbia, 1940. Research on bacterial growth; immunological reactions in tissue culture; local skin reactions to bacterial filtrates (Shwartzman reaction). Book: *Phenomenon of Local Tissue Reactivity and Its Immunological and Clinical Significance*. Hoeber, New York, 1937.

SIMONSEN, Morten [1921–   ]. M.D., Copenhagen. Copenhagen Univ., 1967; Head, Exper. Immunology Inst. Discovered graft-vs-host reaction on chorioallantoic membrane of chick embryo (Simonsen phenomenon); many contributions to transplantation biology, immunogenetics, and tolerance.

SMITH, Richard Thomas [1924–   ]. Born at Oklahoma City. M.D., Tulane, 1956. Univ. Texas, 1957; Univ. Florida, 1958. Many contributions to tolerance; immunopathology; delayed hypersensitivity; organized many symposia.

SMITH, Theobald [1859–1934]. Born at Albany, N.Y. M.D., Albany Med. Coll. Bureau of Animal Industry, U.S. Dept. Agriculture, 1884; Prof. comparative pathology, 1896; Rockefeller Inst., 1915. Isolated agent of Texas cattle fever and other animal diseases; first used dead bacteria to immunize; differentiated human and bovine tubercle bacilli; first reported anaphylaxis in guinea pigs (Theobald Smith phenomenon). Copley medal, 1933. Obit.: *J. Pathol. Bacteriol.* **40,** 621 (1935).

SNELL, George Davis [1903–   ]. Born at Bradford, Mass. D.Sc., Harvard, 1930. Washington Univ., 1933; Jackson Lab., 1936. Definitive work in mouse genetics; invented concept of congenic mice; defined (with Gorer) the H-2 locus; many other contributions to transplantation genetics. Gairdner award, 1976; Nobel prize, 1980. Book: *Histocompatibility* (with Dausset and Nathenson). Academic Press, New York, 1976.

STAVITZKY, Abram Benjamin [1919–   ]. Born at Newark, New Jersey. Ph.D., Univ. Minnesota, 1943; D.V.M., Univ. Penn., 1946. Prof. microbiology, Univ. Penn., 1947; Case Western Reserve, 1983. Studied mechanism of antibody formation; immunity in schistosomiasis.

ŠTERZL, Jaroslav [1925–]. Born at Pilsen. M.D., Charles Univ., Prague. Head, Immunology Dept., Czech Academy of Science Inst. of Microbiology. Many contributions to ontogeny of immune response; cellular reactions in antibody formation; germ-free animal research. Books: *Molecular and Cellular Basis of Antibody Formation*, 1965; *Developmental Aspects of Antibody Formation* (with Říha), 1969.

SULZBERGER, Marion Baldur [1895–1983]. Born at New York. M.D., Harvard; studied dermatology at Zürich and Breslau. Columbia Univ.; Head, Dermatology, Bellevue-N.Y. Univ. Leading investigator of contact allergies; arsphenamine sensitization; desensitization. Obit.: *J. Allergy Clin. Immunol.* **74,** 855 (1983).

SZILARD, Leo [1898–1964]. Born at Budapest. Ph.D., Berlin, 1922; studied physics in Berlin and England. Worked with Fermi in Chicago, 1937; Prof. biophysics, Univ. Chicago, 1946. Discovered nuclear chain reaction; wrote letter with Einstein to Roosevelt leading to American atom bomb project; proposed molecular-genetic theory of antibody formation, 1960. Atoms for Peace award, 1959. Biogr.: *Dict. Sci. Biogr.* **13,** 226 (1976). Obit.: *Biogr. Mem. Natl. Acad. Sci.* **40,** 337 (1969).

TALIAFERRO, William Hay [1895–1973]. Born at Portsmouth, Virginia. Ph.D., Johns Hopkins. Univ. Chicago, 1924. Long-time editor *J. Infect. Dis.* Studied effect of X rays on immune response; role of spleen; early worker on immunology of parasitic diseases. Obit.: *J. Infect. Dis.* **130,** 312 (1974).

TALMAGE, David Wilson [1919–]. Born at Kwangju, Korea. M.D., Washington Univ., 1944; worked with Taliaferro in Chicago. Univ. Pittsburgh, 1951; Prof., Univ. Chicago, 1952; Chairman Microbiology, 1963; Dean, 1968; Director, Webb-Waring Inst., Denver, 1973. Studied antibody formation; transplantation; tolerance to cultured allografts; proposed early selection theory of antibody formation, 1957; helped develop Burnet's clonal selection theory, 1959. Book: *The Chemistry of Immunity in Health and Disease* (with Cann), 1961.

THEILER, Max [1899–1972]. Born at Pretoria. Studied at Capetown, Univ. London. Harvard, 1922; Rockefeller Inst., 1930; Yale, 1964. Many contributions to virology; developed vaccine for yellow fever. Nobel prize, 1951. Biogr.: *Nobel Lect. Physiol. Med. 1942–1962,* p. 360. Elsevier, Amsterdam, 1964.

THORBECKE, G. Jeanette [1929–   ]. Born in the Netherlands, M.D., Groningen, 1950. Worked at Groningen, 1948; Leiden, 1956; New York Univ., 1957. Many contributions to antibody formation; role and reactions of lymphoid tissues; immunological tolerance.

TISELIUS, Arne Wilhelm Kaurin [1902–1971]. Born at Stockholm. Educated at Univ. Uppsala. Worked at Univ. Uppsala, 1935; Inst. Advanced Studies, Princeton, 1934; Swedish Natl. Res. Council, 1946; President, Nobel Foundation, 1960. Developed electrophoresis; identified (with Kabat) antibodies as γ globulins; developed synthetic blood plasmas. Nobel prize in chemistry, 1948. Biogr.: *Biogr. Mem. Fellows R. Soc.* **20,** 401 (1974); *Dict. Sci. Biogr.* **13,** 418 (1976); see also *Festschrift: Perspectives in the Biochemistry of Large Molecules,* dedicated to Arne Tiselius on his 60th birthday, 1962. Obit.: *J. Chromatogr.* **65,** 345 (1972).

TOPLEY, William Whiteman Carleton [1887–1944]. M.D., Cambridge, 1918. Taught at Manchester; pathology at St. Thomas' Hosp.; Charing Cross Hosp.; Prof. bacteriology and immunology, London School Tropical Med. Hygiene. Studied immunology of infectious diseases; argued (against Rich) for importance of hypersensitivity for immunity in tuberculosis. Books: *An Outline of Immunity,* 1933; *Principles of Bacteriology and Immunity* (with Wilson), 1936. Obit.: *Br. Med. J.* **1,** 201 (1944).

TURK, John Leslie. M.B., 1953; D.Sc., London, 1967. Worked at London School Hygiene and Tropical Med.; Medical Research Council; Prof. Pathology, Univ. London. Many contributions to delayed hypersensitivity. Books: *Delayed Hypersensitivity,* 1967; *Immunology in Clinical Medicine,* 1969.

UHLENHUTH, Paul Theodore [1870–1957]. Born at Hanover. Director, Bacteriology Dept., Reichsgesundheitsamt, 1906; Prof. Strassburg, 1911; Marburg, 1921. Worked on differentiation of proteins; discovered organ specificity of lens antigens; syphilis and other infectious diseases. Book: *Handbuch für Mikrobiologischen Technik* (with Kraus), 1923. Obit.: *Muench. Med. Wochenschr.* **107,** 1204 (1965).

UHR, Jonathan William [1927–   ]. Born at New York. M.D., New York Univ.; worked with Pappenheimer. Prof. medicine and microbiology, New York Univ.; Chairman, Microbiology, Univ. Texas, Dallas, 1969. Developed (with Salvin and Pappenheimer) method for inducing delayed hypersensitivity to simple proteins; role of antibody in immunoregulation; mechanism of immunoglobulin synthesis and secretion; immunotoxins.

VAN DER SCHEER, James [1888–?]. Born at Padang, Netherlands East Indies. Educated in chemistry, Delft. Rockefeller Inst., 1912; Dupont Corp, 1920; Lederle Labs., 1939. Worked on chemistry of haptens; specificity of antibodies; long-time associate of Landsteiner.

VAN ROOD, John J. [1926–]. Born near Leiden, Holland. Educated at Univ. Leiden. Practiced internal medicine; worked at Dept. Immunohematology and Blood Bank, Univ. Hosp. Many contributions to transplantation immunology and immunogenetics.

VAUGHAN, Victor Clarence [1851–1929]. Born at Mt. Airy, Missouri. M.D., Harvard, 1943. Director, Hygienic Lab., Prof. physiological chemistry, Univ. Michigan. Worked on immunity and allergy; role of cellular toxins. Books: *Ptomaines and Leukomaines* (with Novy), 1888; *Infection and Immunity*, 1915. Obit.: *J. Lab. Clin. Med.* **15,** 307 (1929).

VOISIN, Guy André [1920–]. Born at Paris. M.D., Univ. Paris, 1945; D.Sc., Sorbonne, 1958. Hôpital Saint-Antoine, 1955; Director of Research, Claude Bernard Assoc., 1964; Sci. Director, Immunopathology and Exper. Immunology, INSERM, 1970. First described autoimmune aspermatogenic orchitis, 1952; coined term "immunopathology," 1953; many contributions to autoimmunity, immunopathology, tolerance, immunology of reproduction.

WAKSMAN, Byron Halstead [1919–]. Born at New York. M.D., Univ. Pennsylvania, 1943. Dept. Neuropathology, Harvard, 1949; Bacteriology and Immunology, 1952; Chairman, Microbiology, Yale Univ., 1963; Prof. pathology, 1974; Vice President Res., Natl. Multiple Sclerosis Soc., 1980. Important contributions to histopathology of delayed hypersensitivity and autoimmunity; role of thymus; antileukocyte serum; immunologic tolerance; neuroimmunology. Book: *Atlas of Experimental Immunobiology and Immunopathology*. Yale University Press, New Haven, Connecticut, 1970.

WALDENSTRÖM, Jan Gosta [1906–]. Born at Stockholm. Educated at Uppsala, Cambridge, Munich. Prof. theoretical medicine, Uppsala, 1947; Malmö, 1950; Lund, 1952. Discovered Waldenstrom's macroglobulinemia; many other contributions. Gairdner award, 1966; Ehrlich medal, 1972.

WASSERMANN, August von [1866–1925]. Born at Bamberg, Germany. Studied at Strassburg, Vienna, and Berlin. Worked under Koch at Inst. Infectious Diseases, Berlin; Director Serum Dept.; Director, Inst. Exper. Therapy, Dahlem, 1913. Developed (with Bruck and Neisser) serological test for syphilis (Wassermann reaction). Book: *Handbuch der Pathogenen Mikroorganismen* (with Kolle), 1903. Ennobled, 1910. Biogr.: *Dict. Sci. Biogr.* **14,** 183 (1976). Obit.: *Int. J. Dermatol.* **16,** 526 (1977).

WEIGLE, William Oliver [1927–   ]. Born at Monaca, Pennsylvania. Ph.D., Univ. Pittsburgh, 1956; worked with Dixon. Univ. Pittsburgh, Dept. Pathology, 1955; member, Scripps Clinic Res. Foundation, La Jolla, 1961; Head, Div. Cellular Immunology, 1984. Many contributions to mechanisms of tolerance; autoimmune diseases; immunity and immunopathology.

WELLS, Harry Gideon [1875–1943]. Born at New Haven. M.D., Rush, Chicago, 1898; Ph.D., Univ. Chicago, 1903. Taught at Rush and Chicago. Studied chemical and general pathology. Books: *Chemical Pathology*, 5th Ed. 1925; *The Chemical Aspects of Immunity*. Chem. Catalog Co., New York, 1929. Obit.: *Arch. Pathol.* **36,** 331 (1943).

WHITE, Robert George [1917–1978]. Born at Barwell, England. M.D., Oxford, 1953. Univ. London; Harvard; Prof. and Chairman, Bacteriology and Immunology Dept., Glasgow. Studied cytology of antibody formation; role of germinal centers; described dendritic cells of germinal centers. Book: *Immunology for Students of Medicine* (with Humphrey), 1963.

WIDAL, Georges Fernand Isidore [1862–1929]. Born at Dellys, Algeria. M.D., Paris. Prof., Paris. Developed Widal serodiagnostic test for typhoid. Obit.: *Br. Med. J.* **1,** 134 (1929). See also *Med. Hist.* **7,** 56 (1963).

WIENER, Alexander [1906–1976]. Born at New York. M.D., State Univ. New York, 1930. Head, Blood Transfer Div., Jewish Hosp., 1932; Director, Wiener Labs., 1935; New York Univ., 1961. Discovered Rh factor (with Landsteiner), 1938; described blood groups of chimpanzees; disputed genetics and nomenclature of Rh system with Mollison. Lasker award, 1946. Biogr.: (Festschrift on 65th birthday). *Hematologia* **6,** 7 (1972). Obit.: *Arch. Allergy Appl. Immunol.* **54,** 191 (1977).

WITEBSKY, Ernest [1901–1969]. Born at Frankfurt. Educated at Frankfurt and Heidelberg; studied under Hans Sachs. Inst. für Krebsforschung, Frankfurt, 1929; Mount Sinai Hosp., New York, 1934; Univ. Buffalo, 1936. Worked in blood group serology; transfusion problems; classical demonstration of experimental autoimmune thyroiditis. Biobibliogr.: *First International Convocation on Immunology*. Karger, Basel, 1968.

WOLFF-EISNER, Alfred [1877–1948]. Born at Berlin. M.D., Tübingen, 1901. Worked in Königsberg; Univ. Polyklinik, Berlin. Long-time student of human allergies; first to interpret hay fever as an immunological process; developed ophthalmoreaction for tuberculosis. Books: *Das Heufieber*, 1906; *Handbuch der Serumtherapie und experimentelle Therapie*, 1910. Biogr.: *Ciba Found. Symp.* **11**, 1398 (1951).

WOODRUFF, Michael Francis Addison [1911–]. Born at London. M.D., Melbourne, 1941; D.Sc., 1962. Prof. Surgery, Univ. Otago, Dunedin; Univ. Edinburgh, 1957. Many contributions to transplantation. Lister medal; Royal Soc. medal. Book: *The Transplantation of Tissues and Organs,* 1960.

WRIGHT, Almroth Edward [1861–1947]. Born at Middleton in Teesdale, Yorkshire. M.D., Trinity Coll., Dublin, 1889. Prof. pathology, Army Med. School, Netley, 1892; Inst. Pathology, St. Mary's, London, 1902. Theory of opsonins (with Douglas); developed system of antityphoid inoculations. Books: *Pathology and Treatment of War Wounds*, 1942; *Researches in Clinical Physiology*, 1943; *Studies in Immunology*, 2 vols. 1944. Biogr.: *Br. Med. J.* **ii**, 516 (1961); *Dict. Sci. Biogr.* **15**, 511 (1976). Obit.: *Br. Med. J* **1**, 699 (1947); *Nature (London)* **159**, 731 (1947).

YALOW, Rosalyn Sussman [1921–]. Born at New York. Ph.D. in physics, Univ. Illinois. Hunter Coll., N.Y., 1946; Chief, Radioisotope Service, Veterans Hosp., N.Y., 1950; Chief, Nuclear Med., 1970; Chairman, Dept. Clinical Sci., Montefiore Hosp., 1980. Discovered (with Berson) antibody cause of insulin-resistant diabetes; developed radioimmunoassay for peptide hormones. Nobel prize, 1977.

YERSIN, Alexandre Emile John [1863–1943]. Born at Rougement, Switzerland. Educated at Lausanne, Marburg, and Paris. Pasteur Inst., Paris; Surgeon, French Colonial Army; Director, Pasteur Inst. Nhatrang, Annam. Discovered diphtheria toxin (with Roux), 1888; discovered plague bacillus, Hong Kong, 1894 (independently of Kitasato). Biogr.: *Dict. Sci. Biogr.* **15**, 551 (1976). See also *Hist. Sci. Med.* **7**, 353, 357 (1973). Obit.: *Bacteriol. Rev.* **40**, 633 (1976).

ZINSSER, Hans [1878–1940]. Born at New York. M.D., Columbia Univ., 1903. Prof. bacteriology, Columbia Univ.; Stanford Univ.; Harvard Univ., 1923. Leading student of plague immunology, hypersensitivity; advanced unitarian theory of antibodies; distinguished tuberculin from anaphylactic hypersensitivity. Books: *Microbiology* (with Hiss), 1911 [now in 18th edition]; *Infection and Immunity,* 1914; *Immunity,* 1939. Autobiogr.: *As I Remember Him: The Biography of R. S.,* 1940. Biogr.: *Dict. Sci. Biogr.* **15,** 622 (1976). Obit.: *Science* **92,** 276 (1940).

Glossary

Included below are definitions of the more commonly employed terms in immunology. For additional definitions, the reader is referred to N. J. Herbert and P. C. Wilkerson, A Dictionary of Immunology. *Oxford: Blackwell, 1971.*

Adjuvant. (*ad juvare,* to give assistance to) Any substance that, when administered with antigen, increases the immunogenicity of the antigen.

Affinity. The measure of the binding strength of antigen with an antibody combining site; directly derived from the intrinsic association constant of the interaction.

Agglutinin. An antibody whose fixation onto cells (erythrocytes, bacteria) causes their visible clumping.

Allele. One of a group of genes that may occupy the same locus on a chromosome.

Allergen. Any substance capable of sensitizing for or provoking an allergic reaction.

Allergy. Abnormal reactivity (hypersensitivity) of an individual to an antigen, referring especially to immediate-type hypersensitivities.

Allogeneic. (Gr. *allos,* other; *genos,* race) Of different genetic constitution within the same species.

Allotype. Genetically controlled polymorphic variants of a protein, particularly the characteristic attributable to the existence of different antigenic determinants on immunoglobulins from individuals of the same species.

Anaphylaxis. IgE-mediated hypersensitivity provoked by a second injection of an antigen into a previously sensitized individual, taking its more severe form as systemic anaphylactic shock.

Anti-antibody. An antibody that reacts with antigenic determinants on a molecule that is itself an antibody.

383

Antibody. An immunoglobulin with a specialized combining site that reacts specifically with an antigen. *See also* immunoglobulin.

Antigen. Any substance that provokes the production of specific antibody or immunocyte, or that interacts specifically with these products of the immune response. In the former sense, **immunogen** is the preferred term.

Arthus phenomenon. The dermal inflammatory reaction that occurs shortly after administration of antigen to an animal that possesses precipitating antibodies, as the consequence of previous sensitization with this antigen. The local reaction may include a wheal and erythema, hemorrhage, and necrosis.

Atopy. (Gr. *a,* out of; *topos,* place) An early term to describe the susceptibility of some individuals to immediate-type hypersensitivity to allergens.

Auto-. Derived from self; for example,
autologous: derived from the individual itself.
autoantibody: an antibody formed within the host and interacting with the body's own antigens.
autoantigen: a substance able to induce autoantibody formation within the host.
autoimmune: immunized against a body's own constituents.

Avidity. A measure of the degree of interaction of antigen with antibody, depending not only upon intrinsic affinity but also upon the valence of antigen and antibody and upon other physicochemical parameters.

B cell. (B lymphocyte) A lymphoid cell lineage that differentiates under the influence of the bursa of Fabricius in birds (and its unknown equivalent in mammals) to give rise to antibody-forming cells—in their most mature form, plasma cells.

BCG. (Bacillus Calmette-Guérin) A strain of bovine tubercle bacilli that has lost its virulence by attenuation in serial culture and is utilized in many countries to immunize against tuberculosis infection.

Bence-Jones protein. A monoclonal kappa or lambda light chain often found in the blood or urine of patients with multiple myeloma or Waldenstrom's macroglobulinemia.

Blocking antibody. Any antibody capable of suppressing the biological activity of other antibodies or of T cells, usually by competing with them for the same antigenic epitope.

Carrier. An immunogenic substance to which a hapten (q.v.) must be attached in order to obtain specific antihapten antibodies. The **carrier**

effect is manifested when a hapten on carrier B is unable to stimulate a booster response or skin test in an animal sensitized with that hapten on non-cross-reacting carrier A.

Cell-mediated immunity. (CMI) An immune state mediated by T cells, which may be passively transferred only by these cells and not by serum. CMI includes delayed-type hypersensitivities, the allograft rejection reaction, and killer T cells.

Chimera. (Gr., a monster possessing the parts of different animal species) An organism possessing both its own cells and those of some foreign donor.

Clonal selection theory. A theory of antibody formation (advanced by F. M. Burnet), which postulates that for any given antigenic determinant there is a corresponding set of preformed lymphocytes whose clonal expansion and subsequent reactions may be stimulated by interaction of that antigen with the specific cell membrane receptors that characterize that set of immunocytes.

Clone. A group of cells or organisms reproduced asexually from a single progenitor and having the same genetic constitution.

Complement. A complex system of plasma protein factors and enzymes capable of binding to and being activated by a large number of antigen–antibody systems. Complement plays an essential role in a number of different immunological effector mechanisms, including immune hemolysis, immune bacteriolysis, and anaphylaxis.

Complement fixation test. Technique for the measurement of antibody (or antigen), taking advantage of the ability of antigen–antibody complexes to fix complement nonspecifically. The test is most generally applied to the serodiagnosis of infectious diseases.

Contact hypersensitivity. Delayed-type hypersensitivity caused by the contact of skin with a variety of active chemicals (e.g., poison ivy).

Coombs test. (antiglobulin test) A technique that utilizes a heterologous anti-immunoglobulin antibody to demonstrate the presence (usually on erythrocytes) of nonagglutinating "incomplete" antibodies.

Cross-reaction. Interaction of an antibody with an antigen that was not used in its induction but possesses determinants structurally similar to those of the original immunogen.

Cytophilic antibody. (homocytotropic antibody) Antibody able to affix to the surface of certain cells that possess appropriate receptors. Thus, IgE is cytophilic for basophiles and mast cells; and numerous other antibodies bind to macrophages that possess receptors for their Fc moieties.

Delayed-type hypersensitivity. (DTH) T cell-mediated hypersensitivity that develops 24 to 48 hours after exposure to antigen (in contrast to immediate-type hypersensitivity), e.g., the tuberculin test, poison ivy dermatitis.

Desensitization. The suppression of a clinical allergic state by the administration of repeated and increasing doses of the offending allergen. Suppression is generally due to the development of blocking antibodies, which compete for the allergen with specific IgE antibody.

Domain. The homologous regions on immunoglobulin chains that confer immunological specificity (the variable regions) and other biological properties (the constant regions). Light chains possess one variable and one constant domain, whereas heavy chains possess one variable and three constant domains.

Epitope. The specific combining site on an antigen molecule that interacts with antibody or with immunocyte receptors.

Freund's adjuvant. A water-oil emulsion in which antigen is mixed to enhance its immunogenicity.
 complete Freund's adjuvant. (CFA) One containing killed mycobacteria to enhance the response further.
 incomplete Freund's adjuvant. One that lacks the added mycobacteria.

Genotype. The complete set of genetic material (genes) possessed by an individual.

Germinal center. (also called secondary follicles or nodules) The highly organized aggregation of T and B lymphocytes, lymphoblasts, and macrophages that develops within the primary follicles of lymphoid organs in response to antigenic stimulation.

Graft-versus-host reaction. (GVH) The severe systemic or local reaction that occurs when allogeneic lymphocytes are administered to a host who is immunosuppressed or otherwise genetically incapable of rejecting these cells.

Hapten. (Gr. *aptain,* to grasp) Any substance, usually of low molecular weight, that is incapable by itself of stimulating antibody formation but is able to react with antibody once formed. A hapten becomes immunogenic only when attached to an immunogenic carrier.

Helper T cell. An antigen-specific T lymphocyte that cooperates with B cells in the production of antibodies or with other T cells in various manifestations of cell-mediated immunity.

Hemagglutination. The clumping of erythrocytes, usually by specific antibody. Hemagglutination may also occur in response to bacterial or virus-derived substances or to plant lectins such as phytohemagglutinin.

Hetero-. (Gr., other) Most often employed in the past to indicate an origin from another species, as in **heteroantibody, heterogeneic,** and **heterograft;** now replaced in this sense by the prefix **xeno-.**

Histocompatibility. The measure of the degree of antigenic similarity between two tissues, usually applied to transplant donor and recipient pairs.

Homo-. Derived from a member of the same species (but one not genetically identical); currently replaced in most usages by the term **allo-,** as in allograft (homograft).

Hybridoma. A hybrid cell line obtained by fusing a B lymphocyte immunized against a defined antigen with a myeloma cell. A continuous culture of identical hybrid cells is thus obtained and is able to produce uniform (monoclonal) antibodies specific for a single antigenic determinant.

Idiotype. (Gr. *idios,* own, private; + *tupos*) The antigenic determinants that characterize the specific combining site of an antibody molecule.

Idiotype network theory. A theory of immunoregulation proposed by Jerne, in which the extent of an immune response (or of tolerance) is determined by the balance of interactions between the specific idiotypes on antibody, their respective anti-idiotypes, and higher levels of anti-idiotype formation.

Immediate hypersensitivity. The group of local or systemic allergic reactions mediated primarily by the interaction of antigen (allergen) with IgE antibodies.

Immune complex. A macromolecular lattice of specifically linked antigen and antibody that may cause tissue damage (e.g., glomerulonephritis, arthritis) when deposited in certain tissues.

Immune response (Ir) **genes.** A group of genes in the I region of the mouse MHC that control the level of immune response to certain antigenic determinants.

Immunity. (L. *immunitas,* exemption) The protection of an organism against infectious agents or toxic antigens afforded by a variety of predominantly specific humoral and cellular factors.
acquired immunity. The specific protection against pathogens or toxins afforded by a known prior exposure through infection or immunization.

natural immunity. Those specific and nonspecific factors that protect against infection in the absence of known prior exposure to the pathogenic agent.

Immunofluorescence. A method in which antibodies coupled to fluorescent molecules are employed as histochemical markers to identify and/or localize antigens or antibodies, by examination in the ultraviolet microscope.

Immunogenicity. The measure of the ability of an antigen to induce a humoral or cellular immune response.

Immunoglobulin. (Ig) A general term referring to all serum globulins that possess antibody activity. Immunoglobulins are symmetrical molecules composed of two heavy and two light chains and are presently divided into five classes whose involvement in physiological functions depend upon the nature of the heavy chain component: IgM, IgD, IgG, IgA, and IgE.

Immunological memory. The term applied to denote the ability of an individual (or of its immunocompetent cells) to give a heightened and more rapid response to the second exposure to an antigen, sometimes even long after the primary immunization. This second response is often called an anamnestic response.

Immunological paralysis. The state of specific immunological unresponsiveness to a polysaccharide antigen that results from prior exposure to large doses of this antigen. Paralysis is probably distinguishable in mechanism from immunological tolerance.

Immunological tolerance. The reduction or complete elimination of the ability of an individual to respond specifically to an antigen. This may occur naturally to most self-antigens or be induced experimentally following the administration of very high or very low doses of that antigen, most usually to the fetus or neonate.

Immunosuppression. The diminution or elimination of immune responses (generally nonspecific) by drug treatment, irradiation, or other causes, e.g, HIV infection in AIDS.

Instruction theory. Those theories of antibody formation that postulate that the information for the production of specific antibodies is derived from the antigen itself.

Interleukins. A group of pharmacologically active substances (cytokines) that stimulate lymphoid cells.
  Interleukin 1. (IL-1) A lymphocyte activating factor (LAF) produced by activated macrophages.
  Interleukin 2. (IL-2) A soluble mediator produced by T cells that

activate other T cells, formally known as T cell growth factor (TCGF) and thymocyte stimulating factor (TSF).

ISO-. (Gr. *isos,* equal) Derived from an animal of identical genetic constitution, and applied generally to highly inbred strains of experimental animals. **Syn-** is now the preferred form.

Isologous. Describing a genetically identical inbred line.

Isoantibody. Original term for an antibody that is formed in an individual and binds to an antigen (e.g., blood group antigen) from another individual from the same species.

Lectin. An agent derived from plants or animals that displays carbohydrate binding and thus antibody-like activity toward animal cells. Most lectins agglutinate erythrocytes, but some also stimulate lymphoid cells.

Lymphokine. A factor released during the activation of lymphocytes (usually following interaction with antigen or with other signal molecules) that affects other cells, e.g., MIF, Il-2, lymphotoxin.

Major histocompatibility complex. (MHC) The multigene region on chromosome 6 of the human and chromosome 17 of the mouse that encodes for a variety of immunologically important functions. These include class I antigens (which define transplantation incompatibility, MHC-restricted antigen-recognition mechanisms important for the function of cytotoxic T cells, and HLA-associated disease predilections) and class II antigens (which mediate immunoregulatory cooperative events and cell maturation signals, immune response genes, the fourth component of complement, and other products).

Migration inhibition factor. (MIF) A protein factor that is liberated by the interaction of sensitized lymphocytes with specific antigen and inhibits the normal migration of macrophages.

Mixed lymphocyte reaction. (MLR) The proliferative response of lymphocytes (measured by radioactive thymidine incorporation into newly formed DNA or the generation of Il-2) when stimulated by allogeneic lymphocytes. In a one-way MLR, one of the two populations is prevented from responding to stimulation by chemical or radiation pretreatment.

Multiple Myeloma. A malignant tumor of B lymphocytes, accompanied by hyperproduction of a monoclonal immunoglobulin and often by Bence-Jones proteinuria.

Natural antibody. Any antibody found in the serum of an individual who has had no apparent previous experience of the corresponding antigen.

Opsonin. (Gr. *opsonein,* to render palatable) A serum antibody whose binding to bacteria or other particles facilitates their phagocytosis by macrophages.

Organ specificity. A term describing antigens that occur only within certain tissues (e.g., lens, thyroid, brain), and whose specific antibodies cross-react with the corresponding antigens in a wide range of other even distantly related species.

Paratope. The combining site on antibody, complementary to the epitope on antigen.

Phagocytosis. The ingestion by a cell of another cell or particle.

Phenotype. Those overt characteristics of an individual that reflect the portion of the genotype that is expressed.

Polyclonal activation. The stimulation of entire populations or subsets of lymphocytes without regard for their antigenic specificities.

Precipitin reaction. The visible combination of antigen and specific antibody, forming a sediment in the test tube and distinct linear aggregates in agar double diffusion.

Reaginic antibody. A former term for those antibodies that mediate immediate hypersensitivity reactions.

Rheumatoid factor. The anti-immunoglobulin antibodies found primarily in patients with rheumatoid arthritis.

Secretory immunoglobulin. The dimeric form of IgA (with an added "secretory piece") that constitutes the major antibody response of mucosal surfaces and their attached excretory glands.

Serum sickness. The set of systemic and local clinical symptoms that appears a week or two after the first injection of large doses of heterologous serum, due to the formation of immune complexes.

Suppressor T cells. A subset of T cells that exerts downward regulation of the functions of B cells or of other T cells.

Surveillance. (immunological) The suggestion by Lewis Thomas that one of the principal functions of the immune system is, through its normal lymphocyte traffic, to detect and destroy abnormal cells that develop in the body through somatic mutation or malignant transformation.

Syngeneic. The term applied to individuals who are genetically identical [e.g., uniovular twins or genetically pure (inbred) strains of animals].

T cell. Those lymphocytes that differentiate under thymic control and possess distinctive cell surface markers, subsets of which serve as helper or suppressor cells in immunoregulation or as effector cells in cell-mediated immunity.

Transfer factor. A low-molecular-weight dialyzable substance, originally described by H. Sherwood Lawrence, that is obtained from sensitized T lymphocytes and is capable of transferring antigen-specific delayed-type hypersensitivity to naive recipients.

Tuberculin test. Diagnostic test for tuberculosis, involving a delayed hypersensitivity response to the intradermal injection of a purified protein derivative (PPD) isolated from cultures of tubercle bacillus.

Vaccine. (L. *vaccus,* cow) Originally, the cowpox vaccine (vaccinia virus) used for Jennerian inoculation to induce immunity against smallpox. Current usage extends the term to any prophylactic immunization.

Xenogeneic. Any material originating from a different species.

Name Index

Subject Index

407